PSYCHIATRY – THEORY, APPLICATIONS AND TREATMENTS

BORDERLINE PERSONALITY DISORDER

Psychiatry – Theory, Applications and Treatments

Additional books and e-books in this series can be found
on Nova's website under the Series tab.

PSYCHIATRY – THEORY, APPLICATIONS AND TREATMENTS

BORDERLINE PERSONALITY DISORDER

CHARLES M LEPKOWSKY
EDITOR

nova
Medicine & Health
New York

Additional color graphics may be available in the e-book version of this book.

Library of Congress Cataloging-in-Publication Data

ISBN: 978-1-53618-021-3

Library of Congress Control Number: 2020938062

Published by Nova Science Publishers, Inc. † New York

CONTENTS

Preface **vii**

Acknowledgments **xi**

Chapter 1 A History and Conceptualization of Borderline Personality Diagnosis **1**
Kathryn M. Chun and Lindsey J. Nelson

Chapter 2 Defining Borderline Personality Disorder **19**
Ronald B. Brooks

Chapter 3 Biological Correlates of Borderline Personality Disorder **65**
Nanako Negome-Kapur

Chapter 4 Evidence-Based Models of Treatment for Borderline Personality Disorder **93**
Chi-Sing Li, Robert J. Lugar, Reade Dowda, Diane Smedley and Yu-Fen Lin

Chapter 5 Object Relations Theory and Borderline Personality Disorder **133**
Erik G. Jul

Chapter 6 Treatment of Borderline Personality Disorder using Dialectical Behavior Therapy **163**
Joanna L. Fava and Madelaine Ellberger

Chapter 7 Constructionist Approaches to Treating Borderline Personality Disorder **205**
Stephen Bacon

Chapter 8 The Stigma of Borderline Personality Disorder **241**
Charles M. Lepkowsky

Afterword **281**

About the Editor **283**

Index **285**

PREFACE

Borderline Personality Disorder is widely recognized as one of the most challenging diagnoses for mental health practitioners. Difficulty understanding the motives and behaviors of people assigned the "borderline" diagnosis have given rise to a long history of negative characterizations of "borderline patients." These include beliefs that borderline patients are invasive, consuming, manipulative, controlling, unpredictable, volatile, and high-risk. Practitioners are often warned not to treat more than one borderline patient at one time because they are "difficult," to expect borderline patients to engage in boundary crossings or violations, to seek consultation during treatment, and to be wary that although the borderline patient might idealize the therapist one day, they are just as likely to demonize the therapist the next. Many mental health practitioners simply decline to work with borderline patients, considering them too much work and too unlikely to make significant improvements through psychotherapy.

Borderline Personality Disorder has a long history. For over a century, various models have been generated for conceptualizing, assessing, and treating Borderline Personality Disorder. These include Psychoanalytic, Object Relations, Cognitive-Behavioral, Dialectical Behavior Therapy, Constructionist, Evidence-Based, and Biological perspectives. Inclusion in the Diagnostic and Statistical Manual of the American Psychiatric Association (DSM) has shaped the development and evolution of current diagnostic criteria, making them more specific and behavior-based. During the last decade, Borderline Personality Disorder has emerged into the awareness of American mainstream media and culture, perhaps increasing stigmatization of people assigned the diagnosis. Recent developments in the understanding of trauma and its neurological correlates, as well as the identification of biological differences in people diagnosed with Borderline Personality Disorder, have produced new questions regarding the etiology and differential diagnosis of Borderline Personality Disorder.

Perhaps the most controversial diagnosis in the current nosology, Borderline Personality Disorder merits exploration and explanation. The book you are about to read represents the mutual efforts of seasoned practicing mental health professionals and doctoral psychology program faculty with over two centuries of combined clinical experience assessing and treating Borderline Personality Disorder. The chapters ahead describe the history of the concept of borderline personality functioning, its applications in the development of a formal diagnosis, how that diagnosis varies according to the theoretical framework in which it is applied, and how the diagnosis has evolved over time. The most prominent theoretical models for conceptualization, assessment, and treatment of Borderline Personality Disorder are explained in detail, including the evolution of the current diagnostic criteria employed in the fifth Edition of the Diagnostic and Statistical Manual of the American Psychiatric Association (DSM 5).

The incorporation of Borderline Personality Disorder into the common American lexicon is discussed, from self-help books to characterizations in the media, with special attention to the influence these characterizations have had on popular thinking, including stigmatization of the person bearing the diagnosis. The consequent effects on the person, their families and friends, and even the mental health practitioners treating them are also considered.

The influences of the DSM system and value-based reimbursement on conceptualization of diagnosis and treatment are also discussed, with attention to the tensions between clinical and fiscally-driven decision-making. Research findings demonstrating biological differences in people diagnosed with Borderline Personality Disorder are described, along with their implications for differential diagnosis and the potential role of historical trauma. Evidence-Based models of treatment are reviewed in detail. Current conceptualizations of the Borderline Personality Disorder diagnosis are discussed, including the possibility that there might be more than one type of Borderline Personality Disorder. Nontraditional models of Borderline Personality Disorder are reviewed, including Constructionist perspectives. Future directions for research, conceptualization, assessment and treatment of Borderline Personality Disorder are explored, including potential DSM changes.

Borderline Personality Disorder provides a comprehensive, in-depth analysis of the history, conceptualization, treatment, and current body of research addressing the Borderline Personality Disorder diagnosis. This book is intended to serve as a useful reference text for practicing mental health professionals, and as a powerful and concise source of information for doctoral level psychology students.

Charles M. Lepkowsky, PhD
Editor

ACKNOWLEDGMENTS

The editor wishes to thank the theorists, psychotherapists and medical professionals whose invaluable insights and ingenuity led to the conceptualization of Borderline Personality Disorder as a unique clinical entity, diagnostic criteria that have evolved over time to more accurately define the condition, and through whose tireless efforts effective treatment methods have been developed.

The editor also wishes to express gratitude and appreciation to Sheldon Berkowitz, PhD, Julie R. Price, PsyD and Betsy Usher PsyD for their time and helpful feedback, and to the chapter authors, whose time, dedication, and professional expertise in the assessment, diagnosis and treatment of Borderline Personality Disorder have made this book possible.

In: Borderline Personality Disorder
Editor: Charles M. Lepkowsky
ISBN: 978-1-53618-021-3

Chapter 1

A History and Conceptualization of Borderline Personality Diagnosis

Kathryn M. Chun[1,*], PhD and Lindsey J. Nelson[2]
[1]Hawaii School of Professional Psychology
at Chaminade University Honolulu, Hawaii, US
[2]Texas Woman's University, Denton, Texas, US

Abstract

The Borderline Personality Disorder (BPD) diagnosis has evolved with the field of psychology and the process of psychological diagnosis. Cultural and historical factors have played a significant role in the conceptualization of internal states and interpersonal interactions associated with BPD. Although different psychological theories have emerged with a variety of explanations for the etiology of BPD, over time there has been growing general agreement about observable symptoms that inform the diagnosis.

Keywords: Freud, personality structure, ego defense mechanisms, ego psychology, object relations theory

---

* Corresponding Author's E-mail: kathryn.chun@chaminade.edu.

INTRODUCTION

Borderline Personality Disorder (BPD) is considered a complex psychological condition, difficult to treat due to its complex symptom presentation. The symptoms of BPD involve extreme mood swings, perceptual disturbances in interpersonal interactions, and emotional and behavioral reactivity that frequently eventuate in personal and/or interpersonal crises. Early psychological theorists had no specific framework for a single diagnosis encompassing all of these symptoms. The notion that multiple symptoms might be attributable to a single disorder is, however, not unique to BPD, nor a recent phenomenon. In 1684, Bonet first conceptualized *folie maniac-melancolique* to signify multiple moods within one diagnosis (Millon et al., 2004).

Psychological theories evolve in the context of political and cultural milieu that influence their underlying values and assumptions. Within the field of psychology, changes in location and era have had significant impact on the conceptualization of the borderline diagnosis. During the late 19th century, Vienna, Austria was a center of European culture during a time of advancement in technology and sociopolitical thought, emphasizing the value and experience of the individual. It was during this period and in this place that Freud developed the theory and practice of psychoanalysis. In the context of early industrial age dynamic technology including steam engines and hydraulic drives, combined with the sociopolitical emphasis on individual experience, Freud's psychodynamic model was conceived in terms of internal drives, the inevitability of their dynamic forces, and their interface with society.

Freud's original psychoanalytic model specified two categories of psychological functioning: the neurotic and the psychotic (Freud, n.d.). Neuroses were considered treatable or "analyzable" conditions, often falling within the realm of acceptable social functioning. Psychoses were thought to encompass beliefs and behaviors beyond the realm of acceptable social functioning, and were considered untreatable (Freud, n.d.; Mitchell & Black, 1995). BPD symptomatology did not fit within the definition of neurosis or psychosis, seeming to fall somewhere along the border between the two.

During the late 19th century, theorists including Sigmund Freud, Karl Kahlbaum, and Emil Kraeplin began to describe a condition that was somewhere between what was considered analyzable and nonanalyzable, leading to the use of the term "borderline" in the 1930's (Nelson, 2019; Rosanoff, 1938; Stern, 1938).

With the rise of fascism, Freud moved his family and his practice to London, England (Bettelheim, 1989). Fascism challenged Western European beliefs about individual experience, human thought and behavior. The inherent optimism underlying psychological thought during the early industrial age was overshadowed by questions about humanity's potential for destruction, and what combinations of internal and external factors might contribute to psychological illness. Subsequent changes in the milieu were reflected in novel psychological theories and treatment approaches.

Psychoanalytic Perspectives on Borderline Symptoms

Sigmund Freud (1920a) explained neuroses and psychoses in his theory of drives. Neurotic symptoms were described as manifestations of ego defense mechanisms. He contended that patient resistance in treatment serves the purpose of preserving symptoms (neurotic ego defenses) in order to protect the ego from annihilation (Freud, 1920b). Within this model, the individual with Borderline Personality Disorder can be seen as resisting the elimination of symptoms in order to preserve conscious or unconscious ego defenses. London (1946) believed that psychosis evolved out of neurosis, so that neurotic obsessions "absorbed" by the psyche end up becoming psychotic delusions.

With the rise of industrialization and urbanization in the early twentieth century, Harry Stack Sullivan introduced interpersonal psychoanalysis. In contrast to Freudian psychology's emphasis on drives, Sullivan suggested that interactions between the individual and the environment produce the experience of anxiety (Sullivan, 1953). Drawing responsibility for symptom evolution out of the intrapsychic state into the interpersonal realm is consistent with more recent theories of BPD that recognize the influence of trauma and other early interpersonal events for having an impact on the development and expression of the disorder (Mitchell & Black, 1995).

In the 1930s, Freud's focus on drives lost ground to an increasing interest in interpersonal interactions and their influence on mental and emotional experience, and ego psychology evolved as a specific area of theory and practice. Rosanoff (1938) strove to better define "undiagnosed psychoses," including borderline behaviors that cross over between manic-depressive and schizophrenic groups, with symptom descriptions that are consistent with current Borderline Personality Disorder symptom criteria. During the same year, Stern (1938) specifically described Borderline Personality Disorder as a condition between neurosis and psychosis (Paris, 2015; Stern, 1938).

The post-war era and efforts to understand the holocaust spurred an interest in social psychology and spirituality. Frankl suggested that a person's wholeness is dependent on the integration of the somatic, the psychic, and the spiritual. A lack of integration was thought to result in a 'disrupted' human being. Frankl suggested that symptoms can be either psychogenic, leading to neurosis, or somatogenic, leading to psychosis, and that borderline symptoms might have origins in both realms (Frankl, 1938). Thorne (1955) highlighted diagnostic uncertainty for symptoms between those considered to be part of "normality" and those in the "mental disorder" category. The diagnostic categories of that time demonstrate the transition from previous attribution of mental illness to somatic ailments to psychogenic origin, which would later be linked to brain structure and functional links to psychological symptoms, specifically including BPD.

The first Diagnostic and Statistical Manual (DSM), published by the American Psychiatric Association in 1952, was psychoanalytically influenced. Conscious and unconscious reactions to psychological, social, and biological factors were thought to result in mental disorders (American Psychiatric Association, 1952). The DSM-II eliminated the term "reaction" from its classification system (American Psychiatric Association, 1994). Aronson (1985) found themes in borderline literature that involve four different descriptions of what comprises "borderline," including borderline schizophrenia, borderline affective disorder, borderline personality disorder, and borderline as a psychostructural level of functioning. Exploration of the specific symptoms involved in dysfunctional personality features led to the eventual labeling of the cluster of symptoms in the diagnostic term "Borderline Personality Disorder" in the DSM, 3rd Edition (DSM-III, 1980). DSM-III introduced the multi-axial diagnostic system, differentiating personality disorder (Axis II) from acute clinical symptom syndromes (Axis I). DSM-III strove to base diagnoses on "methodological innovations, including explicit diagnostic criteria, a multiaxial system, and a descriptive approach that attempted to be neutral with respect to theories of etiology" (American Psychiatric Association, 1994, pp. xvii-xviii) and eliminated the psychoanalytic definitions of symptoms. DSM-III brought the understanding of borderline symptomology closer to what it is today.

Psychodynamic and Object Relations Perspectives on Borderline Symptoms

Almost 40 years after Stern's 1938 description of BPD symptoms, Stone (1976) described the "Borderline Syndrome" to include complications with constitution and coping that are neither fully neurotic as the "common" characteristic nor psychotic as the individual who is not perceiving within the bounds of reality. Freud's view of neurosis relied largely on the influence of the pre-Oedipal mother-attachment (Mahler, 1975; Mitchell, 1974; Reich & Stone, 1976). Subsequent ego psychologists believed that simultaneous contradictory feeling states split the ego into self-parts, as expressed in the thinking of self-psychologist Heinz Kohut and ego psychologist and developmental object relations theorist Otto Kernberg. McWilliams (1994) states that identity confusion is prevalent in borderline personality patients, who have an inconsistent concept of self. Those with borderline personality organization are thought to employ primitive ego defenses including denial, projective identification, and splitting.

Object relations theorists believed that satisfaction or frustration of the infant's libidinal drive for the mother are internalized as good or bad object representations of the mother (Fairbairn, 1952). When disparate internalizations remain unintegrated, splitting occurs, producing borderline symptoms. In Erik Erikson's theory, interruption in the earliest ego stage of trust versus mistrust interferes with ego development. Erik Erikson's developmental stage theory of the late-1960s held that people with neurotic symptoms achieved the basic trust and basic autonomy stages, but the sense of identity and initiative stages were still in progress. With identity integration disruption in the borderline individual, this stage of identity development is also considered undeveloped (Eriksen, 1975). During the 1960's, the Viet Nam war, economic and racial tensions, and a growing distrust of the government contributed to psychological thought that incorporated trust and relationships with parents (authority) as key concepts.

In a shift of borderline personality conceptualization, Otto Kernberg emphasized reality testing and ego integration as critical ends within the diagnosis and identifiers of psychotic, borderline, and neurotic structural levels. Although borderline patients are able to engage in reality testing while psychotic patients are not able to do so, borderline patients do not have the ego integration of neurotic patients. Kernberg asserted that maternal expression of aggression results in splitting as the child attempts to negotiate the need for the idealized mother with the frightening experience of the mother by separating the experiences, resulting in identity diffusion that is characteristic of Borderline Personality Disorder (Ensink, Biberdzic, Normandin, & Clarkin, 2015; Kernberg, 1967).

Some BPD symptoms remained unaffected by psychoanalysis, so modifications were made to both the theory and therapy applied to BPD. BPD individuals were eventually viewed as possessing a weakened and damaged self from self-object and self-interactions that resulted in a self-disorder (Kohut & Wolf, 1978). Kohut and Wolf (1978) explained that primary self-disorders include psychoses, which are now explained as the experiential and behavioral manifestations of a lack of defensive structure protecting the self from damage, or borderline states, which they described involve a defensive structure covering the central defect to the self that is permanent but protected and treatable. This "chronic characterological defense" results from intrusion by the parental self-object interfering with the childhood need to develop an autonomous self. Another primary self-disorder is the narcissistic personality disorder, conceptualized as a temporary distortion of self (Kohut & Wolf, 1978).

Feminist Psychological Perspectives on Borderline Diagnosis

In the mid-1970s, Juliet Mitchell asserted that the feminist movement needed to consider the patriarchal perspective of psychoanalysis instead of rejecting it outright, including R. D. Laing's The Divided Self (Laing, 1959). Laing suggested that "neurotic" and "psychotic" states blend. Psychosis rejects the reality of the present and lives in hallucinations and delusions, but this rejection can be expressed in neuroticism, perhaps as what we now call BPD, when "a neurosis may conceal a psychosis" (Mitchell, J., 1974, p. 266). Because 75% of those diagnosed with BPD are females, understanding the implications of symptom development and perceptions of these symptoms is relevant from a feminist psychology perspective.

Attachment Theory and Borderline Symptoms

A currently predominant explanation of BPD arose from John Bowlby's attachment theory of the 1970s, which in turn developed out of the attachment ideas of psychoanalytic theory combined with more recent developmental psychopathology theory (Bowlby, 1969). Bowlby's theory posited that infants form affective-cognitive schemata of the self and others through repeated interactions with their attachment figures, which results in personality development organization and impacts future relationships. This theory was demonstrated in Mary Ainsworth's classic study on infant attachment in response to mothers versus strangers. When the infant's needs are repeatedly unmet, future expectations of relationships with others consequently suffer. Insecure, fearful avoidant, and preoccupied attachment, then, can result in the development of the psychopathology present in BPD, including unstable, intense interpersonal relationships, feelings of emptiness, bursts of rage, chronic fears of abandonment and intolerance for being alone, and an unstable sense of self (Levy, 2005). Levy, Johnson and Clouthier et al., (2015) also asserted that other personality disorders are also related to attachment disruption and the loneliness and fears of abandonment characteristic of the experience of the individual with BPD. They assert that attachment theory integrates the positions of cognitive, behavioral, psychodynamic, and interpersonal theories. The link between attachment theory and understanding BPD is consistent with earlier recognition of the relationship between early trauma in the infant-caregiver relationship and emotional dysregulation.

Further research of this relationship was conducted by Godbout, Daspe, Runtz, Cyr and Briere (2019) regarding gender differences in attachment related to borderline personality-related symptoms (BPRS). They found that BPRS in women was associated with maternal and paternal maltreatment. An indirect association was found between BPRS in women and paternal maltreatment through attachment anxiety. BPRS in men, however, was associated only with paternal maltreatment. Maternal maltreatment was indirectly associated with BPRS through attachment anxiety (Godbout et al., 2019). Research regarding attachment has shifted into greater detail toward distinctions between etiology, symptom presentation, and associations between experience and reactions.

Conceptual leanings in psychology have shifted with political times and countries of origin, as have theoretical understandings of borderline symptoms. The movement from psychoanalytical theory to psychodynamic theory and then object relations theory evolved as theorists and historical factors influenced additional aspects of symptoms and how human minds are understood. A need for structure and predictability led to the rise of behavioral theory. The information-processing models used in code-breaking during the second world war evolved into computer processing models, giving rise to cognitive theory and its predominance in the 1970's. During the 1980's, behavioral and cognitive influences on theory merged, leading to the development of cognitive-behavioral theory.

Behavioral and Biosocial Theory Perspectives on Borderline Symptoms

Dialectical Behavior Therapy (DBT) is a cognitive-behavioral model that reflects the integration of social perception with active behavioral change. DBT was based on the biosocial model that innate emotional vulnerability as a child, combined with an invalidating social environment, can give rise to borderline traits (Linehan, 1993; Linehan & Schmidt, 1995). Linehan (1993) also adapted "mindfulness" and radical acceptance, critical components of DBT, out of Zen meditation techniques, consistent with a time of cultural fusion in various disciplines. In DBT the focus is on integration into a unified whole that includes acceptance of differences and polarities (Heard & Linehan, 1994), actively seeking to combine the split parts that have been identified from the beginnings of theoretical conceptualizations of BPD. Crowell, Beauchaine and Linehan (2009) elaborated on Linehan's 1993 biosocial developmental model of BPD, suggesting that environmental risk factors strengthen the likelihood of early biological vulnerabilities being expressed in the extreme emotional, behavioral, and cognitive dysregulation of BPD. The family influence on impulsivity and emotional lability is compounded by environmental factors. This notion brings the understanding of BPD to a wider context than the origins of understanding the symptoms through an internal focus. The concept that environmental factors exacerbate risk and can, perhaps, be mitigated through intervention suggests an introduction of the external world contributing to symptom expression.

In testing the biosocial theory upon which DBT is based, Gill and Warburton (2014) found that emotional dysregulation predicted borderline personality traits, but also found that emotional vulnerability and invalidating parenting independently predicted emotional dysregulation, but without interactive effects. Swenson and Choi-Kain (2015) also used the DBT treatment standard and compared it to Mentalization-Based Treatment (MBT), explaining that with their differing origins (psychoanalysis, attachment theory and research, and developmental psychopathology for

MBT; acceptance-based approaches, behavioral science, and dialectical philosophy for DBT) and different approaches, MBT can complement DBT, again demonstrating an integrative approach to the treatment style. Support has also been found for MBT instead of traditional psychodynamic treatment approaches in treating BPD (Kvarstein, Pederson, Urnes, Hummelen, Wilberg, & Karterud, 2015).

Blending Theories in Understanding BPD

The Theory of Mind of the late 20th century with Kernberg's identity integration explanation and mentalization of the early 21st century examines BPD from a cognitive perspective that includes neuropsychological involvement resulting from trauma. Kernberg contended that theory of motivation requires the theory of drives to explain the affect activation that occurs in extremes of excessive affect or inadequate affect (Kernberg, 1967). Adolescents with BPD have immature cognitive and emotional development from disorganized early attachment relationships and are unable to manage their sexual development and risks related to development, resulting in disturbances in self-representation. BPD in adolescents arises from genetic risk and early adversity via insufficient parenting and maltreatment, complicated by identity, mentalization, and attentional control impairment (Ensink et al., 2015). Ensink et al. (2015) also include that the recognition of ego defenses of splitting and identity diffusion, and analyses of personality organization and self and other representations remain crucial to understanding interpersonal functioning in BPD. Ghiasi, Mohammadi, and Zarrinfar (2016) also found support for the use of suppression in those with BPD, which enhances the physiological response of emotion interpersonally, and supported the importance of Theory of Mind, attachment styles, and emotion regulation as important in predicting BPD risk.

Recent research has found support for identity diffusion as a significant feature of Borderline Personality Disorder (BPD) in adolescents, which is commensurate with its place among the diagnostic criteria in the Fifth

Edition of the Diagnostic and Statistical Manual of Mental Health Disorders, or DSM-5 (Lind, Vanwoerden, Penner, and Sharp, 2019; American Psychiatric Association, 2013). The disturbed sense of self that is inherent in identity diffusion is also consistent with early perspectives on borderline symptoms. Psychoanalytic and neuroscientific theory combined to provide the basis of a Rational Affective Theory for understanding personality disorders, proposed as a treatment framework for highly suicidal patients, including those with BPD (Mizen, 2014).

DSM Evolution and BPD Diagnosis

The first and second editions of the Diagnostic and Statistical Manual of Mental Disorders (DSM) held a psychoanalytic focus that did not include BPD as a diagnosis, in large part due to the belief that it was an untreatable disorder. This perspective derived from psychoanalytic expectations that the BPD patient would continue to view the therapist as unreconcilable bad and good objects. BPD was first included in DSM-III in 1980, when the DSM moved away from psychoanalytic theory toward a more behavioral basis for assigning diagnoses. Following the inclusion of BPD in DSM-III, there was a significant increase in research on BPD (Gunderson, 2009). By the time that DSM-IV was published in 1994, the clinical perspective toward BPD shifted to viewing it as a disorder that is treatable through structured intervention. This shift engendered the growth of self-help and family/friends support groups to envision life beyond the crisis symptoms of BPD, with increased recognition of the effectiveness of interventions on symptom reduction. This reconceptualization of BPD as a treatable disorder with a more favorable prognosis led to widening of the scope of symptoms included in the BPD diagnosis, including recognition of higher functioning BPD individuals.

In the DSM-IV, BPD was located under Axis II, Cluster B of dramatic-emotional disorders with antisocial, histrionic, and narcissistic personality disorders. The DSM-5 (2013) also categorizes these personality disorders together as dramatic, emotional, or erratic. In contrast, those personality disorders described as odd or eccentric are combined in Cluster A, while those described as anxious or fearful are clustered together in Cluster C. The three-cluster diagnostic categorization is consistent with the early descriptions of psychosis and neurosis adjusting to include the middle ground of borderline symptoms that have both psychotic and neurotic features.

The specific symptom criteria for BPD has remained consistent from the DSM-IV through the DSM-5, specifying that the individual must have "a pervasive pattern of instability of interpersonal relationships, self-image, and affects, and marked impulsivity beginning by early adulthood and present in a variety of contexts, as indicated by five (or more) of the following: frantic efforts to avoid real or imagined abandonment; a pattern of unstable and intense interpersonal relationships characterized by alternating between extremes of idealization and devaluation; identity disturbance: markedly and persistently unstable self-image or sense of self; impulsivity in at least two areas that are potentially self-damaging (e.g., spending, sex, substance abuse, reckless driving, binge eating); recurrent suicidal behavior, gestures, or threats, or self-mutilating behavior; affective instability due to a marked reactivity of mood (e.g., intense episodic dysphoria, irritability, or anxiety usually lasting a few hours and only rarely more than a few days); chronic feelings of emptiness; inappropriate, intense anger or difficulty controlling anger (e.g., frequent displays of temper, constant anger, recurrent physical fights); and/or transient, stress-related paranoid ideation or severe dissociative symptoms" (DSM-5, p. 663). It should be noted that nowhere in this definition are the older terms of neurosis or psychosis, although it can be argued that the outdated understanding of these terms is implied in the symptom descriptions.

Hughes, Crowell, Uyeji and Coan (2012) used Coan's social baseline theory and explained that frontolimbic neural links that arise from early attachment are also implicated in adult attachment and co-regulation occurs at all developmental levels. Disruption of this social baseline interferes with critical neural links that support healthy attachment and can lead to the emotional dysregulation and interpersonal interaction impairment present in BPD. More recently, DeShong, Grant and Mullins-Sweatt (2019) returned to earlier theory of neuroticism in conjunction with BPD and, using the 2008 emotional cascade model of Selby, Anestis and Joiner (2008), showed that neuroticism predicted rumination and engagement in maladaptive behaviors after one month.

Summary and Conclusion

The movement away from psychoanalytic terminology toward observable behaviors as the basis for diagnosis continues. The contributions of the neurological perspective have been strengthened by advancements in brain imaging technology. Observable neurological changes in response to treatment suggest greater plasticity in BPD than was previously believed. The exploration of BPD and the course of its symptoms continues in greater detail with the emphasis on outcome research.

References

American Psychiatric Association. (19852). *Diagnostic and statistical manual of mental health disorders*. Washington, D.C.: Author.

American Psychiatric Association. (1980). *Diagnostic and statistical manual of mental health disorders* (3rd ed.). Washington, D.C.: Author.

American Psychiatric Association. (1994). *Diagnostic and statistical manual of mental health disorders (4th edition)*. Washington, D.C.: Author.

American Psychiatric Association. (2000). *Diagnostic and statistical manual of mental health disorders (4th ed., text revision)*. Washington, D.C.: Author.

American Psychiatric Association. (2013). *Diagnostic and statistical manual of mental health disorders (5th ed.)*. Arlington, VA: American Psychiatric Association.

Aronson, T. A. (1985). Historical perspectives on the borderline concept: A review and critique. *Psychiatry: Journal for the Study of Interpersonal*

Processes, 48(3), 209-222. http://dx.doi.org/10.1080/00332747.1985.11024282

Bettelheim, B. (1989). *Freud's Vienna & Other Essays*. New York: Alfred A. Knopf, Inc.

Bowlby, J. (1969). *Attachment*. London: Tavistock Publications.

Crowell, S. E., Beauchaine, T. P., & Linehan, M. M. (2009). A biosocial developmental model of borderline personality: elaborating and extending Linehan's theory. *Psychological Bulletin, 135*(3), 495-510. http://dx.doi.org/10.1037/a0015616

DeShong, H. L., Grant, D. M., & Mullins-Sweatt, S. N. (2019, March 21). Precursors of the Emotional Cascade Model of Borderline Personality Disorder: The Role of Neuroticism, Childhood Emotional Vulnerability, and Parental Invalidation. *Personality Disorders: Theory, Research, and Treatment*. Advance online publication. http://dx.doi.org/10.1037/per0000330

Ellman, S.J. (1991). *Freud's Technique Papers*. Northvale, NJ: Jason Aronson Inc.

Ensink, K., Biberdzic, M., Normandin, L., & Clarkin, J. (2015). A developmental psychopathology and neurobiological model of borderline personality disorder in adolescence. *Journal of Infant, Child, and Adolescent Psychotherapy, 14*, 46-69. http://dx.doi.org/10.1080/15289168.2015.1007715

Erikson, E. H. (1975). *Life history and the historical moment*. New York: Norton.

Fairbairn, W. R. D. (1952). *Psychoanalytic Studies of the Personality*. London and New York: Routledge.

Frankl, V. E. (1948). *The Unconscious God*. New York: Simon and Schuster.

Freud, S. (n.d.). *The Standard Edition of the Complete Psychological Works of Sigmund Freud*. Translated by James Strachey. 24 vols. London: Hogarth, 1953–74.

Freud, S. (1920a). Resistance and suppression. In *A General Introduction to Psychoanalysis*. New York, NY, US: Horace Liveright, pp. 248-261. http://dx.doi.org/10.1037/10667-018

Freud, S. (1920b). Traumatic fixation – the unconscious. In *A General Introduction to Psychoanalysis.* New York, NY, US: Horace Liveright, pp. 236-247. http://dx.doi.org/10.1037/10667-017

Ghiasi, H., Mohammadi, A., & Zarrinfar, P. (2016). An investigation into the roles of theory of mind, emotion regulation, and attachment styles in predicting the traits of borderline personality disorder. *Iran Journal of Psychiatry, 11*(4), 206-213. Retrieved from https://www.ncbi.nlm.nih.gov/pmc/articles/PMC5206322/

Gill, D. & Warburton, W. (2014). An investigation of the biosocial model of borderline personality disorder. *Journal of Clinical Psychology, 70*, 866-873. http://dx.doi.org/10.1002/jclp.22074

Gill, D., Warburton, W., & Sweller, N. (2018). The development of borderline personality disorder: beyond the biosocial model. *Journal of Evidence-Based Psychotherapies, 18*(2), 55-75. http://dx.doi.org/10.24193/jebp.2018.2.14

Godbout, N., Daspe, M. E., Runtz M., Cyr, G., & Briere, J. (2019). Childhood maltreatment, attachment, and borderline personality-related symptoms: gender-specific structural equation models. *Psychological Trauma: Theory, Research, Practice, and Policy, 11*(1), 90-98. http://dx.doi.org/10.1037/tra0000403

Gunderson, J. G. (2009). Borderline personality disorder: ontogeny of a diagnosis. *American Journal of Psychiatry, 166*(5), 530-539. http://dx.doi.org/10.1176/appi.ajp.2009.08121825

Hughes, A. E., Crowell, S. E., Uyeji, L., & Coan, J. A. (2012). A developmental neuroscience of borderline pathology: emotion dysregulation and social baseline theory. *Journal of Abnormal Child Psychology, 40*(1), 21-33. http://dx.doi.org/10.1007/s10802-011-9555-x

Kernberg, O. F. (1967). Borderline personality organization. *J Am Psychoanal Assoc, 15*(3), 641-685. http://dx.doi.org/doi.org/10.1177/000306516701500309

Kernberg, O. F. (2004). Borderline personality disorder and borderline personality organization: psychopathology and psychotherapy. In Magnavita, J. J. (Ed.), *Handbook of Personality Disorders* (pp. 92-119).

Hoboken, NJ: John Wiley & Sons, Inc. Retrieved from https://search.ebscohost.com/login.aspx?direct=true&db=psyh&AN=2004-13688-005&site=ehost-live

Kohut, H. & Wolf, E.S. (1978). The disorders of the self and their treatment: an outline. *The International Journal of Psychoanalysis, 59*(4), 413-425. Retrieved from http://www.sakkyndig.com/psykologi/artvit/kohut1978.pdf

Kvarstein, E. H. et al., (2015). Changing from a traditional psychodynamic treatment programme to mentalization-based treatment for patients with borderline personality disorder – Does it make a difference? *Psychology and Psychotherapy: Theory, Research and Practice, 88*(1), 71-86. http://dx.doi.org/10.1111/papt.12036

Laing, R. D. (1959). *The divided self: An existential study in sanity and madness.* London: Tavistock Publications.

Levy, K. N. (2005). The implications of attachment theory and research for understanding borderline personality disorder. *Development and Psychopathology, 17*(4), 959-986. http://dx.doi.org/10.1017/S0954579405050455

Levy, K. N., Johnson, B. N., Clouthier, T. L., Scala, J. W., & Temes, C. M. (2015). An attachment theoretical framework for personality disorders. *Canadian Psychology, 56*(2), 197-207. http://dx.doi.org/10.1037/cap0000025

Lind, M., Vanwoerden, S., Penner, F., & Sharp, C. (2019, April 29). Inpatient Adolescents with Borderline Personality Disorder Features: Identity Diffusion and Narrative Incoherence. *Personality Disorders: Theory, Research, and Treatment*. Advance online publication. http://dx.doi.org/10.1037/per0000338

Linehan, M. (1993). *Cognitive-behavioral treatment of borderline personality disorder*. New York: The Guilford Press.

Linehan, M. M. & Schmidt, H. III (1995). The dialectics of effective treatment of borderline personality disorder. In *Theories of Behavior Therapy: Exploring Behavior Change*, edited by O'Donohue, W. T. & Krasner, L., American Psychological Association, pp. 553-584. http://dx.doi.org/10.1037/10169-020

London, L. S. (1946). The libido in the borderline neuroses. In *Libido and delusion, Enlarged 2nd ed.*, Washington, D.C., US: Mental Therapy Publications, pp. 47-48. http://dx.doi.org/10.1037/14662-004.

Mahler, M. S. (1975). *The Psychological Birth of the Human Infant*. London: Routledge. http://dx.doi.org/10.4324/9780429482915

McWilliams, N. (1994). *Psychoanalytic Diagnosis*. New York: The Guilford Press.

Millon, T., Grossman, S., Millon, C., Meagher, S., & Ramnath, R. (2004). The borderline personality disorder. In T. Millon, S. Grossman, C. Meagher, & R. Ramnath (Eds.), *Personality disorders in modern life, 2nd ed.* (pp. 417-516). Hoboken, NJ: John Wiley & Sons, Inc.

Mitchell, J. (1974). *Psychoanalysis and Feminism: A Radical Reassessment of Freudian Psychoanalysis.* New York: Basic Books.

Mitchell, S. A. & Black, M. J. (1995). *Freud and Beyond: A History of Modern Psychoanalytic Thought.* New York: Basic Books.

Mizen, C. S. (2014). Towards a relational affective theory of personality disorder. *Psychoanalytic Psychotherapy, 28*(4), 357-378. http://dx.doi.org/10.1080/02668734.2014.975154

Nelson, L. J. (2018). *Attitudes among psychologists working with borderline personality disorder* (Doctoral dissertation). Retrieved from AU E-Dissertations. Honolulu, HI: Argosy University Hawai`i..

Paris, J. (2015). Borderline personality disorder. In American Psychological Association (Ed.), *A Concise Guide to Personality Disorders,* American Psychological Association, pp. 73-89. http://dx.doi.org/10.1037/14642-007

Rosanoff, A. J. (1938, reprinted 1947). Mixed, transitional, borderline, and miscellaneous groups. In *Manual of Psychiatry and Mental Hygiene, 7th ed.,* Hoboken, NJ, US: John Wiley & Sons, Inc., pp. 644-653. http://dx.doi.org/10.1037/11375-026

Selby, E. A., Anestis, M. D. & Joiner, T. F. (2008). Understanding the relationship between emotional and behavioral dysregulation: Emotional cascades. *Behaviour Research and Therapy, 46*(5), 593-611. http://dx.doi.org/10.1016/j.brat.2008.02.002

Stern, A. (1938). Psychoanalytic investigation of and therapy in the borderline group of neuroses. *The Psychoanalytic Quarterly, 7*, 467-489. http://dx.doi.org/10.1080/21674086.1938.11925367

Stone, M. H. (1977). The borderline syndrome: evolution of the term, genetic aspects, and prognosis. *American Journal of Psychotherapy, 31*(3), 345-365. Retrieved from https://search.ebscohost.com/login.aspx?direct=true&db=psyh&AN=1979-01215-001&site=ehost-live

Sullivan, H. S. (1953). *The interpersonal theory of psychiatry*. New York: W. W. Norton & Co.

Swenson, C. R. & Choi-Kain, L. W. (2015). Mentalization and dialectical behavior therapy. *American Journal of Psychotherapy, 69*(2), 199-217. Retrieved from https://search.ebscohost.com/login.aspx?direct=true&db=psyh&AN=2015-32680-008&site=ehost-live

Thorne, F. C. (1955). Diagnostic classifications. In *Principles of Psychological Examining: A Systematic Textbook of Applied Integrative Psychology*. Brandon, VT, US: *Journal of Clinical Psychology*, pp. 83-109. http://dx.doi.org/10.1037/13896-005

In: Borderline Personality Disorder
Editor: Charles M. Lepkowsky
ISBN: 978-1-53618-021-3

Chapter 2

DEFINING BORDERLINE PERSONALITY DISORDER

Ronald B. Brooks**, PhD
Independent Practice, Santa Barbara, California, US

ABSTRACT

The development of diagnostic criteria for Borderline Personality Disorder (BPD) has been a slow and controversial process. Competing theoretical and nosological considerations have resulted in compromise rather than clarity of the diagnosis. A detailed description of the evolution and current advancement of the diagnostic criteria for BPD is presented.

Keywords: borderline personality disorder, DSM-5 diagnostic criteria, alternative model for personality disorders

---

* Corresponding Author's E-mail: dr.brookspsychologicalservices@hushmail.com.

INTRODUCTION

Borderline Personality Disorder (BPD) is the most frequently diagnosed personality disorder in mental health settings (Trull, Stepp, & Durrett, 2003). The prevalence of BPD in the general population is estimated to range from one to two percent (American Psychiatric Association, 2013; Ellison, Rosenstein, Morgan, & Zimmerman, 2018; Torgersen, Kringlen, & Cramer, 2001), 20 percent of psychiatric inpatients, and 10 percent of psychiatric outpatients (Zimmerman, Rothschild, & Chelminski, 2005). The BPD rate of suicide is estimated at 50 times that encountered in the general adult population (Pompili, Girardi, Ruberto, & Ruberto, 2005) with suicide completed in 8 to 10% of those with BPD (American Psychiatric Association, 2013). There is an overrepresentation of women, who account for over 70 percent of BPD diagnoses in clinical settings (Paris, 2010).

The initial onset of symptoms is typically in late adolescence, with prodromal symptoms identified in early adolescence and symptoms of emotional dysregulation sometimes observed in childhood (Stepp, 2012; Stepp, Keenan, Hipwell, & Krueger, 2014). The impact of this condition upon the individual, their family, the workplace environment and other points of interaction is often severe (Pompili, Girardi, Roberto, & Tatarelli, 2005). There is a temporal summation of the emotional turmoil that surrounds the daily activities of these individuals that is marked by mood instability, chronic feelings of inadequacy, frequent bouts of depression, rage and a piercing sense of helplessness to modulate their emotions, direct their life course and use active mastery to allow their feelings to work for them rather than on them. The emotional swings from baseline to depression, despair, and oftentimes rageful affect, frequently co-occur with elevated levels of hypervigilance and fears that others will think less of them, disparage their character or accomplishments, and ultimately reject or abandon them. Poorly controlled emotions color the perceptions of people with BPD, laying fertile ground for misinterpretations and distortions of the intent and actions of others until proven differently through various tests of caring and fidelity (American Psychiatric Association, 2013).

The BPD person's emotional waves seek outlet and typically overcome fragile defenses, often releasing an outpouring of impulsive, sensation-seeking and unfortunately harmful behavior that is typically self-directed and marked by episodes of dissociation, derealization and numbness that is countered with acts of self-harm to help them "feel alive" again. In this backdrop, their friends, family, and mental health professionals often misread, misunderstand, and misapply various strategies to ameliorate and contain the emotional pain and risk for self-injury for individuals with untreated or poorly treated BPD. This mission is often confounded by the misdiagnosis of the condition, which shares many features and a biological diathesis with other conditions, such as bipolar disorder and major depressive disorder (Fowler, Madan, Allen, Oldman, & Frueh, 2019; Gunderson & Lyons-Ruth, 2008; Perez-Rodriguez et al., 2018). Treatment efficacy is dependent upon a thoughtful and individualized approach to specific symptoms and clusters of symptoms, while understanding the biopsychosocial precipitants, context, and long-term course of the symptom constellations.

History of Diagnostic Criteria for Borderline Personality Disorder

The diagnostic criteria for BPD have evolved toward the development of a polythetic diagnostic system, in which criteria are based on shared characteristics commonly occurring in members of a group, no one of which is essential for membership in that group. The initial diagnostic formulation of BPD was first described by Stern (1938) who portrayed these individuals as treatment resistant and unresponsive to psychoanalytic techniques designed to retrospectively reconstruct early life experiences and personality organization. Stern (1938) characterized these individuals as resistive to change, masochistic and hypersensitive to and protective against the perceived threats from others. Stern (1938, p. 471) described a "psychic bleeding" in the face of stressful or threatening situations. He outlined prototypic features of BPD that had their origins in early childhood events leading to recurring periods of "psychic rigidity" (Stern, 1938, p. 472). He detailed 10 features and the mechanisms of actions that were designed to help preserve and protect the brittle defenses of these individuals. They include: "narcissism", "psychic bleeding", "inordinate hypersensitivity", "psychic and body rigidity – the rigid personality", "negative therapeutic reactions", "constitutionally rooted in feelings of inferiority"; "masochism", "a state of deep organic insecurity or anxiety", "the use of projection mechanisms" and difficulties in reality testing, particularly in interpersonal relationships" (Stern, 1938, p. 468).

At that time in psychoanalytic theory there were two classifications, neurosis and psychosis. The concept of borderline fell somewhere between these points without crossing the boundary into overt psychotic process (Kernberg, 1967; Stern, 1938). Stern's work was followed by a series of psychoanalysts who refined the concept. The Diagnostic and Statistical Manual of the American Psychiatric Association, First Edition (DSM-I) (American Psychiatric Association, 1952) and DSM-II (American Psychiatric Association, 1968) assumed that all symptoms were correlated and were present before the diagnosis could be established. The classical system assumed that all criteria were mutually inclusive and homogeneous (Ohio State Notes, 2001). Neither DSM-I or DSM-II included BPD as a diagnosis, because BPD was not considered a treatable condition.

Knight (1953) characterized the symptom as borderline states and Grinker (1968) reframed it as a borderline syndrome. The reformulation of the diagnosis of BPD followed the work of Kernberg (1967), who conceptualized it as borderline personality organization and Gunderson and Singer (1975) who reviewed the existing literature and offered six features that they felt represented a condition that laid the foundation for its inclusion and structure in DSM III (American Psychiatric Association, 1980). This reformulation transformed BPD from its theoretical origins as a state between neurosis and psychosis into a distinctly separate diagnostic entity that was not a precursor to psychosis and did not include the unusual and odd thoughts and behaviors of schizotypal personality disorder (Spitzer, Endicott, & Gibbon, 1979).

The behavioral descriptors offered by Spitzer et al. (1979) provided a more refined basis for a polythetic diagnostic nomenclature that outlined multiple ways in which the diagnostic threshold can be satisfied. This allowed for a number of heterogeneous symptoms to be included within a diagnosis without requiring that all symptoms be present before diagnostic criteria was met. This change represents an important shift in the conceptualization of diagnosis from the systems used in DSM-I (American Psychiatric Association, 1952) and DSM-II (American Psychiatric Association, 1968), which required that all symptoms were present before the diagnosis could be established.

The shift to the polythetic classification system of DSM-III (American Psychiatric Association, 1980) broadened the global conceptualization of BPD, with the potential for many combinations of heterogeneous symptoms contributing to the diagnosis, at the same time providing greater sensitivity and specificity for membership in the diagnosis. Diagnostic sensitivity is the ability of a feature to accurately identify those with the diagnosis, which is the true positive rate. Specificity is the ability of the feature to correctly identify those without the disorder, which is the true negative rate. Sensitivity and specificity are inversely proportional to each other. This balance in the DSM-III created an opportunity to question the inclusion criteria and the relative importance or weighting of each symptom. DSM-III included 265 disorders and provided a first attempt to rely on available research in establishing the diagnoses (Ohio State Notes, 2001). It was descriptive in its characterization of symptoms and behaviors and sought to avoid the influence of any one theoretical model.

The American psychiatric community at that time divided into relatively distinct camps of psychoanalytic theoreticians and a biological model of psychiatry. Criticisms of the DSM-III diagnostic system populated the research that followed, most notably the low interrater reliability of diagnostic agreement. Spitzer and Fleiss (1974) provided kappa (k) values for several diagnostic groupings. Adequate reliability coefficients were obtained for just three categories: mental deficiency (.72), organic brain syndrome (.77) and alcoholism (.71). Reliability levels for psychosis (.55) and schizophrenia were "fair" (Spitzer & Fleiss, 1974, p. 344). Kappa values were low for most other diagnoses. Threats to reliability and interrater agreement were ascribed to criterion variance and information variance. Criterion variance is associated with different raters using a nonstandard set of criteria. Information variance involves uncertain and typically nonstandard ways in which information is obtained, often leading to a varying database used to describe a set of behaviors (Ohio State Notes, 2001).

Clarkin, Widiger, Francis, Hurt, & Gilmore (1993) emphasized that the classical system requires that all symptoms have a true positive hit rate of 100 percent. The variance among diagnostic symptoms only occurs in their negative rates, which is the percentage of those without the diagnosis that do not have the symptom. The polythetic system allows for wide differences in the presence or absence of the diagnostic criteria, as long as the required five of eight symptoms can be supported in the diagnosis. This provided for varying levels of positive rates and diagnostic efficiency among the symptoms (Cantor, Smith, French, & Messich, 1980; Clarkin et al., 1983). This concept would hold true for other DSM-III diagnoses as well. The inherent strength of a flexible grouping of symptoms is qualified by its weakness. On what basis do we establish the relative importance of any one or any combination of symptoms within a diagnosis (Clarkin et al., 1983)? Francis (1982) indicates that there is no empirical basis for understanding the weighted value of any symptom versus another and the lack of efficiency weights in the polythetic classification system detracts from our confidence in the sturdiness of each symptom within a diagnosis.

Greater knowledge about the relative weighting of the symptom would provide diagnostic clarity and better inform treatment planning and decision-making. Clarkin et al. (1983) argued that a symptom with a lower positive hit rate may become more important and yield higher diagnostic efficiency when combined with other symptoms. Their study established the positive hit rate of the diagnosis with varying combinations of clusters of symptoms. The combination of any two symptoms combined for a positive hit rate of 50%. The authors note that the diagnosis of borderline personality could be established with confidence in their sample with two diagnostic criteria: identity disturbance and unstable/intense relationships. The sensitivity of the symptoms in the sample population was 60%. The combination was not present in any of the comparative group of other personality disorder subjects. This yielded a specificity of 100%. Clarkin et al. (1983) contend that the feature of identity disturbance is a weak predictor of the diagnosis, but an important predictor when paired with unstable/intense relationships.

In a similar study, Rusch, Guastello, and Mason (1992) found significant intercorrelations among two clusters of BPD features. The first group was designated the volatility component and included unstable interpersonal relationships, behavioral impulsivity and inappropriate anger. The second grouping involved features of self-harm and unpredictability that included affective instability and acts of self-mutilation. The interrater reliability of coefficients for seven of the eight diagnostic criteria were strong, ranging from .77 to .89, while symptom eight, fear of abandonment, showed a reliability coefficient of .61. The mean inter-judge reliability of .81 provides overall confidence in this aspect of the methodology. The study showed only mild intercorrelations among individual symptoms. However, when three features were clustered together the diagnosis was identified in 82 of the 89 cases. The symptoms included comprise the Self-Destructive Unpredictability (SDU) factor, which involved affective instability and self-mutilating acts, with reliability coefficients of .99 and .52, respectively. The results provide confidence in the inter-rater reliability of the diagnosis of BPD and relatively robust positive predictive power that the diagnosis of BPD is present when criteria for the SDU were met (Rusch et al., 1992).

DSM-III diagnostic criteria for BPD remained unchanged in DSM-III-R (American Psychiatric Association, 1987), but added a ninth criterion in DSM-IV: "Transient, stress-related paranoid ideation or severe dissociative symptoms" (American Psychiatric Association, 1994, p. 663). Questions have been raised in the literature and by clinicians concerning the assignment of membership of symptoms to BPD. There is considerable diagnostic overlap and comorbidity among several other diagnoses that raises concerns about the reliability of the diagnosis (Clarkin et al., 1983; Rusch et al., 1992).

Sanislow et al. (2002) examined the factor structure of DSM-IV criteria for BPD using confirmatory factor analysis. Three homogeneous clusters of symptoms were identified and empirically supported. The first group was disturbed relatedness and involved diagnostic features of unstable relationships, identity disturbance, chronic feelings of emptiness and stress-related paranoid ideation. The second group was labeled behavioral dysregulation and involved features of impulsivity in two areas including suicidality and self-mutilation. The results supported the unitary model or one-factor model of the diagnosis and showed significantly greater support for the three-factor model, which was replicated by a panel of interviewers who were blind to the study diagnosis in a two year follow-up after the baseline rating with the DSM-IV Diagnostic Interview for DSM-IV Personality Disorders. Other researchers have attempted to increase clinical unity and diagnostic accuracy by categorically grouping items based on shared features or intercorrelation of symptoms (Sanislow et al., 2002).

The work of Zanarini (2019) and Zittel, Conklin, and Westen (2005) provides support for a two-factor model of BPD symptom clusters including intense inner pain in individuals with BPD persisting over the lifetime, and a second characteristic with hallmark symptoms of suicidality, self-mutilation, suicidality and impulsive acting-out risk-taking behavior. Skodol et al. (2002) provided three phenotypes for BPD: affective instability, impulsivity and disturbed relationships that has gained wide acceptance in the literature.

Alternative Model for DSM-5 Personality Disorders

All nine BPD criteria were retained for DSM-5 (American Psychiatric Association, 2013) with an important distinction between two parallel systems of classification. The polythetic categorical system in place since the establishment of the DSM-III has continued and a dimensional system of personality traits listed as the Alternative DSM-5 Model for Personality Disorders has been added. This hybrid model allows for further study, validation and comparison of two competing conceptualizations of BPD that share many similarities in their behavioral descriptors of symptoms. The new dimensional model proposed established a continuum of personality traits that is reported to provide a more empirically supported system of understanding personality factors that range from normal to pathological conditions (Widiger, Crego, Rojas, & Oltmanns, 2018).

The dimensional model of five pathological personality traits or five-factor model (FFM) yields new insight into personality factors and a platform for testing the validity and reliability for specific personality traits and recent research provides support for its continued clinical investigation. However, the usefulness in clinical settings may be of uncertain value, particularly when formulating treatment planning in concert with other mental health professionals who rely upon symptom specificity and a common understanding of diagnostic features in order to assess risk factors, pharmacological intervention and treatment disposition for differential diagnosis and assessment for inpatient versus outpatient care. Meehan, Clarkin, and Lenzenweger (2018a) indicate that the personality traits comprising the underlying dimensional structure are unclear and represent an ordinal measurement of patient self-report that is reliant upon the Personality Inventory for DSM-5 (PID-5). Self-report measures in clinical research are often fraught with threats to validity as subject rater bias combines with inaccuracies inherent in retrospective self-analysis, as well as simple misunderstandings of questionnaire items by subjects. A review of the literature documented challenges in the early construction of self-report personality inventories among subjects with comorbid anxiety disorders and personality disorders (Brooks, Baltazar, & Munjack, 1989). More recent studies provide robust support for the PID-5, which is considered to be a highly reliable and valid instrument (Calvo, Valero, Saez-Francas, Gutierrez, Casas, & Ferrer, 2016; Krueger, Derringer, Markon, Watson, & Skodol, 2012), and for the dimensional model for personality disorder diagnoses (Anderson, Snider, Sellborn, & Krueger, 2013; Krueger & Hopwood, 2014; Morey & Skodol, 2013; Widiger et al., 2018; Wright, Hopwood, & Zanarini, 2015). Widiger et al. (2018) and Clark (2007) contend that the FFM is the most useful dimensional model of personality organization. They provide five domains of personality traits including:

neuroticism, extraversion, openness, agreeableness and conscientiousness. Widiger et al. (2018) suggest that the personality make-up of individuals in mental health settings may be more similar rather than dissimilar to individuals who have not sought treatment for problematic personality traits.

The proposed BPD criteria in the DSM-5 Alternative Model for Personality Disorders involve two clusters of personality traits. In Criterion A, the four areas include: “identity”, “self-direction”, “empathy” and “intimacy” (American Psychiatric Association, 2013, p. 766). Individuals who satisfy two or more of the criteria may show an inconsistent self-image marked by frequent negative self-reference, feelings of emptiness and intense anxiety often leading to stress-related dissociative states. These individuals frequently have poor planning and organization skills and difficulty establishing goals and maintaining a set of values while planning for the future. They often experience high levels of interpersonal sensitivity, are easily slighted and may experience intense emotions that cloud their ability to recognize the feelings and needs of others. Relationships with others are often conflictual and marked by intense emotions, mistrust, requests for support and preoccupation with fears of abandonment. Periods of idealization and devaluation co-vary with excessive involvement often followed by withdrawal (American Psychiatric Association, 2013).

Individuals who meet threshold criteria for Criterion B must satisfy four or more of seven personality traits including at least one of the following three traits: “impulsivity”, “risk taking” or “hostility”. The remaining four personality traits include: “emotional lability”, “anxiousness”, “separation insecurity” and “depressivity” (American Psychiatric Association, 2013, p. 766). They often experience mood instability marked by intense feelings and reactions that appear out of proportion to the situation. There is frequently a high level of anxiety, negativity, excessive apprehension about past events and threats from future negative outcomes. These individuals are often apprehensive, uncomfortable with poorly defined circumstances and complain of fears of personality disintegration and loss of control. They often ruminate and worry about separation from important relationships and are concerned that they may become overly dependent upon others and lose their ability to maintain their individuation and self-identity. There are frequent feelings of sadness, hopelessness, negative outlook for the future, chronic feelings of inadequacy, low self-worth and suicidal ideation, intent and plan (American Psychiatric Association, 2013).

Impulsive acts of disinhibition may occur without thinking through the consequences of their behavior. Individuals with BPD will experience a compelling need to act upon a thought or feeling and they are prone to self-harm under emotional stress. Risk-taking behavior is associated with disinhibition and poor impulse controls. They often risk situations that may cause them great harm and they display an inadequate appreciation of the danger they may place themselves in. The personality trait of hostility, an aspect of antagonism, is often marked by chronic feelings of anger and irritability typically precipitated by perceived slights and insults that are often minor in comparison to the emotional response exhibited by these individuals (American Psychiatric Association, 2013; Chapman, 2019).

The DSM-5 Alternative Model for Personality Disorders provides an increasingly evidence-based approach for understanding personality traits. The application of this classification system in clinical settings remains unclear until it is known how well mental health professionals can operationalize the dimensional model to describe their patients' affect and patterns of behavior (Meehan, Clarkin, & Lenzenweger, 2018a). The system in place for classifying and treating individuals with BPD at this time remains the DSM-5 categorical model with nine diagnostic criteria and associated features. This chapter will primarily focus on the DSM-5 classification system and its definition and understanding of BPD.

Definitions of DSM-5 Diagnostic Criteria for Borderline Personality Disorder

Definitions of the nine DSM-5 diagnostic criteria of BPD involves an understanding of each symptom and in combination within clusters of symptoms and their contextual expression at varying levels of intensity. BPD falls within Cluster B of DSM-5 Personality Disorders that also includes: antisocial personality disorder, narcissistic personality disorder and histrionic personality disorder. DSM-5 describes the condition as a pervasive pattern of unstable relationships, self-image, and affects, impulsive acts with onset typically in early adulthood that is best characterized by five or more of the nine diagnostic features (American Psychiatric Association, 2013).

> Diagnostic Criterion 1 involves: “Frantic efforts to avoid real or imagined abandonment” (American Psychiatric Association, 2013, p. 663).

Individuals with BPD are fearful that others in close relationships, work settings and social groups will withdraw from and oftentimes abandon them based upon some inherent flaw or vulnerability that is prone to discovery. At other times, their sense of low self-worth is projected outwards at others who they fear will ultimately reject them. The risk for rejection is often minimal or nonexistent and is an expression of catastrophic thoughts emanating from cognitive distortions and exaggerated levels of rejection sensitivity. These are painful moments for individuals with BPD and those caught up during these times of desperation and intense efforts to hold onto another and test and retest their fidelity to them (American Psychiatric Association, 2013).

Individuals with BPD may repeatedly call, text, email or physically track the location of another individual in an effort to gain pledges of loyalty and reassurance that are intended to but typically do not fill the emotional void and fear of abandonment resulting in personality disintegration. Fears of abandonment are often triggered by minor environmental events, such as the availability of a partner or friend on a demand basis (American Psychiatric Association, 2013; Gunderson & Lyons-Ruth, 2008). The ensuing painful affect compromises otherwise adequate judgment with no clear path for resolution. This pattern repeats itself among both new and established relationships. Individuals with BPD often become overly close and self-disclosing as they seek comfort and solace in the pseudo-intimacy of an early encounter or friendship. Poor boundaries between themselves and others creates uncertainty and anxious attempts to understand just how much another individual cares for them and under what situations they may leave them. (American Psychiatric Association, 2013, p. 663).

In psychotherapy, these individuals may demand additional time in session and after hour emergency calls for reassurance. They may ask for personal information, or will sit too close or far away from the therapist. There is an array of treatment strategies and practical steps in daily living that provide structure and clear boundaries that support the separation and individuation of individuals in all relationships. Porous boundaries between self and others are tested until some limit and sense of certainty is reached. Consistent boundaries provide safety and a reference point for stability within a relationship that builds over time and decreases frantic efforts to avoid real or imagined abandonment.

> Diagnostic Criterion 2: "A pattern of unstable and intense interpersonal relationships characterized by alternating between extremes of idealization and devaluation" (American Psychiatric Association, 2013, p. 663).

As noted in Criterion 1, fears of abandonment are driven by chronic feelings of inadequacy and fears that if they become close to another they will ultimately be rejected and suffer great emotional harm. The cognitive distortions, overgeneralized thinking and catastrophic processes create an emotional vulnerability that lends itself to intense interpersonal relationships with shifts from idealization to devaluation of another. Overly close relationships are attempts to gain from another what they are unable to provide for themselves. This merging of identities requires a suspension of critical judgment and over estimation of the attributes of another, resulting in an idealistic, rather than realistic appraisal of that individual's character and strengths. Idealization depends upon an unequal relationship where one individual has claim to superior value and worth than the other. This pedestal of power is precarious as idols and idealized figures typically have the same chinks in the armor that the rest of us have. Their perch above someone can be toppled by the supplicants growing sense of unease and fear that they will be cast out of the light they share and left to stumble on their own in the darkness of uncertain identity and self-worth. Small transgressions or omissions of praise by the idealized figure result in fears of rejection and the protective mechanism of devaluation. The all-or-nothing basis for affiliation is untenable, unstable and marked by intense emotional reactions that are experienced as all-encompassing or all-rejecting. Within a family, perceived rejection by one parent can lead to the devaluation of that figure and the over identification with and idealization of the other parent (Masterson, 1981).

Academic and employment situations often involve less intense but dynamically parallel patterns. A graduate student may feel devastated by a professor's constructive criticisms and suggestions. That faculty member may become devalued and another faculty member is idealized in order to stem a rising sense of inadequacy precipitated by well-intentioned comments to expand upon or improve the quality of their academic effort.

> Diagnostic Criterion 3: "Identity disturbance: markedly and persistently unstable self-image or sense of self" (American Psychiatric Association, 2013, p. 663).

Criterion 3 blends elements of diagnostic criteria 1 and 2. DSM-5 (American Psychiatric Association, 2013) indicates that the toxicogenic effects of intense unstable relationships and the often crippling belief that they are less than others hampers the ability of individuals with BPD to establish and maintain academic and career goals and fulfill promises to themselves for a more developed and integrated persona. They are challenged by the complexities of interpersonal relationships and exhibit poor social judgment and problem-solving ability in both overlearned and novel social situations. The inability to tolerate minor frustrations and gain emotional distance from disappointing encounters disables their cognitive controls and fluid reasoning ability as they pay attention to the greater emotional stimulus of intense fear of failure. Individuals with BPD may recognize but feel helpless to modulate their emotions and meet the demands of employment, academic and social situations. They may leave work, school or social groups before risking failure and change direction in their life course, and employment goals. All individuals strive for sense of meaning and self-identity in their careers and in significant relationships. Without this, we are adrift without a future and lead life experientially rather than purposely. The inability to pursue and stay with a career is a frequent outcome among many individuals with BPD. This likely explains why so many feel they have so little to look back upon as personal accomplishments (American Psychiatric Association, 2013)

Many individuals with BPD have a history of traumatic childhood experiences and report a family environment that was unstable and unpredictable (Chapman, 2019). One or more family members may have shown symptoms of BPD, major depression or bipolar I or II disorder. Comorbidity for these conditions is significantly higher than in the general population (Shah & Zanarini, 2018) and may in part be explained by a genetic vulnerability (Amad, Ramoz, Thomas, Jadri, & Gorwood, 2014). The chaotic behavior in these families does not lend itself to positive role modeling and the internalization of aspirational aspects of the parental figure into themselves. The parental imperative to provide care for a child is often set aside in order to stem the rising tide of emotional pain and personality fragmentation that is the common experience of individuals with BPD. A child is a reflection of their parents' behavior and subject to the vicissitudes of emotional crises and the absence of pathways to manage their emotions, express ideas and progress along the developmental continuum feeling safe, cared for and confident in their ability to make thoughtful and reasonable decisions that create, rather than cripple, a strong and stable sense of self.

> Diagnostic Criterion 4: "Impulsivity in at least two areas that are potentially self-damaging (e.g., spending, sex, substance abuse, reckless driving, binge eating)." Suicidal and self-mutilating behavior is excluded and included in Criterion 5 (American Psychiatric Association, 2013, p. 663).

There is a growing body of literature describing the initial onset, clinical course and outcome of impulsive and self-destructive behaviors with origins in adolescence followed by a brief period of respite and resurgence of symptoms in the early 20s in a subgroup of adolescents. However, the long-term course of symptoms for most adolescents is a gradual decline in the intensity and frequency of occurrence (Sharp, Vanwoerden, & Wall, 2018). Studies by Álvarez-Tomás, Ruiz, Guilera and Bados (2018), Temes and Zanarini, (2018) and Zanarini, (2019) indicate a high rate of symptom reduction for this cluster of BPD features in comparison to the improving but persistently troubling symptoms of negative affect and emotional lability throughout the lifetime. Long-term prospective studies, such as the CLPS (McGlashon et al., 2000) and MSAD (Zanarini, 2019) show encouraging results that most symptoms of impulsiveness, self-destructive acts and self-harm will show a gradual course of improvement over the lifespan.

Biskin (2018) indicates that improved symptomology does not consistently translate into higher functioning and employability with similar findings noted by Esquivillas et al. (2018). Impulsive and self-harm behavior is often a protective mechanism that at its core has a goal of softening painful affect, which individuals with BPD often feel helpless to lessen in any other way (Zanarini, 2019). They may intermingle or shift from one behavior to another and invoke the outrage, empathy and containment efforts of others that proffer a limiting factor to their seemingly endless spiral of self-defeating behavior. The impulsive and crisis-laden external acts mirror their inner chaos and follow a cascading course that is often harmful to self and others. Inpatient psychiatric treatment is a frequent outcome and provides a structure and limit-setting for individuals who are unable to provide that safety mechanism for themselves (Zimmerman, Rothschild, & Chelminski, 2005). Polysubstance abuse, risk-taking in sexual encounters, gambling, excessive spending of money, reckless driving and the binge eating of bulimia nervosa are self-directed behaviors that often leave emotional scars. The intent is to dampen intrusive negative thoughts and affect by changing their emotional state from despair to excitability and their self-image from incapable to powerful. Sexual encounters may involve approach-avoidance behaviors and submission or domination, while reckless driving mitigates feelings of helplessness with brief flashes of invincibility as they barrel down the road at seemingly impossible speeds. Binge eating provides instant comfort followed by acts designed to maintain an idealized body image (American Psychiatric Association, 2013).

> Diagnostic Criterion 5: "Recurrent suicidal behavior, gestures, or threats, or self-mutilating behavior" (American Psychiatric Association, 2013, p. 663).

A plethora of research has been devoted to studying suicidal behavior and self-mutilating acts, including non-suicidal self-injury (Guinea et al., 2019; Hankin & Adela, 2011; Nokar et al., 2016; Pompili, Girardi, Ruberto, & Tataelli, 2005; Sarhan, et al., 2019; Taylor et al., 2018). Suicidal behaviors occur at a high rate among individuals diagnosed with BPD. Klonsky and Mueuhlenkamp (2007) found that 13% to 23% of community dwelling adolescents reported a history of non-suicidal self-injury while Cooper (2005) indicates that there is a 30 times increased risk factor for completing suicide, compared to those who had never committed self-destructive acts. Both adolescents and adults present for evaluation and treatment in hospital emergency rooms. Nearly 50% of those evaluated that are diagnosed with BPD (Biskin, 2013). Adults diagnosed with BPD were found to have a high prevalence rate of suicidality of approximately 50% and completion rates ranging from 3% to 10% (Zanarini et al., 2008) and 8% to 10% (American Psychiatric Association, 2013).

Comorbid major depression was thought to increase the risk of suicide among individuals with BPD (Zeng et al., 2015). Risk factors for suicidal behavior and self-mutilative acts are typically precipitated by the loss or threatened loss of another with concomitant fears of disintegration of self, following the real or misconstrued threat of abandonment. The speed of deterioration and personality disorganization is remarkable, often unpredictable, and can be dangerous in that painful affect seeks relief with an impaired regard for safety or the capacity to see a situation through until a better day. The essential goal of non-suicidal self-injury is mood stabilization, affect regulation and avoidance of inner pain. (Klonsky & Muehlenkamp, 2007; Taylor et al., 2018).

Individuals with BPD may display many intellectual gifts, and at times a charming persona, but emotional resiliency is not one of their most common assets. The most concerning factor is that individuals with BPD have a 10% rate of completed suicide, which is 50 times greater than the general population (Paris & Zweig-Frank, 2001). They often make multiple attempts and undergo repeated hospitalizations before terminating their life (Paris, 2019). Every care and consideration should be extended to anyone who feels unable to bring themselves out of this level of despair and contemplates any form of self-harm or risk-taking behavior that purposely, or accidentally on purpose, may lead to the most unfortunate of circumstances.

> Diagnostic Criterion 6: "Affective instability due to a marked reactivity of mood, e.g., intense episodic dysphoria, irritability, or anxiety usually lasting a few hours and only rarely more than a few days" (American Psychiatric Association, 2015, p. 663).

The American Psychiatric Association (2013) characterizes affective instability as a fluctuating state of poorly filtered emotions resulting from a heightened emotional state of protective physiological arousal involving a fear reaction of acute anxiety, anger and dysphoria. The onset may be gradual but is often sudden and catches others unaware and unprepared for the torrent of emotions and the dramatic presentation that often follows. The duration is typically a few hours but on rare occasions may languish for a few days. Individuals with BPD feel incapable of tempering their emotions as they sort through the possibilities of why some event has occurred. An emotional switch is thrown as they latch on to the worst rather than the most probable cause of a negative event. There is a heightened arousal in preparation for the most threatening rather than most likely possibility. This feels seems safer to them rather than tolerating some level of ambiguity. There are a number of theoretical paradigms that have been offered to explain this state of mental and emotional decompensation. Linehan's (1993) biosocial model suggests that behavioral skill deficits result from an emotionally sensitive temperament that is worsened by negative and invalidating experiences from a critical and rejecting childhood environment.

There is a growing body of evidence that supports a neurobiological model for BPD where a genetic predisposition for affective dysregulation is sparked by environmental factors (Carpenter, Tomko, Trull, & Boomsma, 2013; Zanarini, 2019; Perez-Rodriguez, 2018), which precipitates an affective startle response (Perez-Rodriguez et al. 2018; Cuthbert et al., 1998). An intriguing discussion by Perez-Rodriguez et al. (2018) suggests that there are elevated levels of alexithymia in individuals with BPD where emotional responses are intensified and the recognition and understanding of those responses is minimal or "blunted", resulting in an "impairment in emotional interoception" (p. 636). Alexithymia is a Greek word suggestive of an impaired ability to recognize emotions. Darios, Zakzanis and Ruocco (2012) reviewed a series of 10 studies examining recognition of facial emotions. Patients with BPD, compared to non-clinical control subjects, showed significant difficulty recognizing neutral facial expressions, and to a lesser degree, correctly identifying facial emotions of anger and disgust.

Although there are no specific risk genes or molecular pathways that have been identified for BPD there appears to be growing evidence of a genetic predisposition as well as an interpersonal hypersensitivity, which has been described by several studies (Amad, Ramoz, Thomas, Jardi, & Gorwood, 2014; Amad, Ramoz, Peyre, Thomas, & Gorwood, 2019; Gunderson & Lyons-Ruth, 2008). The psychobiological models and genetic precursors for development of many psychiatric conditions is a burgeoning area of research into complex and overdetermined factors of the interplay between emotions, cognitions and their expression and development in response to environmental factors and changes over time.

> Diagnostic Criterion 7: "Chronic feelings of emptiness" (American Psychiatric Association, 2013, p. 663).

Chronic feelings of emptiness are not well defined in the literature and show a paucity of research. It appears more clinically descriptive than empirically-based. DSM-5 characterizes this feature in two sentences:

"Individuals with BPD may be troubled by chronic feelings of emptiness. Easily bored, they may constantly seek something to do" (American Psychiatric Association, 2013, p. 663). This leaves us questioning: What is the subjective experience of persistent feelings of emptiness? Elsner, Broadbear and Rao (2018, p. 89) offer a table of somatic experiences and existential experiences of chronic emptiness provided by patients. Several of the somatic experiences include: "I feel like there is a hole inside me from the front of me right through to my back"; "I feel hollow-a true emptiness, a void, where my heart is"; "I feel hollow, like a shell." Existential experiences of chronic emptiness include statements such as: "hopelessness and existential nihilism"; "a sense of purposelessness"; "There's always something missing--I'm looking for something that's not there." There are perhaps two distinct descriptors that stand out from the rest. Individuals with BPD may experience emotional distress that is somaticized if there is internal pain or discomfort. This is the "void". It may be precipitated by separation from another and difficulty tolerating any ambiguity in the relationship. This is likely associated with an uncertain sense of self and identity disturbance (Elsner et al. 2018, p. 89). The existential experiences of chronic emptiness described by Elsner et al. (2018) may represent an immature or partially developed emotional core and personality structure in a world where competency and accomplishment in a career are defining factors in one's work role and self-identity. The value of our efforts is less existential and more practical in that they are byproducts of our ability to engage in successful career-oriented tasks.

> Diagnostic Criterion 8: "Inappropriate, intense anger or difficulty controlling anger, (e.g., frequent displays of temper, constant anger, recurrent physical fights)" (American Psychiatric Association, 2013, p. 663).

Often in concert with affective instability, inappropriate and intense displays of anger are common among individuals with BPD. Cognitive distortions of the intent of others, rejection sensitivity and fears of abandonment usher in shifts from baseline to temper outbursts, and at times physical altercations with others (American Psychiatric Association, 2013). Affective instability is often intense dysphoria and negativism turned inwards. Criterion 8 is the other side of the emotional coin where depressive affect and negative self-referents are projected outwards with targeted displays of anger against others. DSM-5 suggests that this is often followed by periods of remorse, self-reproach and guilty recriminations that further confirm their core identity as broken and inferior. There is a progression in the formation of emotional dysregulation where poorly defined situations evoke emotional responses that trigger emotions that belong to an earlier time, but are displaced upon the current situation or person. The pain of the moment is an old familiar feeling that touches an open wound and unleashes a cascade of intertwined thoughts and emotions that are preserved, reinforced over time, and are now attributed to the current situation in place of the actual event or intended outcome by another. In this context, the logic of a strong response to a minor issue unveils itself. The angry, yet protective response, originating from the past was a survival tool at some point in time, but like a blunt tool, its indiscriminate use produces less than optimal results.

The emotional vulnerability conceptualized by Linehan (1993) in her biosocial model provides an explanation for readily observed behavioral correlates of intense dysphoria, anger and their behavioral correlates among many individuals with BPD. Chapman (2019) reviewed the literature and reports additive factors that provide a more integrated model. Beauchaine, Hinsaw and Bridge (2019), Chapman (2019), Crowell, Beauchaine and Linehan (2009) suggest that trait impulsivity is a genetic predisposition that compromises an individual's ability to cope with the toxicogenic effects of an invalidating and negative childhood environment. The emotionally harmful behavior of the parents or caretakers echoes in the responses of the child in escalating rhythm with each other. Crowell et al. (2009) indicate that there is an intermittent reinforcement of negative affect, emotional dyscontrol, and at times emotional and physical abuse and neglect. The combined factors of inheritable genetic vulnerability and harmful childhood environments may be potentiated by stressors in late adolescence and early adulthood that confirm past transgressions against an individual and propel them down a path of devolving rather than evolving integration of cognitive and emotional controls with an expanded set of values and positive and self-image. Painful affect gives way to impulsive emotionally-driven decision-making. Helping these individuals to understand the validity of their emotions, the logic in their intent, and the potential for a different interpretation of themselves offers hope for the future in small, but in the end highly successful gradients of personal development.

> Diagnostic Criterion 9: "Transient, stress-related paranoid ideation or severe dissociative symptoms" (American Psychiatric Association, 2013, p. 663).

Disturbed thought processes are common among individuals with BPD (Zanarini, 2019; Zanarini, Frankenburg, Wedig, & Fitzmaurice, 2013). Three primary areas of impaired cognition involving 17 types of disturbed thought processes were identified by Zanarini et al. (2013) in a 16-year retrospective study. The three clusters of impaired thought processes involved: (1) nonpsychotic ideation including unusual or odd thoughts, perceptual experiences and non-delusional paranoia; (2) psychotic thought processes that approach but did not break with reality; (3) individuals with brief episodes of overt psychotic thought processes. Subjects in the study further divided into five groups. The results indicated that 80% of individuals with BPD reported unusual or odd thinking, 76% acknowledged disturbed sensory perceptual experiences and 87% were found to have some form of paranoia that did not reach the level of delusional thought processes. All three types of impaired cognition were found in significantly greater numbers among individuals with BPD than with a comparison group of other individuals with other personality disorders. Despite a notable decline in the presence of symptoms at two-year intervals over the course of 16 years, the prevalence of the three types of impaired cognition remained high with 37% reporting odd thinking, 26% acknowledged disturbed sensory perceptual experiences and 43% endorsed paranoia that was nondelusional. An important finding of the study was that thought processes approaching psychosis were common at the start of the study with a prevalence rate of 57%, but showed significant improvement after 16 years with a rate of not greater than 7%. The third finding of the study was that overt psychotic experiences were rare and included brief episodes of delusional thought processes and hallucinations. Zanarini (2019) states that the quasi-psychotic symptoms may be related to severe depression or the resurgence of a physical memory triggered by some reminder of past physical abuse, sexual abuse or other traumatic currents from the distant or recent past.

Cognitive slippage in the form of suspicious and paranoid ideation is typically brief, situation specific, and follows either brief or prolonged exposure to stressful events and/or perceived threats (American Psychiatric Association, 2013). The feared circumstances involves times when individuals with BPD feel criticized, shamed or humiliated by others, or, when loss of status within a group or organization is threatened. Baer, Peters, Eisenlohr-Moul, Geiger, and Sauer (2012) indicate that there is a selective bias toward negative memories and excessive self and other criticism that rests upon inaccurate representations of an interaction or event. Fears of withdrawal and abandonment by others weakens the structure of otherwise intact reality testing, as greater weight is given to low probability occurrences that carry the most painful outcomes. Thought processes involve overgeneralized thinking and cognitive distortions of the content and intent of communication from others or times in which neutral facial expressions are misinterpreted as anger (Shin, Goldstein, & Pick, 2019), or reading expressionless faces with emotion that is not there (Meehan, Clarkin, & Lenzenweger, 2018b; Meehan et al., 2017), or failing to recognize emotion, particularly those that have a negativity bias or intense sensitivity to negatively-tinged affect (Morey, 2014). An individual may question what hidden meaning there is to someone else's words and whether they are critical of them or against them based upon little or no evidence.

The American Psychiatric Association (2013) indicates that stressful events may trigger painful memories and their accompanying negative affect and negative thought patterns. Ruminative thoughts and intolerable levels of emotional pain may cause someone to shut down emotionally, become numb, detach themselves from feelings, and sometimes from reality.

They may experience dissociative symptoms that interrupt the integration of cognitive processing, affective organization, sensory perceptual experiences, memory and motor functioning. The onset may be sudden, debilitating and involve feelings of acute anxiety that give way to depersonalization, detachment from self and others and feeling suspended outside of, and looking down upon themselves. Visual perceptions of oneself and others may appear distorted for facial images, body image, and at times, a shrinking appearance to the fingers and extremities.

The intense negative thoughts and painful affect that precipitate the symptoms is often associated with current, recent or past emotional, physical or sexual trauma. The antecedents may accrue from childhood or adult abuse, bullying or traumatic experiences, including those that meet diagnostic criteria for posttraumatic stress disorder. Symptoms of dissociation are common among individuals with BPD, particularly those who are victims of trauma (Perez-Rodriguez et al., 2018).

The more severe the traumatic experience the greater the symptomatology and lower the functioning and remission rates with sexual abuse for adults occurring at higher rates than for other individuals with personality disorders (Aquino Ferreira, Pereira, Benevides, & Melo, 2018). A meta-analysis of research from 1997 to 2017 yielded 40 studies that found sexual abuse, violence or victimization in childhood and suggested that these factors placed children at risk for the development of BPD (Aquino Ferreira et al., 2018). A different perspective is proposed by Hiraoka, Crouch, Reo, Wagner, Milner, & Skowronski (2019) and Lieb, Zanarini, Schmalh, Linehan, & Bohus (2004) who report a high incidence of childhood sexual abuse but no direct causal link between sexual abuse in childhood and BPD. Further study of these and other risk factors is indicated. There is a growing interest in the genetic predisposition (Amad et al., 2014; Mistry, Escott-Price, Florio, Smith, & Zammit, 2019) and the neurobiology of this condition (Perez-Rodriguez et al., 2018).

Differential Diagnosis of Borderline Personality Disorder

Differential diagnosis of BPD from primary mood disorders, such as depression, bipolar I disorder and bipolar II disorder is a difficult task for most clinicians and requires a lengthy process of clinical interviewing, behavioral observations and history-taking from the patient, with information often gained from family members or partners. BPD is distinguished from depression in a number of ways. The course of affective symptoms is driven by reactions to environmental stressors, where mood declines at the prospect of a negative event and/or fears of rejection and can quickly return to baseline when a state of homeostasis is restored. Individuals in the midst of a major depression or persistent depressive disorder may or may not react to favorable news, and the extent and duration of their improvement is slight and brief. The depressive state remains unremitting until it runs its course or responds to pharmacologic and/or psychotherapeutic interventions over several months, and not several hours (Gunderson & Phillips, 1991).

DSM-5 includes several physiological symptoms of major depression that are not among the diagnostic criteria for BPD. If they do occur, it is as a comorbid depression. The symptoms include psychomotor retardation where an individual's body feels like lead or weighed down. It is difficult to rise in the morning and movement is slow with easy fatigability and excessive tiredness from everyday tasks. Depressive mood shows little variation and is distinct from the mood swings and the volatile and the turbulent affective presentation of individuals with BPD (Paris, 2018). The disorders are also differentiated by the quality of the affective dysphoria described by DSM-5 Criterion 7 as "chronic feelings of emptiness" and the expression of the dysphoria in Criterion 3, as an identity disturbance with a "persistently unstable self-image", and Criterion 6, which includes "intense episodic dysphoria" (American Psychiatric Association, 2013, p. 663).

The impact of intense dysphoria may be seen in all nine DSM-5 symptoms. It drives the "frantic efforts of individuals to avoid real or imagined abandonment" in Criterion 1 and forms the basis for a "pattern of unstable relationships" in Criterion 2, which often leads to the impulsive "self-damaging" acts of Criterion 4, the "recurrent suicidal behavior" of Criterion 5 and the "intense anger" and rageful outbursts described in Criterion 8. The severe dissociative symptoms, suspiciousness and paranoid ideation listed in Criterion 9 is a result of anxious and depressive thoughts and feelings that bend reality as intense affect compromises cognitive controls (American Psychiatric Association, 2013, p. 663).

The variability in mood characteristic of BPD is similar to but distinct from bipolar I disorder or bipolar II disorder. Paris (2018, p. 576) indicates that some researchers have questioned whether BPD is a form of "soft bipolarity." Akiskal (2003) indicates that there is considerable interest in regarding borderline personality as a mood disorder with subthreshold symptoms of bipolar disorder. A review of the DSM-5 diagnostic criteria yields some marked distinctions between these conditions. A manic episode involves a period of elevated or irritable mood and increased energy or activity that is present for most of the day for at least one week and often longer. Mood swings from the manic to depressive states typically average three months for each phase of the disorder (Paris & Zweig-Frank, 2001). The mood disorder is severe and causes significant impairment often resulting in hospitalization and/or an inability to adequately function at work and in social interactions (American Psychiatric Association, 2013). This may occur among patients with BPD, but it does not almost always occur, as it does with a severe manic or depressive phase of bipolar I disorder. Bipolar II disorder is a less severe condition than bipolar I disorder, but still requires an extended period of elevated, expansive or irritable mood with increased energy and often goal-directed activity that is typically unproductive and abnormal. The mood disturbance must be present for at least four days. Symptoms are observable nearly every day for most of the day and represent a dramatic change in behavior. The mood swings that are characteristic of those with BPD are listed in DSM-5 as "intense episodic dysphoria, or anxiety usually lasting a few hours and rarely more than a few days". The affective instability and mood swings are precipitated by environmental factors, most often involving fear of rejection or abandonment from another in an important relationship (American Psychiatric Association, 2013, p. 663).

The differentiation of BPD from other DSM-5 personality disorders is complicated by the diagnostic overlap that is described in the literature (Clarkin et al., 1983; Wright, Hopwood, & Zanarini, 2015). Careful review of symptoms by an experienced clinician generally decides the matter, although the interview process and history-taking is often extensive. BPD is included in Cluster B personality disorders. It shares the symptoms of irritable mood and angry displays of emotion that is also present among those with either antisocial personality disorder or narcissistic personality disorder. However, the level of intensity is often more pronounced and frequently followed by periods of remorse among patients with BPD. Individuals with antisocial personality disorder have little or no remorse and those with narcissistic personality disorder have an inflated sense of self-worth that is easily distinguishable from the poor self-image and negative self-referents that are prototypic features of BPD noted in DSM-5 (American Psychiatric Association, 2013).

Criterion 5, of schizotypal personality disorder is: "Suspiciousness or paranoid ideation" (American Psychiatric Association, 2013, p. 663). It is the experience of this author that the presentation of patients with this disorder is strikingly different from BPD. They do not show the intense and dramatic affective displays and are instead characterized by an unusual display of odd verbalizations, thought processes and behaviors that is often subtle and can include the "odd beliefs", "magical thinking" and "superstitious" beliefs noted in Criterion 2 of schizotypal personality disorder (American Psychiatric Association, 2013, p. 663). Criterion 8 indicates that there is an absence of close friends and little desire for interpersonal connections, other than with family members. Individuals with BPD seek out and cling to others. They have elevated levels of rejection-sensitivity and fears of abandonment.

Adolescent Presentation of Borderline Personality Disorder Symptoms

There has been considerable research devoted to discovering the presence or absence of BPD. The discussion is complicated by transient symptoms of emotional dysregulation and impulsive, sensation-seeking proclivities that are often present and then fade over the course of development (Dahl, 2004; Steinberg & Morris, 2001). Clinical understanding is also guided by brain development from neuroscience and the expected developmental trajectories that are ushered in at the onset of adolescence and are integrated in predictable pathways throughout early adulthood. There is increased production of white matter, synaptic pruning of underused grey matter and increased connectivity and integration among all areas of the brain. An increased production of dopamine along partially formed pathways from limbic, striatal and prefrontal cortex areas can impair the judgement and reasoning ability of a 13 year old that seemed well-mannered and quite reasonable at 11 years of age (Casey, Jones, & Hare, 2008; Wahlstrom, Collins, White, & Luciana, 2010). The poorly contained upsurge of dopamine produces a period of "hot cognition" that often leads to poorly planned, emotionally-laden and impulse-driven behavior (Dahl, 2004, p. 19). The dorsal lateral prefrontal cortex is one of the last regions of the brain to mature, typically in early adulthood. It is involved with controlling impulses (Giedd, 2004). Poor cognitive controls over emotions increases the propensity for ill-considered actions and a heightened risk for self and other destructive acts (Casey et al., 2008). The morbidity risk in adolescence increases by 200% (Dahl, 2004).

However, most adolescents are well-adjusted and up to 80% do not give way to impulsive and destructive behavior during this developmental stage (Casey et al. 2008; Dahl, 2004). Care should be given to separate the normal development of adolescents from early markers of BPD. Winsper et al. (2016) caution researchers not to confuse the short-lived dysfunctional personality traits often present in adolescence with prodromal or fully established symptoms of adolescent BPD. Their review of the literature cites numerous studies that highlight the risk factors of stigmatizing an adolescent with a diagnosis that carries a negative association. They also warn of missing the diagnosis and the opportunity to lessen the symptoms and provide relief to an adolescent who is in intense emotional distress. The results of their literature review and meta-analysis indicate a consistency of symptom presentation among adolescents and adults who were found to have the disorder. They support the assignment of the diagnosis for this age cohort. DSM-5 states that the features of the disorder must be present for at least one year for an adolescent.

Prevalence rates within the general population of different countries and within different studies show significant variation (Guile, Boissel, Alaux-Cantin, & Garny de La Riviére, 2018; Sharp, Vanwoerdden, & Wall 2018). The prevalence rate among studies in the United States was generally lower at 1% (Zanarini et al., 2011). Guile et al. (2018) reviewed a series of studies and concluded that a cautious estimation of prevalence rates in the general populations worldwide is 3%. Different sampling and data gathering methods likely contribute to the variance in prevalence rates.

A large study of community dwelling children and adolescents was conducted in the Children in the Community Study (CIC) (Cohen, Crawford, Johnson, & Kasen, 2005). This was a retrospective study that tracked the development of 800 children and adolescents with an earliest age of 9. The study was conducted over 20 years. The results found evidence for the presence of BPD in early adolescence, with increased symptomology in mid-adolescence that declined by late adolescence. This mirrors the trajectory of brain maturation proffered by neuroscience (Anderson, 2016; Casey, Jones, & Hare 2008; Dahl, 2004; Van Duijvenvoorde, Peters, & Braams, 2016; Wahlstrom et al., 2010). Twenty-one percent of the study subjects in the CIC study were rated at higher levels for personality disorder traits in early adulthood supporting the thesis that the symptoms are stable over time and that the diagnosis is often present in adolescence (Sharp et al., 2018).

Longitudinal Course of Borderline Personality Disorder

BPD was previously considered an unremittingly, severe and disabling condition that was largely treatment resistant. A growing body of literature suggests that the prognosis is more favorable with a gradual course of symptom reduction, and at times, remission of many features of this disorder. Temes and Zanarini (2018) outline a series of longitudinal and follow-back studies that track the symptom constellation of patients with this disorder. Many studies reviewed showed methodological flaws that detracted from their findings. There have been two large studies with stricter methodologies that yield encouraging results for the long-term pattern of symptoms and reconstitution of functioning in areas of interpersonal functioning and employability. The McClean Study of Adult Development (MSAD) was initiated in 1992 and continues to this date. Ratings of symptoms have occurred every two years. The study reports that 99% of patients with BPD showed symptom remission at some point, with a duration of at least two years, when checked at the 16 year follow-up (Zanarini, Frankenburg, Reich, & Fitzmaurice, 2012). Sixty percent of patients with the disorder obtained a Global Assessment of Functioning (GAF) scale rating of 61, which is considered adequate functioning, at year 16 follow-up (Zanarini et al., 2012). Identical values were found at the 20 year assessment (Zanarini, Temes, Frankenburg, Reich, & Fitzmaurice, 2018). Closer examination of the data in the same study showed that 39% of BPD patients were rated with a Global Assessment of Functioning Scale score (GAF) of 71.

This higher level of functioning was associated with the absence of a co-occurring disorder that impaired important areas of functioning. The improvement, while encouraging, was well below that shown in a comparative group of patients with other personality disorders. Seventy-three percent of that group showed a GAF score of 71 or higher and had no comorbid disorders that significantly impaired their functioning. Zanarini (2019) points out that the rate of recovery in the MSAD study decreased over time with 88% showing recovery at the eight year follow-up with just an 11% of additional subjects at this same level over the course of the next 11 years. It is possible that this second group may have had more significant symptoms and/or experienced less support and more negative events at different points of the study. Relapse rates two years after a two year remission was low at 16%. The relapse rate after 14 years was 36%. Cumulative rates of symptom remission were studied at year 16 of the study. Survival analyses were implemented. The median cumulative recurrence rate was 75% following two years of remission and 56% after four years of symptom remission (Zanarini, 2019). The study found that the more serious or acute symptoms were more likely to remit than the affective disorder features of BPD. Of particular interest are data suggesting that recovery rates were not specifically tied to treatment. Only a paucity of study subjects were in treatment at McClean Medical Center. Most subjects were served by community-based treatment services with an unknown level of effectiveness. Zanarini (2019, p. 76) draws some important conclusions from the MSAD study and points out that professionals now have a "cognitive map" of the course of BPD. Acute symptoms may be more amenable to treatment and show the greatest improvement over time. Twelve symptoms fell in this category. Several of the more crisis-oriented symptoms included: affective instability, impulsive acts of self-harm, suicide attempts, turbulent relationships, quasi-psychotic cognitions, regressions and countertransference problems. These symptoms and all others in the group significantly improved throughout the lifespan. The 12 temperamental or affective symptoms showed a slower and shallower rate of recovery. Several of the more impactful symptoms include: a pervasive course of major depression, persistent feelings of helplessness, hopelessness and worthlessness, chronic anxiety, difficulty being alone, unusual or odd thought process and perceptual experiences and frequent displays of anger and acts of anger.

The Collaborative Longitudinal Personality Disorders Study (CLPS) conducted by McGlashan et al. (2000) was initiated in 1996 with reassessment of individuals with BPD on an annual basis over the course of 10 years. At the 10-year mark, 85% of study participants were in symptom remission for at least 12 months in the 10 year follow-up study by Gunderson et al. (2011). The results showed that 21% of subjects had a GAF rating of 71 or higher, while 48% of a comparison group of other personality disorder patients in Cluster C obtained a GAF score of 71 or higher (Gunderson et al., 2001; Temes & Zanarini, (2018).

Recovery rates are important indicators of long-term functioning. The MSAD study also informs us of specific symptoms that show promise of improvement and those that are resistant to change. Affective symptoms of depression, anger, anxiety, chronic loneliness/emptiness and helplessness, hopelessness and worthlessness continued to dominate the clinical presentation at the six year follow-up. Significantly lower levels of impulsive symptoms were found at this same time marker. Suicide attempts and self-mutilation had reduced for 81% of patients at the start of the study and fell to 25% at the six year follow-up (Zanarini, 2019).

Summary and Conclusion

The evolution of more behaviorally based diagnostic criteria have made it possible to treat BPD with greater precision and effectiveness. Data suggest that the personality traits of BPD may show greater plasticity and less "psychic rigidity" than Stern (1938, p. 472) first postulated. The trajectory of symptom development is now better understood with individuals achieving both brief and long-term reduction in symptoms and improved psychosocial functioning. The impulsive acts of desperation that cause alarm and disrupt lives are tempered by the benefits of time, supportive relationships, evidence-based interventions and improved skills in navigating the emotions and thought processes that at one time threatened to destroy self-identity and put at risk significant accomplishments and relationships.

REFERENCES

Akiskal, H. (2003). Demystifying borderline personality: critique of the concept and unorthodox reflections on its natural kinship with the bipolar spectrum. *Acta Psychiatry Scandinavia,* 110, 401-407. http://dx.doi.org/10.1111/j.1600-0447.2004.00461.x

Álvarez-Tomás, I., Ruiz, J., Guilera, G. & Bados, A. (2019). Long-term clinical and functional course of borderline personality disorder: a meta-analysis of prospective studies. *European Psychiatry 56,* 75-83. http://dx.doi.org/10.1016/j eurpsy.2018.10.010

Amad, A., Ramoz, N., Thomas, P., Jardi, R. & Gorwood, P. (2014). Genetics of borderline personality disorder: Systematic review and proposal of an integrative model. *Neuroscience and Biobehavioral Reviews, 40,* 6-19. http://dx. doi.org/10.1016/j.neubiorev.2014.01.003

Amad, A., Ramoz, N., Peyre, H., Thomas, P., & Gorwood, P. (2019). FKBP5 gene variants and borderline personality disorder. *Journal of Affective Disorders, 248,* 26-28. http://dx.doi.org/10.1016/j.jad. 2019.01.025

American Psychiatric Association. (1952). *Diagnostic and statistical manual of mental disorders* (1st ed.). Washington, DC.: Author.

American Psychiatric Association. (1964). *Diagnostic and statistical manual of mental disorders* (2nd ed.). Washington, DC.: Author.

American Psychiatric Association. (1980). *Diagnostic and statistical manual of mental disorders* (3rd ed.). Washington, D. C.: Author.

American Psychiatric Association. (1994). *Diagnostic and statistical manual of mental disorders* (4th ed.). Washington, D. C.: Author .

American Psychiatric Association. (2000). *Diagnostic and statistical manual of mental disorders* (4th ed., text revision). Washington, D. C.: Author.

American Psychiatric Association. (2013). *Diagnostic and statistical manual of mental health disorders* (5th ed.). Washington, D. C.: Author.

Anderson, J., Snyder, S., Selborn, M., Krueger, R. & Hopwood, C. (2014). A comparison of the DSM-5 section II and section III personality disorder structures. *Psychiatry Research,* 216, 363-372. http://dx.doi.org/10.1016/jpsychres. 2014.01.007

Anderson, S. (2016). Commentary on the special issue on the adolescent brain: Adolescence, trajectories, and the importance of prevention. *Neuroscience and Biobehavioral Reviews, 70,*329-333. http://dx.doi. org/10.1016/j.neubiorev. 2016.07.012

Aquino Ferreira, L., Henrique Queroz Pereira, F., Luna Neri Benevides, A. M. & Carvalho Aguilar Melo, M. (2018). Borderline personality disorder and sexual abuse: A systematic review. *Psychiatry Research, 262,* 70-77. http://dx.doi.org/10.1016/j.psychres.2018.01043

Aquino Ferreira, L. F., Pereira, F. H., Benevides, A. M. & Melo, M. C. (2018). Borderline personality disorder and sexual abuse: A systematic review. *Psychiatry Research, 262,* 70-77. http://dx.doi.org/10.1016/ j.psych.2018.01.043

Baer, B. A., Peters, J. R., Eisenlohr-Mohl, T. A., Geiger, P. J. & Shannon, E. S. (2012). Emotion-related cognitive processes in borderline personality disorder: A review of the empirical literature. *Clinical Psychology Review, 32*, 359-369. http:/dx.doi.org/10.1016/j.cpr. 2012.03

Bassir Nia, A., Evelleth, M. C., Gabbay, J. M., Hassan, Y. J., Zhang, B. & Mercedes Perez-Rodriguez, M. (2018). Past, present, and future of genetic research in borderline personality disorder. *Current Opinion in Psychology, 21*, 60-68. http://dx.doi.org/10.1016/jcopsych.2017.09. 002

Beauchaine, T. P., Hinshaw, S. P. & Bridger, J. A. (2019) Nonsuicidal self-injury and suicidal behaviors in girls: The case for targeted prevention in preadolescence. *Clinical Psychological Science, 7,* 643-667. http://dx.doi.org/10.1177/2167702618818474

Biskin, R. S. (2015). The lifetime course of borderline personality disorder. *Canadian Journal of Psychiatry, 60,* 303-308. www.TheCJP.ca

Biskin, R. S. & Paris, J. (2012). Diagnosing borderline personality disorder. *Canadian Journal of Psychiatry, 6,* 1789-1794. http://dx.doi.org/ 10.1503/cmaj.090618

Brooks, R. B., Baltazar, P. L. & Munjack, D. J. (1989). Co-occurrence of Personality Disorder with panic disorder, social phobia and generalized anxiety disorder: A review of the literature. *Journal of Anxiety Disorders, 3,* 259-286. http://dx.doi,org/10.1016/0887-185(89)90018-2

Calvo, N., Valero, S., Sáez-Francàs, N., Gutiérrez, F., Casas, M. & Ferrer, M. (2016). *Comprehensive Psychiatry, 70,* 105-111. http://dx.doi:10. 1016/jcomp.psych2016.07.002

Cantor, N., Smith, E., French, R., & Mezzich, J. (1980). Psychiatric diagnosis as prototype categorization. *Journal of Abnormal Psychology 89,* 181-193. http://dx.doi.org/10.1037/10021-843X89.2.181

Carpenter, R. W., Tomko, R. L., Trull, T. J. & Boomsma, D. I. (2013). Gene-environment studies and borderline personality disorder. *Current Psychiatry Reports, 15,* 336. http://dx.doi.org/10.1007/s11920-012-0336-1

Casey, B. J., Jones, M. J. & Hare, T. A. (2008). *Annals of the New York Academy of Sciences, 1124,* 111-126. http://dx.doi.org/10.1196/ annals.1440.010

Chapman, A. (2019). Borderline personality disorder. *Development and Psychopathology,* 1-14. http:/dx.doi.org/10.1017/S0954579419000658

Clark, L. A. (2007). Assessment and diagnosis of personality disorder: Perennial issues and an emerging reconceptualization. *Annual Review of Psychology, 58,* 227-257. http://dx.doi.org/10.1046/annurev. psych57. 102904.190200

Clarkin, J. F., Widiger, T. A., Frances, A., Hurt, S. W. & Gilmore, M. 1 (1983). Prototypic typology and the borderline personality disorder. *Journal of Abnormal Psychology, 92,* 263-275. http://dx.doi.org/ 10.1037/0021-843X.92.3.263

Cohen, P. Crawford, T. N., Johnson, J. G. & Kasen, S. (2005). The children in the community study of developmental course of personality disorder. *Journal of Personality Disorders*, 19, 466-486. http://dx.doi.org/ 10.1052/pedi.2005.19.5.466

Cooper, J. (2005). Suicide after deliberate self-harm: A 4-year cohort study. *American Journal of Psychiatry, 162,* 297-303. http://dx.doi.org/ 10.1176/appi.ajp.162.2.297

Crowell, S. E., Beauchaine, T. P. & Linehan, M. M. (2009). A biosocial biological model of borderline personality: Elaborating and extending Linehan's theory. *Psychological Bulletin, 135,* 495-510. http://dx.doi./org/10.1037/a0015616

Cuthbart, B. N., Schupp, H. T., Bradley, M. & McManis, M. (1998). Probing affective pictures. *Psychophysiology, 35,* 344-347.

Dahl, R. E. (2004). Adolescent brain development-keynote address. *Annals New York Academy of Sciences, 1021,* 1-22. http://dx.doi.org/10.1196/annals.1308.001

Daros, A. R., Zakzanis, K. K. & Ruocco, A. C. (2012). Facial recognition in borderline personality disorder. *Psychological Medicine, 43,* 1953-1963. http://dx.doi.org/10/1017/S0033291712002607

Ellison, W. D., Rosenstein, L. K., Morgan, T. A. & Zimmerman, M. (2018). Community and clinical epidemiology of borderline personality disorder. *Psychiatric Clinics of North America, 41,* 561-573. http://dx.doi.org/10.1016/j.psc.2018.07.008

Elsner, D., Broadbear, J. H. & Rao, S. (2018). What is the clinical significance of chronic emptiness in borderline personality disorder? *Australasian Psychiatry, 26,* 88-91. http://dx.doi.org/10.1177/1039856217734674

Esguevillas, A., Diaz-Caneja, C. M., Arango, C., Del Rey-Mejias, A. L., Bernardo, E. G., Delgado, C. & …Carrasco, J. L. (2018). Personality organization and its association with clinical and functional features in borderline personality disorder. *Psychiatry Research, 262,* 393-399. http://dx.doi.org/10.1016/j.psyres.2013.09.013

Few, L. R., Miller, J. D., Rothbaum, A. O., Meller, A., Maples, J., Terry, D. P. &…MacKillop, J. (2013). Examination of the section III DSM-5 diagnostic system for personality disorders in an outpatient clinical sample. *Journal of Abnormal Psychology*, 122, 1057-1069. http://dx.doi.org/:10.1037/a0034878

Fowler, J. C., Madan, A., Allen, J. G., Oldham, J. M. & Frueh, C. C. (2019). Differentiating bipolar disorder: Diagnostic accuracy of the difficulty in emotion regulation scale and personality inventory for DSM-5. *Journal of Affective Disorder, 245,* 856-860. http://dx.doi.org/10.1016/j.jad.2018.11.079

Francis, A. (1982). Categorical and dimensional systems of personality diagnosis: A comparison. *Comprehensive Psychiatry* 23, 516-527. Grune & Stratton, Inc. 0010- 440X/82/2306/003$2. 00/0

Giedd, J. N. (2004). Structural magnetic resonance imaging of the adolescent brain. *Annals of New York Academy of Sciences, 1021,* 77-85. http://dx.doi.org/10.1196/annals.1308.009

Ghinea, D., Koenig, J., Parzer, P., Brunner, R., Carli, V., Hoven, C. W. &…Kaess, M. (2019). Longitudinal development of risk-taking and self-injurious behavior in association with late adolescent borderline personality disorder symptoms. *Psychiatry Research, 273,* 127-133. http://dx.doi.org/10.1016/j.psychres.2019.01.010

Grinker, R. R. (1968). *The borderline syndrome: a behavioral study of Ego-functions.* New Haven: Yale University Press. https://yalebooks.yale.edu

Guile, J. M., Boissel, L., Alaux-Cantin, S. & Garney de La Riviére, S. (2018). Borderline personality disorder in adolescents: prevalence, diagnosis, and treatment strategies. *Adolescent Health, Medicine and Therapeutics, 9,* 199-210. www.dovepress.com

Gunderson, J. G. & Phillips, K. A. (1991). A current view of the interface between borderline personality disorder and depression. *American Journal of Psychiatry, 148,* 967-965. http://dx.doi.org/10.1176/ajp.148.8.967

Gunderson, J. G., & Lyon Ruth. (2008). BPD's interpersonal hypersensitivity phenotype: A gene-environment developmental model. *Journal of Personality Disorders, 22,* 22-41. http://dx.doi10.1521/pedi.2008.22.1.22

Gunderson, J. G. & Singer, M. T. (1975). Defining borderline patients: An overview. *American Journal of Psychiatry*, 132, 1-10. http://dx.doi:10.1176/ajp.132.1.1

Gunderson, J. G., Stout, R. L., McGlashan, T. H., Shea, M. T., Morey, L. C., Grilo, C. M…Skodol, A. E. (2011). Ten-year course of borderline personality disorder: psychopathology and function form the

Collaborative Longitudinal Personality Disorders Study.*Archives of General Psychiatry, 68,* 827-837. http://dx.doi.org/10.1001/archgenpsychiatry.2011.37

Hankin, B. L. & Abela, J. R. (2011). Nonsuicidal self-injury in adolescence: Prospective rates and risk factors in a 2 ½ year longitudinal study. *Psychiatry Research, 186*, 65-70. http://dx.doi.10.1016/j.psychres.2010.07.056

Hecht, K. F., Cicchetti, D., Rogosch, F. A., Crick, N. R. (2014). Borderline features in childhood: The role of subtype, developmental timing, and chronicity of child maltreatment. *Development and Psychopathology, 26,* 805-815. http://dx. doi.10.1017/S0954579414000406

Hiraoka, R., Crouch, J. L., Reo, G., Wagner, M. F., Milner, J. S. & Skowronski, J. J. (2016). Borderline personality features and emotion regulation deficits are associated with child physical abuse potential. *Child Abuse and Neglect, 52,* 177-184. http://dx.doi.org/10.1016/j.chiabu.2015.10.023

Kernberg, O. (1967). Borderline personality disorder organization. *Journal of American Psychoanalytic Association,* 15, 641-685. http://doi/10.1177/000306516701500309

Kernberg, O. (1984). *Object Relations Theory and Clinical Psychoanalysis.* New York: Jason Aronson, Inc. rowman.com

Kernberg, O. (2018). What's next? A clinical overview. *Psychiatric Clinics of North America, 41, xvii-xxii.* http://dx. doi.org/10. 1016/j. psc. 2018. 08. 003

Klonsky, E. D. & Muelenkamp, J. J. (2007). Self-injury: A research review for the practicioner. *Journal of Clinical Psychology,* 63, 1045-1056. http://dx.doi.org/10.1002/jclp. 20412

Knight, R. P. (1953). Borderline States. *Bulletin Menninger Clinic, 1,* 1-12. psc@periodicals.com

Krueger, R. F. (2013). Personality disorders are the vanguard of the post-5. 0 Era. *Personality Disorders, Theory, Research and Treatment, 4,* 355-362. http://dx.doi:10.1037/per0000028

Krueger, R. F., Derringer, J., Markon, K. E., Watson, D. & Skodol, A. (2012). Initial construction of a maladaptive personality trait model and inventory for DSM-5. *Psychological Medicine, 42,* 1879-1890.http://dx.doi.org/10.1017/S0033291711002674

Kuo, J. R., Khoury, J. E., Metcalfe, R., Fitzpatrick, S. & Goodwill, A. (2015). An examination of the relationship between childhood emotional abuse and borderline personality disorder features: The role of difficulties with emotion regulation. *Child Abuse and Neglect, 39,* 147-155. http://dx.doi.org/10.1016/j.chiabu.2014.08.008

Lieb, K., Zanarini, M. C., Schmahl, C., Linehan, M. M. & Bohus, M. (2004). Borderline personality disorder. *Lancet, 364,* 453-461. http://dx. doi.org/10/1016/S0140-676(04)-6736

Masterson, J. F. (1981). *The Narcissistic and Borderline Disorders*. New York: Brunner/Mazel, Publishers. http://dx.doi.org/10.176/ajp. 139.101366

McGlashan, T. H., Grilo, C. M., Skodol, A. E., Gunderson, J. G., Shea, M. T., Morey, L. C. &…Stout, R. L. (2001).The Collaborative Longitudinal Personality Disorders Study: baseline Axis I/II and II/III diagnostic co-occurrence. *Acta Psychiatry Scandinavica, 102,* 256-264. http://dx.doi:10.1034/j.1600-0447.2000.102004256.x

Meehan, K. B., Clarkin, J. F. & Lenzenweger, M. F. (2018a). Conceptual models of borderline personality disorder, part 1. *Psychiatric Clinics of North America, 41,* 536-548. http://dx.doi.org/10/1016/j.psc.2018. 08.001

Meehan, K. B., Clarkin, J. F. & Lenzenweger, M. F. (2018b). Conceptual models of borderline personality disorder, part 2. *Psychiatric Clinics of North America, 41,* 535-548. http://dx.doi.org/10.1016/j.psc.2018. 08.002

Meehan, K. B., DePanfilis, C., Cain, N. M. Antonucci, C., Soliana, A. & Clarkin, J. F. & Sambataro, F. (2017). Facial emotion recognition and borderline personality pathology. *Psychiatric Research. 255,* 347-354. http://dx.doi:10.1016/jjpsyres.2017.05.042

Morey, L. C. & Skodol, A. E. (2013). Convergence between DSM-IV-TR and DSM-5 diagnostic models for personality disorder: Evaluation of strategies for establishing diagnostic thresholds. *Journal of Psychiatric*

Practice, 19, 179-193. http://dx.doi.org/10.1097/01.pra.0000430502.78833.06

Morey, L. C. (2014). Borderline features are associated with inaccurate trait estimation. *Borderline Personality Disorder and Emotional Dysregulation, 1*, 1-6. http://dx.doi:10.1186/20516673-1-4

Nakar, O., Brunner, R., Schilling, O., Chanen, A., Fischer, G., Parzer, P.,… Kaess, M. (2016). Developmental trajectories of self-injurious behavior and substance misuse and their association with adolescent borderline personality pathology. *Journal of Affective Disorders, 197,* 231-238. http://dx.doi.org/10.1016/j. jad.2016.03.02

Ohio State Notes. (2001). *History of the Diagnostic and Statistical Manual of Mental Disorder.* Retrieved from: http://tpb.psy.ohiostate.edu/5681/notes/dsm/01.htm#Spitzer

Oldham, J. M. (2018). DSM models of personality disorders. *Current Opinion in Psychology, 21,* 86-88. http://dx.doi.org/10.1016/j.copsyc.2017.09.010

Paris, J. (2010). Estimating the prevalence of personality disorders in the community. *Journal of Personality Disorders, 24*, 405-411. http://dx.doi.org/10.1521/pedi.2010.24.4.405

Paris, J. (2018). Differential diagnosis of borderline personality disorder. *Psychiatric Clinic of North America, 41,* 575-582. http://dx.doi.org/10.1016/j.psc.2018.07.001

Paris, J. (2019). Suicidality in borderline personality disorder. *Medicina, 55,* 1-6. http://dx.doi.10.3390/medicina55060223

Paris, J. & Zweig-Frank, H. (2001). A 27-year follow-up of patients with borderline personality disorder. *Comprehensive Psychiatry, 42,* 482-487. http://dx.doi.org/10.1053/comp.2001.26271

Perez-Rodriguez, M. M., Bulbena-Cabre, A., Nia, A. B., Zipursky, G., Goodman, M. & New, A. S. (2018). The neurobiology of borderline personality disorder. *Psychiatric Clinics of North America, 41,* 633-650. http://dx.doi.org/10.1016/j.psc.2018.07.012

Pompili, M., Girardi, P., Ruberto, A & Tatarelli, R. (2005). Suicide in borderline personality disorder: a meta-analysis. *Nordic Journal of Psychiatry, 59,* 319-323. http://dx. doi.org/10.1018039480500320025

Reardon, K. W., Mercadante, E. J. & Tackett, J. L. (2018). The assessment of personality disorder: methodological, developmental, and contextual considerations. *Current opinion in Psychology, 21,* 39-43. http://dx.doi.org/10.1016/j.copsyc.2017.09.004

Rusch, K. M., Guastello, S. J. & Mason, P. T. (1992). Differentiating symptom clusters of borderline personality disorder. *Journal of Clinical Psychology, 48,* 730-738. http://dx.doi.org/10.1002/10974679(199211)48:6,30::AIDJCLP2270480606,3.0.CO;2-V

Russell, J. J., Moskowitz, D. S. & Zuroff, D. C., Sookman, D. & Paris, J. (2007). Stability and variability of affective experience and interpersonal behavior disorder. *Journal of Abnormal Psychology, 116,* 578-588. http://dx.doi.org/10.1037/0021-843X.116.3.578

Sanislow, C. A., Grilo, C. M., Morey, L. C., Bender, E. S., Skodal, A. E., Gunderson, J. G. &…McGlashoan, T. H. (2002). Confirmatory factor analysis of DSM-IV criteria for borderline personality disorder: Findings from the collaborative longitudinal personality disorder study. *American Journal of Psychiatry, 159,* 284-290. http://dx.doi.org/10.1176/appi.ajp.159.2.297

Sarhan, Z. A., El Shinnawy, H. A., Eltawil, M. E., Elnawawy, Y., Rashad, W., Mohammedf, M. S. (2019). Global functioning and suicide risk in patients with depression and comorbid borderline personality disorder. Neurology, *Psychiatry and Brain Research, 31,* 37-42. http://dx.doi.org/10.1016/j.npbr.2019.01.001

Shah, Ravi & Zanarini, M. C. (2018). Comorbidity of borderline personality disorder - Current status and future directions. *Psychiatric Clinics of North America, 41,* 583 – 593. http://dx.doi.org/10.1016/j.psc.2018.07.009

Sharp, C., Ha, C. Michonski, J., Venta, a. & Carbone, C. (2012). *Comprehensive Psychiatry, 53,* 765-774. http://dx.doi.org/10.1016/jcomprpsych.2011.12.003

Sharp, C. Vanwoerden, S. & Wall, K. (2018). Adolescence as a sensitive period for the development of personality disorder. *Psychiatric Clinics of North America, 41,* 669-683. http://dx.doi.org.10/1016/j.psc.2018.07.004

Shin, G. I., Goldstein, H. L. & Pick, S. (2018). Evidence for subjective emotional numbing following induced acute disassociation. *Behavior Research and Therapy, 119,* 1-6. http://dx. doi.org/10.1016/j.brat. 2019.05.004

Skodol, A. E., Siever, L., Livesley, W. J., Gunderson, J. G., Pfohl, B. & Widiger, T. A. (2002). The borderline diagnosis II: Biology, genetics, and clinical course. *Biological Psychiatry, 5,* 951-963. http://dx.doi. org/10.1016/S00063223(02)01325-2

Sosic-Vasic, Z., Eberhardt, J., Bosch, J. E., Dommes, L., Labek, K., Buchheim, A. & Viviani, R. (2019). Mirror neuron activations in encoding of psychic pain in borderline personality Disorder. *NeuroImage: Clinical, 22,* 1-8. http://dx.doi.org/10.1016/j.niel. 2019.101737

Spitzer, R., Endicott, J. & Gibbon, M. (1979). Crossing the border into borderline personality and borderline schizophrenia. *Archives of General Psychiatry, 36,* 17-24. http://dx.doi.org/10.1001/archpsyc. 1979.01780010023001

Spitzer, R. L. & Fleiss, J. L. (1974). A re-analysis of the reliability of psychiatric diagnosis. British Journal of Psychiatry*, 125,* 341-7. http://doi.org/10.1192/bjp.125.4.341

Steinberg, L. & Morris, A. S. (2001). Adolescent development. *Annual Review of Psychology, 52,* 83-110. http://dx.doi.org/10.1146/annurev. psych.52.11.83

Stepp, S. D. (2012). Development of borderline personality disorder in adolescents and young adulthood: Introduction to the special edition. *Journal of Abnormal Child Psychology, 40,* 1-8. http://dx.doi.org/ 10.1007s10902011-9594-3

Stepp, S. D., Keenan, K., Hipwell, A. E. & Krueger, R. F. (2014). The impact of childhood temperament on the development of borderline personality disorder symptoms over the course of adolescence. *Borderline Personality Disorder and Emotion Dysregulation, 1,* 1-10. bpded.com/content/1/1/18

Stern, Adolph (1938). Psychoanalytic investigation of and therapy in the border line group of neuroses. *The Psychoanalytic Quarterly, 7,* 467-489. http://dx.doi.org/0.1080/21674086.1938119.11925367

Taylor, P. J., Jomar, K., Dhingra, K., Forrester, R., Shahmalak, U. & Dickson, J. M. (2018). A meta-analysis of the prevalence of different functions of non-suicidal self-injury. *Journal of Affective Disorders, 227,* 759- 769. http://dx.doi.org/10.1016/j.jad.2017.11.073

Temes, C. M. & Zanarini, M. C. (2018). The longitudinal course of borderline personality disorder. *Psychiatric Clinics of North America, 41,* 685-4. http://dx.doi.org/10/1016/j.psc.2018.07.002

Torgersen, S., Kringlen, E. & Cramer, V. (2001). The prevalence of personality disorders in acommunity sample. *Archives of General Psychiatry, 58,* 590-596. http//dx.doi.org/10.1001/archpsych.58.6.590

Trull, T. J., Stepp, S. E. & Durrett, C. A. (2003). Research on borderline personality disorder: An update. *Current Opinion in Psychiatry, 16,* 77-82. http://dx.doi.org/10.1097/01.yco.000-0049398.78338.f7

Van Dijke, A., Hopman, J. A. & Ford, J. D. (2018). Affect dysregulation, adult attachment problems, and disassociation mediate the relationship between childhood trauma borderline personality symptoms in adulthood. *European Journal of Trauma and Dissociation, 2,* 91 – 99. http://dx.doi.org/10.1016/j.ejtd.2017.11.002

Van Duijvenvoorde, A. C., Peters, S., Braams, B. R. & Crone, E. A. (2016). What motivates adolescence? Neural responses to rewards and their influence on adolescents' risk-taking, learning, and cognitive control. *Neuroscience and Biobehavioral Reviews, 70,* 135-147. https://dx.doi.org/10.1016/j.nuebiorev.2016.06.037

Wahlstrom, D., Collins, P., White, T. & Luciana, M. (2010). Developmental changes in dopamine neurotransmission in adolescents: behavioral implications and issues in assessment. *Brain and Cognition, 72,* 146-159. http://dx. doi.org/10.1016/j.bandc.2009.10.013

Watters, C. A., Bagby, R. M. & Selbom, M. (2019). Meta-Analysis to Derive an Empirically Based Set of Personality Facet Criteria for the Alternative DSM-5 Model for Personality Disorders. *Personality*

Disorders: Theory, Research, and Treatment, 10, 97-104. http://dx.doi.org/10.1037/per0000307

Widiger, T. A., Crego, C., Rojas, S. L. & Oltmanns, J. R. (2018). Basic personality model. *Current Opinion in Psychology, 21,* 18-22. http://dx.doi.org/10.1016/j.copsyc.2017.09.007

Winsper, C. (2018). The aetiology of borderline personality disorder (BPD): contemporary theories and putative mechanisms. *Current Opinion in Psychology, 21,* 105-110. http://dx. doi.org/10.1016/j.copsyc.2017.10.005

Winsper, C., Lereya, S. T., Marwaha, S., Thompson, A., Eyden, j. & Singh, Swaran. (2016). The aetiological and psychopathological validity of borderline personality disorder and youth: A systematic review and meta-analysis. *Clinical Psychology Review, 44,* 13-24. http://dx.doi.org/j.cpr.2015.12.001

Wright, A. G., Hopwood, C. J. & Zanarini, M. C. (2015). Associations between changes in normal personality traits and borderline personality disorder symptoms over 16 years. *Personality Disorders, Theory, Research, and Treatment, 6,* 1-11. http://dx.doi.org/10.1037/per0000092.supp

Zanarini, M. (2019). *In the fullness of time.* New York: Oxford University Press. global.group.com

Zanarini, M. C., Frankenburg, F. R., Reich, D. B. & Fitzmaurice, G. M. (2012). Attainment and stability of sustained symptom remission and recovery among borderline personality disorder patients and axis II comparison subjects: A 16-year prospective follow-up study. *American Journal of Psychiatry,* 167, 476-483. http://dx.doi.org/101176/appi.ajp.2011.11101550

Zanarini, M. C., Frankenburg, F. R., Wedig, M. M. & Fitzmaurice, G. M. (2013). Cognitive experiences reported by patients with borderline personality disorder and axis II comparison subjects: a 16-year perspective follow-up study. *American Journal of Psychiatry, 170,* 671-679. http://dx.doi.org/10.1176/appi.ajp.2013.13010055

Zanarini, M. C., Horwood, J., Wolke, D., Waylen, A., Fitzmaurice, G & Grant, B. F. (2011). Prevalence of DSM-IV borderline personality disorder in two community samples: 6,330English 11-year olds and 34, 653 American adults. *Journal of Personality Disorder, 25,* 607-619. http:/dx.doi.org/10.1521/ped.2011.25.5.607

Zanarini, M. C., Temes, C. M., Frankenburg, F. R., Reich, D. B. & Fitzmaurice, G. M. (2018). Description and prediction of time-to-adjustment of excellent recovery for borderline personality disorder patients followed prospectively for 20 years. *Psychiatry Research, 262,* 40-45. http://dx.doi.org/10.106/j.psychres.2018.01.034

Zeng, R., Cohen, I. J., Tanis, T., Qizilbash, A. Lapattyuk, Y., Yaseen, Z. S.,…Galynker, I. (2015). Assessing the contribution of borderline personality disorder and features to suicide risk in psychiatric inpatients with bipolar disorder, major depression and schizoaffective disorder. *Psychiatric Research, 226,* 361-367. http:/dx.doi.org/ 10.1016/j.psychres.2015.01.020

Zimmerman, M., Rothschild, I. & Chelminski, I. (2005). The prevalence of DSM-IV personality disorders in psychiatric outpatients. *American Journal of Psychiatry, 162*, 1911-1918. http://dx.doi.org/10.1176/ appi.ajp.162.10.1911

Zittel Conklin, C. & Westen, D. (2005). Borderline personality disorder in clinical practice. *American Journal of Psychiatry, 162,* 867-875. http://dx.doi.org/appi.ajp.162.5.867

In: Borderline Personality Disorder
Editor: Charles M. Lepkowsky
ISBN: 978-1-53618-021-3

Chapter 3

Biological Correlates of Borderline Personality Disorder

Nanako Negome-Kapur* [*], *PsyD
4C Medical Group, Phoenix, Arizona, US

Abstract

Neuroimaging studies have paved the way for providing a better understanding of the neurobiological underpinnings of Borderline Personality Disorder (BPD). Research is summarized demonstrating observable neurobiological correlates of BPD. Included is a review of methodologies including neuroimaging of BPD, functional brain imaging studies in BPD, genetic studies and BPD, and molecular genetic research in BPD, and discussion of the use of these methodologies to measure changes in brain structure and function as quantifiable effects of psychotherapy on BPD.

Keywords: neuroimaging, borderline personality disorder, genetic and molecular genetic research

---

* Corresponding Author's E-mail: n.negome_kapur@me.com.

BPD and Emotional Dysregulation: Early Conceptualization

Over the past century, various models have been generated in an effort to understand Borderline Personality Disorder (BPD), conceptualize its etiology, and make specific recommendations for effective treatment. The term "borderline" was proposed by early theorists who suggested that there are people who fall between the border of 'neurosis' and 'psychosis' (Rosanoff, 1938; Stern, 1938). In the current literature, BPD is characterized by disturbed emotional processing, emotional dysregulation, difficulty with impulse control including suicidality or self-harming behavior, distorted self-image, cognitive disturbances including dissociations, and difficulties with interpersonal relationships (American Psychiatric Association, 2013; Leichsenring, Leibing, Kruse, New, & Leweke, 2011; Lieb, Zanarini, Schmahl, Linehan, & Bohus, 2004).

Historically, BPD research mainly explored psychological aspects of the disorder, including psychosocial stressors, characteristic behaviors, and risk factors, with early life stressors having strong association with BPD (O'Neill & Frodl, 2012), but none of those studies produced conclusive evidence in support of a single-cause theory. Considering the heterogeneity of the disorder, there most likely are multiple factors involved in the development of BPD, with individual differences (Asnaani et al., 2007; Wingenfled et al., 2010). Currently prominent theories posit early life trauma(s), such as childhood abuse or maternal separation, genetics, neurobiological alterations, or a combination of these stressors, along with environmental or adverse psychosocial stressors, as factors contributing to the development of BPD (Goodman et al., 2004; Steele & Siever, 2010).

Neurobiological Bases of BPD

In the last decade, there has been rapid expansion in the number of research studies seeking potential neurobiological underpinnings of BPD

(Krause-Utz, Winter, Liedtfeld, & Schmahl, 2014). This body of research is based on the hope that studying and clarifying the biological and molecular basis for BPD will lead to a more thorough understanding of the etiology and functional components of the disorder, which might in turn lead to more effective treatments for BPD (Pier, Marin, Wilsnack, & Goodman, 2016).

NEUROIMAGING IN BPD

Neuroimaging has revealed differences in structure and function in the brains of individuals diagnosed with BPD, when compared with a non-BPD population (Krause-Utz, Winter, Liedfeld, & Schmahl, 2014). Various Magnetic Resonance Imaging MRI techniques have become most commonly used methods in neuroimaging studies of adult psychopathologies, because they are widely available and non-invasive (Horga, Kaur, & Peterson, 2014). MRI is also widely utilized because it can examine the brain across multiple modalities (e.g., brain structure, changes in blood flow, concentrations of chemical metabolites or neurotransmitters, and nerve fiber integrity). Positron emission tomography (PET) has also been used to investigate neurotransmitter systems in the brains. Previous neuroimaging studies examining neurobiological differences in people diagnosed with post-traumatic stress disorder (PTSD) paved the way for similar research in BPD (O'Neill & Frodl, 2012).

The corticolimbic system is frequently studied in BPD research (Pier, Marin, Wilsnack, & Goodman, 2016). The corticolimbic system consists of dorsolateral prefrontal cortex (DLPFC), anterior cingulate cortex (ACC), amygdala, and the hippocampus. The amygdala is considered crucial in neuroimaging studies of individuals with BPD because it is involved with emotional processing, especially the initiation of the stress and fear responses (Davis & Whalen, 2001; Ochsner & Gross, 2007; Phillips, Drevets, Rauch, & Lane, 2003). The hippocampus, located next to the amygdala, is another crucial area for BPD studies. The hippocampus is known for memory consolidation and declarative memory.

Brodmann areas (BAs) are broad regions of the cerebral cortex defined by its cytoarchitecture or organization of cells (Zilles, 2018). In brain studies of BPD patients, some BAs have been looked at (e.g., BA 24, 25, 32) because they are connected to the amygdala and the ortibofrontal cortex among other regions. Some BAs are known for salience of emotional and motivational information and regulation of emotional responses (Bush, Luu, & Posner, 2000). The Dorsolateral prefrontal cortex (DLPFC) and anterior cingulate cortex (ACC) are parts of the prefrontal cortex, an area known for goal directed behavior, cognitive control, executive functioning, and regulation of impulses and emotions (Krause-Utz, Frost, Winter, & Elzinga, 2017). The DLPFC is important for motivation and executive functioning (Pier, Marin, Wilsnack, & Goodman, 2016). The ACC plays a role in emotional regulation, response inhibition, and arousal modulation (Krause-Utz, Frost, Winter, & Elginga, 2017; Wingenfeld, Spitzer, Rullkotter, & Lowe, 2010). In addition to DLPFC and ACC, the orbitofrontal cortex (OFC) is another area often studied for BPD research. The OFC plays a crucial role in the coding of rewards (e.g., the subjective value of rewards) and the ability to flexibly change behavior and decision according to shifting situations (Gottfried, 2003; Sescousse, Caldu, Segura, & Dreher, 2013). The OFC also plays a crucial role in integrating sensory and emotional information (Berridge & Kringelbach, 2008).

In a meta-analysis of 22 previous studies, the hippocampus was most consistently found to exhibit structural alterations in BPD patients (O'Neill & Frodl, 2012). Previous studies has found that there was significant bilateral hippocampus reduction in BPD patients compared to non-BPD subjects (Brambilla, Soloff, Sala, Nicoletti, Keshavan, & Soares, 2004; Schmahl et al., 2008; Schmahl, Vermetten, Elzinga, & Bremner, 2003). Other studies have found overall reduced volumes in the hippocampus and the amygdala (Nunes, Wenzel, Borges, Porto, Caminha, de Oliveira, 2009). Similarly, studies investigating gray and white matters of the brain found that BPD patients had overall reduced gray matter concentration in ventral cingulate gyrus and several regions of the medial temporal cortex, which includes the hippocampus, amygdala, parahippocampal gyrus, and uncus compared to non-BPD individuals (Soloff, Nutche, Goradia, & Diwadkar,

2008). Another study looking at the whole-brain microstructure white matter of BPD subjects, instead of focusing on certain areas of the brain, found diffusion alterations in both portico-cortical (superior longitudinal fasciculus) and several portico-subcortical bundles (Quattrini et al., 2019).

Other studies investigated differences in structural gray and white matter volume in BPD patients with comorbid disorders. A few studies have found that BPD patients with comorbid Post Traumatic Stress Disorder (PTSD) or childhood abuse have significantly smaller right and left hippocampal volumes (Brambilla et al., 2004; Schmahl et al., 2008; Schmahl et al., 2003). A similar study seeking structural differences between gray and white matter volumes in the cingulate gyrus of BPD patients and BPD patients with comorbid schizotypal personality disorder found that BPD patients had reduced cingulate gray matter and increased white matter volume in BAs 24 and 31, compared to a standard population sample (Hazlett et al., 2005). BPD patients without comorbid Schizotypal personality disorder had reduced gray matter volume in BA 24, but not BA 31. BPD patients with comorbid Schizotypal personality disorder had reduced gray matter in BAs 24 and 31. The gray matter loss in BA 31 was significantly greater in this subject group. Another study found diminished gray matter concentration in the orbital frontal cortex, temporal, insular, and paralymbic structures of BPD suicide attempters as opposed to BPD non-attempters, which correlated with high and low lethality (Soloff et al., 2013).

Brain structure studies are important because volume reductions in specific regions of the brain or specific brain structures might lead to neurocognitive deficits, dissociative symptoms, and perceptual distortions, which might in turn underlie behavioral instability observed in BPD patients (Brambilla et al., 2004). During stressful times, the amygdala and the hippocampus play an important role in modulating and regulating expression of fear responses (Davidson, Abercrombie, Nitschke, & Putnam, 1999; Davis & Whalen, 2001). Structural differences in these limbic circuits might lead to loss of inhibitory regulations, resulting in disinhibited fear responses and impulsive or aggressive behaviors (Phillips & LeDoux, 1992). The hippocampus is also responsible for monitoring one's emotional state, addressing discrepancies between present perceptions of reality and past representations of autobiographical memories (Soloff et al., 2012). Retrieval of specific and positive autobiographical memories has been shown to be impaired for people who attempt suicide, and is often associated with poor problem solving (Williams & Broadbent, 1986). The hippocampus-orbitomedial prefrontal cortex circuit is believed to be germane in maintaining cognitive-emotional control of behavior (Wall & Messier, 2001). This might help explain why BPD patients engage in self-harming behavior or attempt suicide in the face of high stress at a greater rate than the general population. Suicidal behavior in BPD is often accompanied by perceived rejection, abandonment, or negative social interactions (e.g., social disapproval) (Soloff et al., 2012). Structural differences in the orbital frontal, temporal, insular, and paralympic structures found in BPD patients, who engage in suicidal behaviors, might lead to maladaptive responding when facing high stressful events. BPD patients might have difficulty envisioning positive outcomes based on past experiences and have limited cognitive inhibitory control in stressful social situations, which might increase the likelihood that individuals with BPD will engage in impulsive, aggressive, and/or self-destructive behaviors.

FUNCTIONAL BRAIN IMAGING STUDIES IN BPD

To compliment brain structure studies, there have been a number of functional brain imaging studies. Functional MRI allows researchers to compare patterns of regional brain activities when subjects are either engaged in a specific task (e.g., viewing certain images, visual go/no-go tasks, and/or gambling tasks) or purposefully not engaged in any tasks (e.g., looking at brain at resting state). Previous studies found that when compared to non-BPD controls, BPD patients viewing images with negative connotations or emotional value showed greatest activation in the amygdala (Donegan, 2003; Herpertz et al., 2001; Koenigsberg et al., 2009a; Koenigsberg et al., 2009b; Krause-Utz et al., 2012; Niedtfeld et al., 2010; Minzenberg, Fan, New, Tang, & Siever, 2007; Schulze et al., 2011; Sosic-Vasic et al., 2019) and the insula (Beblo et al., 2006; Krause-Utz et al., 2012;

Niedtfeld et al., 2010; Ruocco, Amirthavasagam, Choi-Kain, & McMain, 2013; Schulze et al., 2011). Compared to control subjects, individuals with BPD also exhibited a slower return to baseline in amygdala activation (Kamphausen et al., 2013). These findings suggest that BPD patients experience more heightened activity in limbic regions than control subjects, especially when processing negative social or emotional loading scenes.

When inhibiting negative versus natural stimuli, BPD patients have also been shown to exhibit higher activity than non-BPD controls in the inferior parietal lobe and frontal eye fields (Zutphen et al., 2019). In a study where participants performed a visual affective go/no-go task, BPD patients were compared to non-BPD patients and cluster C personality disorder groups. Activity in the inferior parietal lobe was positively correlated with the BPD symptom checklist sub-scale for impulsivity.

Functional connectivity studies have also provided information about which brain regions are co-activated or can be looked at correlatively. Three neural networks have demonstrated problematic connectivity in BPD patients, for whom regions of the medial prefrontal cortex and posterior cingulate cortex (responsible for self-referential thinking) are often active at rest, in the absence of goal-directed tasks or activities. The salience network, which includes the orbital frontal insula and dorsal anterior cingulate and the medial temporal lobe network, has been shown to exhibit similar dysfunction in BPD patients. These areas are responsible for processing negative emotions (Pier, Marin, Wilsnack, & Goodman, 2016).

It has also been found that in a region of the brain containing the cortical midline at resting state, patients with BPD displayed increased functional connectivity in the left frontopolar cortex (FPC) and the left insula, but deceased connectivity in the left cuneus (Wolf et al., 2011). Patients with BPD also showed decreased connectivity of the left inferior parietal lobule and the right middle temporal cortex compared to non-BPD subjects. Increased connectivity between the amygdala and a brain region comprising the dorsal insula, orbitofrontal cortex, and the putamen has also been found in BPD patients compared to control subjects at resting state (Krause-Utz et al., 2014).

Four major symptom dimensions of BPD (i.e., affective disturbance, cognitive disturbance, disturbed relationships, and impulsivity) have been shown to correlate with neural activity at resting state. Higher Impulsivity scores in BPD patients were correlated with increased resting state connectivity between the right amygdala and the left hippocampus. When symptom presentation in the Cognitive Disturbance domain had improved with psychotropic medication (i.e., quetiapine), increased positive resting state connectivity between the left amygdala, the left temporal fusiform, and the parahippocampal gyri was observed. Additionally, improvements in the Disturbed Relationships domain were associated with increased resting state connectivity in the right amygdala and the right frontal pole (Schreiner et al., 2019). Compared to control subjects, patients with BPD have also demonstrated a lack of tight coupling in the orbital frontal cortex and the ventral amygdala (New et al., 2007).

fMRI has been used to assess responses in patients with BPD with non-suicidal self-injury (NSSI) and BPD patients without NSSI while performing gambling tasks. Compared to a non-BPD control group and BPD NSSI patients, BPD patients with exhibited increased activation in the orbitofrontal cortex following an unexpected reward. BPD patients with NSSI also showed diminished functional connectivity between the left orbitofrontal cortex and the right parahippocampal gyrus (Vega et al., 2018).

These findings might help explain why BPD patients have difficulty down regulating the amygdala in response to adverse stimuli. Clinically observed emotional hypersensitivity and intense, long lasting emotional reactions in BPD could stem from increased and prolonged activation in the limbic system during high stress or emotionally challenging situations (Kamphause et al., 2013). Some theories seeking neurological underpinnings of aggressiveness (sometimes exhibited in patients with BPD) suggest a failure to control emotional reactivity between the prefrontal cortex, especially the orbital frontal cortex, and the amygdala (Rosell & Siever, 2015).

A link also has been established between dissociative states/traits and altered activity in brain regions (including the amygdala, hippocampus, parahippocampus gyrus, and middle/superior temporal gyrus) involved with emotional processing and memory (Krause-Uts, Frost, Winter & Elzinga, 2017). This might be because the insula plays a role in interception and attention regulation, and the prefrontal cortex and the precuneus play a role in self-referential processing, including cognitive control and arousal modulation. BPD patients who also exhibit non-suicidal self-injury (NSSI) might have difficulty updating reward associations of potential choices. Exposure to a painful stimulus (similar to NSSI) can alter emotional regulation processes in BPD patients, possibly by eliciting enhanced negative coupling between the limbic and the para-limbic regions and the prefrontal cortex (Niedtfeld et al., 2012). Self-harming behavior appears to be maintained and reinforced because it is effective at relieving emotional distress (Nock, 2010). At resting state (no tasks), BPD patients exhibited coupling between the amygdala and a region of the brain including the dorsal insula, ortitofrontal cortex, and the putamen when compared to non-BPD controls (Krause-Utz et al., 2014). The putamen is part of the basal ganglia involved with movement control (Packard & Knowlton, 2002), suggesting that this enhanced coupling might play a role in taking action in the face of contempt or disgust (Zeki & Romaya, 2008).

Genetic Studies and BPD

Genetic studies suggest that BPD has a genetic component. A family study investigating the degree to which BPD clusters in family found that the prevalence of BPD among relatives was 14%, compared to 4.9% in family members of controls (Gunderson et al., 2011). Twin studies show heritability of BPD falling between 40% and 70% (Pier, Marin, Wilsnack, & Goodman, 2016). A longitudinal twin sample, which investigated the genetic and environmental influences on the co-development of BPD traits and major depressive disorder (MDD), alcohol use disorder (AUD), and drug use disorder (DUD) from middle adolescent to young adulthood, found a large correlation between an average level of BPD traits and average level of other disorder traits (Bornovalova et al., 2018). It appears there is a greater genetic influence on the correlation between BPD traits and AUD and DUD, but more of an environmental influence correlated with BPD traits and MDD symptoms. There is also strong evidence that the volumetric decreases in the amygdala and hippocampus (more so with hippocampal volume) might serve as ~~an~~ important biological liability markers for BPD (Ruocco, Amirthavasagam, & Zakzanis, 2012).

Molecular Genetic Research in BPD

Some molecular genetic research has focused on specific enzymes in serotonin synthesis (5-hydroxytryptomine (5-HT)), 5-HT receptors, and specific transport genes related to 5-HT (Pier, Marin, Wilsnack, & Goodman, 2016). 5-HT is attained from tryptophan through a process moderated by tryptophan hydroxylase. A neuron-specific enzyme called tryptophan hydroxylase 2 (TPH2) helps produce 5-HT in the central nervous system. A specific THP2 isoform genotype has been associated with higher rates of anxiety, depression, and suicidal behavior. BPD patients exhibit a more prevalent THP2 haplotype than control groups and exhibited higher levels of aggression, emotional lability, and increased suicidal behavior (Perez-Rodriguez, 2010). Specific serotonin receptors genes, specifically polymorphisms in 5HTR2A and 5HTR2C, have also been correlated with BPD (Amad, Ramos, Thomas, Jardri, & Gorwood, 2014). Variations in ~~the~~ 5HT2A receptors have been correlated with suicidal behavior, emotional lability, and impulse control.

Molecular genetic studies have also focused on the polymorphism of the dopamine D4 receptor (DRD4) and the 10/10 dopamine transporter (DAT) (O'Neill & Frodl, 2012). Dopamine is known to play a crucial role in behavioral inhibition and the D4 receptors are observed in brain regions that plays a role in behavioral inhibition (Congdon & Canli, 2008). Suboptimal dopaminergic receptors might lead to impaired inhibitory control. The DAT is a specific protein that is significant in dopamine neurotransmission because it is responsible for removing dopamine from the extracellular space (Bannon, Michelhaugh, Wang, & Sacchetti, 2001). Specific brain regions, such as the striatum, play~~s~~ a role in behavioral inhibition (Aron & Poldrack,

2006; Brown, Manuck, Flory, & Hariri, 2006) and rely on an optimal range of dopamine for optimal functioning (Congdon & Canli, 2008). Having excessive DAT may lead to decreased dopamine levels in the extracellular space, which might be associated with impaired inhibitory control.

EFFECTS OF PSYCHOTHERAPY ON BPD

There has also been considerable research investigating the effect of psychotherapy on the brain. Dialectical Behavioral Therapy (DBT) appears to effect structural and functional changes in the brain of BPD patients. BPD patients who received 12 weeks of DBT residential treatment showed an increase in gray matter volume in the ACC and the orbital part of the inferior frontal gyrus (Mancke et al., 2018). DBT treatment also increased gray matter volume in the superior temporal gyrus and altered the gray matter volume in the angular and supra marginal gyrus. These findings suggests that the increase in ACC gray matter volume with DBT treatment might represent a biological correlate of the effects of therapeutic interventions intended to maintain or regain cognitive control over maladaptive emotions (Mancke et al., 2018).

Significant gains in the activation of specific brain regions have also been observed following months of DBT treatment. After 7 months of treatment, BPD patients showed significant gains in the activation of bilateral middle/inferior frontal gyri during response inhibition (Ruocco et al., 2016). Compared to a control group, BPD patients with behavioral impulsivity (e.g., active self-harm) have demonstrated reduced activation in the lateral arms of the prefrontal cortex responsible for motor inhibitory control (Aron, Robbins, & Poldrack, 2004). Similarly, BPD patients who exhibited the greatest improvements in reduction in self-harm behavior had the lowest activation in the DLPFC prior to treatment, but also demonstrated the greatest increased activation in that area after 7 months of DBT treatment (Ruocco et al., 2016). A similar study found that after twelve months of DBT treatment, BPD patients showed a reduction in overall amygdala activation (Goodman et al., 2014). These findings suggest that DBT treatment promotes structural and functional improvements in brain structures that lead to overall improvement in emotional regulation and behavioral control.

Special Considerations

Although the current literature points to biological differences between BPD and non-BPD populations, there are some limitations worthy of consideration. Despite evidence of structural and functional differences between the brains of people with BPD and other populations, there are some inconsistent or contradictory findings between studies using the same technology and/or theoretically similar procedures (Lis, Greenfield, Henry, Guile, & Dougherty, 2007). Differences in hippocampus volume between BPD patients with comorbid PTSD and control groups have not been have not been universally observed (Schmahl et al., 2009), nor have differences in whole amygdala volume between BPD patients and control subjects (Mancke, Herpertz, Hirjak, Knies, & Bertsch, 2018; Mancke et al., 2018).

It is possible that the inconsistency in findings relates to comorbidity with other disorders commonly found in BPD, such as MDD, PTSD, and alcohol or drug use disorder (Soloff et al., 2008). Some studies included BPD patients with comorbid MDD, PTSD, or other disorders, while other studies excluded BPD patients with comorbid disorders (Lis et al., 2007; O'Neill & Frodl, 2012). It is still unclear from neuroimaging studies whether volumetric and functional differences are purely an endemic function of BPD, or stem from traumatic events in childhood or comorbid PTSD, both of which are common conditions found in BPD (Krause & Schmahl, 2010; Lieb, Zanarini, Schmahl, Linehan, & Bohus, 2004). The question remains whether both BPD and PTSD independently lead to a reduction in amygdala and hippocampus volume, or whether having both disorders comorbidly significantly reduces hippocampal volume (Schmahl, 2008).

BPD patients with MDD might also have structural or functional differences in specific brain areas (Brambilla, Barale, Caverzasi, & Soares, 2002; Soares & Mann, 1997). Decreased hippocampal volumes have been found in studies investigating brain differences with patients with unipolar major depression and control subjects (Bremner et al., 2000; Steffens et al., 2000; Vythilingam et al., 2002). MDD is highly prevalent in patients with BPD. A history of MDD along with childhood trauma together could contribute to hippocampal volume loss (Vythilingam et al., 2002). Comorbid disorders make it difficult to attribute the differences found to one single disorder (Lis et al., 2007). Contradictory amygdala results might also stem from psychotropic medication status at the time of research, because psychotropic medications diminish limbic activity (Pier, Marin, Wilsnack, & Goodman, 2016). Gender might also play a role in brain structural and functional differences in people with BDP. Research has shown that specific emotional states, such as aggression, express themselves through patterns of neural activation that appear gender-specific (Schmahl & Bremner, 2006; Schmahl et al., 2003).

There also appear to be inconsistent findings regarding the relationship between brain structure and functioning. In general, neuroimaging studies still have not yet fully integrated findings from different modalities to explain comprehensively how structural, functional, neurochemical, and connectivity characteristics of the brain relate to one another in any specific psychiatric disorder (Horga, Kaur, & Peterson, 2014). Reduced or increased size of a particular brain region does not necessarily result in decreased or increased function or efficiency, metabolic activity, or blood flow (Diwadkar et al., 2011; Hazlett et al., 2005). Gray and white matter metabolic rates have been observed independent of BA volume. Volume changes in the cingulate might be associated with compromised functioning or disturbance in efficiency of processing, increasing metabolic activity independent of brain volume (Hazlett et al., 2005). Conversely, some structures and functions appear to influence each other mutually, some at the level of single neurons (including dendritic spine structure) and others at the level of neural systems (Lee, Soares, Beique, 2012).

Excluding BPD patients with comorbid disorders or on psychotropic medication might not accurately represent the BPD population, considering the high rate of comorbid MDD, trauma-related disorders and symptoms, and the high percentage of BPD patients using psychotropic medications. Inconsistent sample characteristics across different neuroimaging studies likely contributed to inconsistent findings (Horga, Kaur, & Peterson, 2014). There is also evidence that some neuroimaging studies of psychiatric conditions might have challenges with reproducibility, which is an important condition for establishing validity (Ahmed, Ras, & Seedat, 2012; Hart, Radua, Nakao, Mataix-Cols, & Rubia, 2013; Hulvershorn, Cullen, & Anand, 2011; Stanfield et al., 2008; Valera, Faraone, Murray, & Seidman, 2007). Research that cannot be reproduced has some questionable validity and value (Horga, Kaur, & Peterson, 2014). In addition, neuroimaging studies often use small sample sizes. When sample sizes are small, correlation analyses have to be interpreted with caution, making it difficult to generalize results (Horga, Kaur, & Peterson, 2014; Schmahl et al., 2009).

Neuroimaging studies also tend to be cross-sectional, which introduces additional potential limitations (Horga, Kaur, & Peterson, 2014). Cross-sectional studies by themselves might not distinguish the effects of an illness from its causes, even when study groups are demographically matched to one another. It is difficult to determine which findings reflect core pathophysiological processes, which findings are related to epiphenomenon, and which findings represents adaptation of the nervous system due to the presence of an illness or illnesses (Peterson, 2003). Also, correlational studies does not establish causality. It is extremely difficult to determine whether a particular psychiatric disorder caused brain differences, or whether brain differences caused the psychiatric disorder to manifest in the individual, or whether a third unidentified variable caused both the brain differences and the psychiatric disorder (Horga, Kaur, & Peterson, 2014).

Summary and Conclusion

Neuroimaging studies examining the brains of individuals with BPD and other populations have paved the way for gaining a better understanding of the neurobiological underpinnings of BPD. MRI techniques have become common in neuroimaging studies with adult psychopathologies because they are widely available, non-invasive, and can examine the brain across multiple modalities (Horga, Kaur, & Peterson, 2014). Despite the challenges and limitations with neuroimaging studies, they have proven to be an invaluable tool in advancing our understanding of structural and functional neurological differences between individuals with BPD and non-BPD individuals, causes and effects of specific BPD symptoms, and neurological and behavioral effects of DBT.

In the future, studies with larger samples including both male and female participants might provide more comprehensive and meaningful data to improve our understanding of potential gender differences and the neurological causes and effects of BPD. Larger sample sizes will also help increase statistical power. Future studies might also benefit from comparing BPD patients with comorbid disorders to BPD patients without comorbid disorders, to determine brain differences between BPD patients with and without comorbid disorders. Future neuroimaging studies exploring relationships between brain structure and function will be important for achieving greater understanding of the brain processes of individuals with BPD vary from those of a non-BPD population (Horga, Kaur, & Peterson, 2014).

Longitudinal studies might help determine how the brain is affected by age, how BPD progresses with age, how the effects of treatment are affected by time, and the ongoing effects of pharmacological treatment on the brain (O'Neill & Frodl, 2012). There is evidence that BPD symptoms tend to decline with age, and that the decline in BPD symptoms is related to declines in other symptoms of comorbid psychiatric disorders (Bornovalova, Hicks, Iacono, & McGue, 2009; Gunderson et al., 2008).

Future studies regarding treatment effects on the brain might benefit from parsing out which specific emotional regulation skills and other therapeutic interventions are needed for a particular patient (Goodman et al., 2014). Investigating functional connectivity between the amygdala and other regions, such as the prefrontal and anterior cingulate cortex, might clarify how changes in the amygdala consequent to DBT interact with other brain regions associated with emotional regulation (Etkin, Egner, & Kalisch, 2011; Ochsner, Bunge, Gross, & Gabrieli, 2002). Studies examining the effects of other evidenced-based treatments on specific symptoms of BPD and their neurological correlates might also contribute to further understanding emotional regulatory processes, the neuropathology of BPD, and possibly inform the development of new treatments (Goodman et al., 2014). Targeted, specific neuroimaging studies examining the structural and functional features of BPD and the effects of evidenced-based treatment might lead to the development of better diagnostic tools, more targeted evidenced-based treatment, and specific pharmacological treatment for BPD.

References

Amad, A., Ramos, N., Thomas, P., Jardri, R., & Gorwood, P. (2014). Genetics of borderline personality disorder: systemic review and proposal of an integrative model. *Neuroscience & Biobehavioral Review*, *40*, 6-19. http://dx.doi.org/10.1016/j.neubiorev.2014.01.003.

Ahmed, F., Ras, J., & Seedat, S. (2012). Volumetric structural magnetic resonance imaging findings in pediatric post traumatic stress disorder and obsessive compulsive disorder: a systemic review. *Frontiers in Psychology*, *3*, 368. http://dx.doi.org/10.1016/10.3389/fpsyg.2012.00568.

American Psychiatric Association. (2013). *Diagnostic and statistical manual of mental disorders*, 5th edition. Arlington, VA: American Psychiatric Publication.

Aron, A.R. & Poldrack, R.A. (2006). Cortical and subcortical contributions to stop signal response inhibition: role of the subthalamic nucleus. *Journal of Neuroscience*, *26*(9), 2424-2433. http://dx.doi.org/10.1523/JNEUROSCI.4682-05.2006.

Aron, A.R., Robbins, T.W., & Poldrack, R.A. (2004). Inhibition and the right inferior frontal cortex. *Trends in Cognitive Science*, *8*, 170-177. http://dx.doi.org/10.1016/j.tics.2004.02.010.

Asnaani, A., Chelminski, I., Young, D., & Zimmerman, M. (2007). Heterogeneity of borderline personality disorder: do the numbers of criteria make a difference? *Journal of Personality Disorders*, *21*(6), 615-625. http://dx.doi.org/10.1521/pedi.2007.21.6.615.

Bannon, M.J., Michelhaugh, S.K., Wang, J., & Sacchetti, P. (2001). The human dopamine transporter gene: gene organization, transcriptional regulation, and potential involvement in the neuropsychiatric disorders. *European Neuropsychopharmacology*, *11*(6), 449-455. http://dx.doi.org/10.1016/s0924-977x(01)00122-5.

Beblo, T., Driessen, M., Mertens, M., Wingenfeld, K., Piefke, M., Rullkoetter, N...Woemann, F.G. (2006). Functional MRI correlates of the recall of unresolved life events in borderline personality disorder. *Psychological Medicine*, *36*(6), 845-856. http://dx.doi.org/10.1017/S0033291706007227.

Berridge, K.C. & Kringlebach, M.L. (2008). Affective neuroscience of pleasure: reward in humans and animals. *Psychopharmacology*, *199,* 457-480. http://dx.doi.org/10.1007/s00213-008-1099-6.

Bornovalova, M.A., Hicks, B.M., Iacono, W.G., & McGue, M. (2009). Stability, change, and heritability of borderline personality traits from adolescents to adulthood: a longitudinal twin study. *Development and Psychopathology*, *21*(4), 1335-1353. http://dx.doi.org/10.1017/S0954579409990186, PubMed:19825271.

Bornovalova, M.A., Verhulst, B., Webber, T., McGue, M., Iacono, W.G., & Hicks, B.M. (2018). Genetics and environmental influences on the co-development between borderline personality disorder traits, major depression symptoms, and substance use disorder symptoms from adolescents to young adulthood. *Development and Psychopathology*, *30*(1), 49-65. http://dx.doi.org/10.1017/S0954579417000463.

Brambilla, P., Barale, F., Caverzasi, E., & Soares, J.C. (2002). Anatomical MRI findings in mood and anxiety disorder. *Epidemiologia e Psichiatria Sociale, 11,* 88-99. http://dx.doi.org/10.1017/S1121189X00005558.

Brambilla, P., Soloff, P.H., Sala, M., Nicoletti, M.A., Keshavan, M.S., & Soares, J.C. (2004). Anatomical MRI study of borderline personality disorder patients. *Psychiatry Research*, *131*(2), 125-133. http://dx.doi.org/10.1016/j.pscychresns.2004.04.003.

Bremner, J.D., Narayan, M., Anderson, E.R., Staib, L.H., Miller, H.L., & Charney, D.S. (2000). Hippocampal volume reduction in major depression. *Am J Psychiatry*, *157*, 115-118. http://dx.doi.org/10.1176/ajp.157.1.115.

Brown, S.M., Manuck, S.B., Flory, J.D., & Hariri, A.R. (2006). Neural basis of individual differences in impulsivity: contributions of corticolimbic circuits for behavioral arousal and control. *Emotion*, *6*(2), 239-245. http://dx.doi.org/10.1037/1528-3542.6.2.239.

Bush, G., Luu, P., & Posner, M.I. (2000). Cognitive and emotional influences in anterior cingulate cortex. *Trends in Cognitive Science*, *4*, 215-222. http://dx.doi.org/10.1016/s1364-6613(00)01483-2.

Congdon, E. & Canli, T. (2008). A neurogenetic approach to impulsivity. *Journal of Personality*, *76*(6), 1447-1484. http://dx.doi.org/10.1111/j.1467-6494.2008.00528.x.

Davis, M. & Whalen, P.J. (2001). The amygdala: vigilance and emotion. *Molecular Psychiatry*, *6*, 13-24. http://dx.doi.org/10.1038/sj.mp.4000812.

Davidson, R.J. Abercrombie, H., Nitschke, J.B., & Putnam, K. (1999). Regional brain function, emotion and disorders of emotion. *Current Opinion in Neurobiology*, *9*, 228-234. http://dx.doi.org/10.1016/S0959-4388(99)80032-4.

Diwadkar, V.A., Pruitt, P., Goradia, D., Murphy, E., Bakshi, N., Keshavan, M.S… Benitez, C. Fronto-parietal hypo-activation during working memory independent of structural abnormalities: conjoint fMRI and sMRI analyses in adolescent offspring of schizophrenia patients. *NeuroImage*. *58*, 234-241. http://dx.doi.org/10.1016/j.neuroimage.2011.06.033.

Donegan, N. (2003). Amygdala hyperreactivity in borderline personality disorder: implications for emotional dysregulation. *Biological Psychiatry*, *54*(11), 1284-1293. http://dx.doi.org/10.1016/S0006-3223(03)00636-X.

Etkin, A., Egner, T., & Kalisch, R. (2011). Emotional processing in anterior cingulate and medial prefrontal cortex. *Trends in Cognitive Science*, *15*, 85-93. http://dx.doi.org/10.1016/j.tics.2010.11.004.

Goodman, M., Carpenter, D., Tang, C.Y., Goldstein, K.E., Avedon, J., Fernandez, N…Hazlett, E.A. (2014). Dialectical behavioral therapy alters emotion regulation and amygdala activity in patients with borderline personality disorder. *Journal of Psychiatric Research, 57,* 108-116. http://dx.doi.org/10.1016/j.jpsychires.2014.06.020.

Goodman, M., New, A., & Siever, L. (2004). Trauma, genes, and the neurobiology of personality disorders. *Annals of the New York Academy of Science, 1032,* 104-116. http://dx.doi.org/10.1196/annals.1314.008.

Gottfried, J.A. (2003). Encoding predictive reward value in human amygdala and orbitofrontal cortex. *Science, 301,* 1104-1107. http://dx.doi.org/10.1126/science.1087919.

Gunderson, J.G., Stout, R.L., Sanislow, C.A., Shea, M.T., McGlashan, T.H., Zanarini, M.C…Skodol, A.E. (2008). New episodes and new onsets of major depression in borderline and other personality disorders. *Journal of Affective Disorders. 111*(1), 40-45. http://dx.doi.org/10.1016/j.jad.2008.01.026.

Gunderson, J.G., Zanarini, M.C., Choi-Kain, L.W., Michell, K.S., Jang, K.L., Hudson, J.I. (2011). Family study of borderline personality disorder and its sectors of psychopathology. *Arch Gen Psychiatry, 68,* 753-762. http://dx.doi.org/10.1001/archgenpsychiatry.2011.65.

Hart, H., Radua, J., Nakao, T., Mataix-Cols, D., & Rubia, K. (2013). Meta-analysis of functional magnetic resonance imaging studies of inhibition and attention in attention-deficit/hyperactivity disorder: exploring task-specific, stimulant medication, and age effects. *JAMA Psychiatry, 70,* 185-198. http://dx.doi.org/10.1001/jamapsychiatry.2013.277.

Hazlett, E.A., New, A.S., Newmark, R., Haznedar, M.M., Lo, J.N., Speiser, L.J…Buchsbaum, M.S. (2005). Reduced anterior and posterior cingulate gray atter in borderine personality disorder. *Biological Psychiatry, 58,* 614-623. http://dx.doi.org/10.1016/j.biopsych.2005.04.029.

Herpertz, S.C., Dietrich, T.M., Wenning, B., Krings, T., Erberich, S.G., Willmes, K…Sass, H. (2001). Evidence of abnormal amygdala functioning in borderline personality disorder: a functional MRI study. *Biological Psychiatry, 50*(4), 292-298. http://dx.doi.org/10.1016/S0006-3223(01)01075-7.

Horga, G., Kaur, T., & Peterson, B.S. (2014). Annul research review: current limitations and future directions in MRI studies in child- and adult-onset developmental psychopathologies. *Journal of Child Psychology and Psychiatry*, *55*(6), 659-680. http://dx.doi.org/10.1111/jcpp.12185.

Hulvershorn, L.A., Cullen, K., & Anand, A. (2011). Toward dysfunctional connectivity: a review of neuroimaging findings in pediatric major depressive disorder. *Brain Imaging and Behavior*, *5*, 307-328. http://dx.doi.org/10.1007/s11682-011-9134-3.

Kamphausen, S., Schroder, P., Maier, S., Bader, K., Feige, B., Kaller, C.P…Tuscher, O. (2013). Medial prefrontal dysfunction and prolonged amygdala response during instructed fear processing in borderline personality disorder. *World Journal of Biological Psychiatry*, *4(*4), 307-318. http://dx.doi.org/10.3109/15622975.2012.665174.

Koeningsberg, H.W., Fan, J., Ochsner, K.N., Liu, X., Guise, K.G., Pizzarello, S…Siever, L.J. (2009a). Neural correlates of the use of psychological distancing to regulate responses to negative social cues: a study of patients with borderline personality disorder. *Biological Psychiatry*, *66*(9), 854-863. http://dx.doi.org/10.1016/j.biopsych.2009.06.010.

Koenigsberg, H.W., Siever, L.J., Lee., H., Pizzarello, S., New, A.S., Goodman, M…Prohovnik, I. (2009b). Neural correlates of emotions processing in borderline personality disorder. *Psychiatry Research*, *172*(3), 192-199. http://dx.doi.org/10.1016/j.pscychresns.2008.07.010.

Krause-Uts, A., Frost, R., Winter, D., & Elzinga, B. (2017). Dissociation and alterations in brain function and structure: implications for borderline personality disorder. *Current Psychiatry Reports*, *19*(1). http://dx.doi.org/10.1007/s11920-017-0757-y.

Krause-Utz, A., Oei, N.Y., Niedtfeld, I., Bohus, M., Spinhoven, P., Schmahl, C., & Elzinga, B.M. (2012). Influence of emotional distraction on working memory performance in borderline personality disorder. *Psychological Medicine*, *42*(10), 2181-2192. http://dx.doi.org/10.1017/S0033291712000153.

Krause-Utz, A. & Schmahl, C. (2010). Neurobiological differentiation between borderline patients with and without post-traumatic stress disorder. *European Psychiatry Review*, *3*(2), 63-68.

Krause-Utz, A., Veer, I.M., Rombouts, S.A.R.B., Bohus, M., Schmahl, C., & Elzinga, B.M. (2014). Amygdala and anterior cingulate resting-state functional connectivity in borderline personality disorder patients with a history of interpersonal trauma. *Psychological Medicine*, *44,* 2889-2901. http://dx.doi.org/10.1017/s0033291714000324.

Krause-Utz, A., Winter, D., Niedtfeld, I., & Schmahl, C. (2014). The latest neuroimaging findings in borderline personality disorder. *Current Psychiatry Reports*, *16*(438), 45-55. http://dx.doi.org/10.1007/s11920-014-0438-z.

Lee, K.F., Soares, C., & Beique, J.C. (2012). Examining form and function of dendritic spines. *Neural Plast*, 704103. http://dx.doi.org/10.1155/2012/704103.

Leib, K., Zanarini, M.C., Schmahl, C., Linehan, M.M., & Bohus, M. (2004). Borderline personality disorder. *Lancet*, *364*(9432), 453-461. http://dx.doi.org/10.1016/S0140-6736(04)16770-6.

Leichsenring, F., Leibing, E. Kruse, J. New, A.S., & Leweke, F. (2011). Borderline personality disorder. *Lancet*, *377*(9759), 74-84. http://dx.doi.org/10.1016/S0140-6736(10)61422-5.

Lis, E., Greenfield, B., Henry, M., Guile, J.M., & Dougherty, G. (2007). Neuroimaging and genetics of borderline personality disorder: a review. *Journal of Psychiatry and Neuroscience*, *32*(3), 162-173. PMCID: PMC1863557.

Mancke, F., Herpertz, S.C., Hirjak, D., Knies, R. & Bertsch, K. (2018). Amygdala structure and aggressiveness in borderline personality disorder. *European Archives of Psychiatry and Neuroscience*, *268*, 417-427. http://dx.doi.org/10.1007/s00406-016-0747-9.

Mancke, F., Schmitt, R., Winter, D., Niedtfeld, I., Herpertz, S.C., & Schmahl, C. (2018). Assessing the marks of change: how psychotherapy alters the brain structure in women with borderline personality disorder. *Journal of Psychiatry and Neuroscience*, *43*(3), 171-181. http://dx.doi.org/10.1503/jpn.170132.

Minzenberg, M.J., Fan, J., New, A.S., Tang, C.Y., & Siever, L.J. (2007). Fronto-limbic dysfunction in response to facial emotion in borderline personality disorder: an event-related fMRI study. *Psychiatry Research, 155*(3), 231-243. http://dx.doi.org/10.1016/j.pscychresns.2007.03.006.

New, A.S., Hazlett, E.A., Buchsbaum, M.S., Goodman, M., Mitelman, S.A., Newmark, R…Siever, L.J. (2007). Amygala-prefrontal disconnection in borderline personality disorder. *Neuropsycho-pharmacology, 32*(7), 1629-1640. http://dx.doi.org/10.1038/sj.npp.1301283.

Niedtfled, I., Kirsch, P., Schulze, L., Herpertz, S.C., Bohus, M., & Schmahl, C. (2012). Functional connectivity of pain-mediated affect regulation in borderline personality disorder. *PloS One*, *7*, e33293.

Niedtfeld, I., Schulze, L., Kirsch, P., Herpertz, S.C., Bohus, M., & Schmahl, C. (2010). Affect regulation and pain in borderline personality disorder: a possible link to the understanding of self-injury. *Biological Psychiatry, 68*(4), 383-391. http://dx.doi.org/10.1016/j.biopsych.2010.04.015.

Nock, M.K. (2010). Self-injury. *Annual Review of Clinical Psychology, 6*, 339-363. http://dx.doi.org/10.1146/annurev.clinpsy.121208.131258.

Nunes, P.M., Wenzel, A., Borges, K.T., Porto, C.R., Caminha, R.M., & de Oliveira, I.R. (2009). Volumes of the hippocampus and amygdala in patients with borderline personality disorder: a meta-analysis. *Journal of Personality Disorder, 23*(4), 333-345. http://dx.doi.org/10.1521/pedi.2009.23.4.333.

Ochsner, K.N., Bunge, S.A., Gross, J.J., & Gabrieli, J.D. (2002). Rethinking feelings: an fMRI study of cognitive regulation of emotion. *Journal of Cognitive Neuroscience, 14,* 1215-1229. http://dx.doi.org/10.1162/089892902760807212.

Ochsner, K.N. & Gross, J.J. (2007). The neural architecture of emotion regulation. In J.J. Gross (Ed.), *Handbook of emotions regulation* (pp. 87-109). New York: Guilford Press.

O'Neill, A. & Frodl, T. (2012). Brain structure and function in borderline personality disorder. *Brain Structure and Function, 217*, 767-782. http://dx.doi.org/10.1007/s00429-012-0379-4.

Packard, M.G. & Knowlton, B.J. (2002). Learning and memory functions of the basal ganglia. *Annual Review of Neuroscience*, *25*, 563-593. http://dx.doi.org/10.1146/annurev.neuro.25.112701.142937.

Peterson, B.S. (2003). Conceptual, methodological, and statistical challenges in brain imaging studies of developmentally based psychopathologies. *Development and Psychopathologies*, *15*(3), 811-832. http://dx.doi.org/10.1017/S0954579403000385.

Phillips, M.L., Drevets, W.C., Rauch, S.L., & Lane, R. (2003). Neurobiology of emotion perception. *Biological Psychiatry*, *54*, 504-514. http://dx.doi.org/10.1016/S0006-3223(03)00168-9.

Phillips, R.G. & LeDoux, J.E. (1992). Differential contributions of amygdala and hippocampus to cued and contextual fear conditioning. *Behavioral Neuroscience*, *106*, 274-285. http://dx.doi.org/10.1037/0735-7044.106.2.274.

Pier, K.S., Marin, L.K., Wilsnack, J., & Goodman, M. (2016). The neurobiology of borderline personality disorder. *Psychiatric Times*, *33*(3). Retrieved from https://www.psychiatrictimes.com/special-reports/neurobiology-borderline-personality-disorder.

Quattrini, G., Marizzoni, M., Magni, L.R., Magnaldi, S., Lanfredi, M., Rossi, G., Frisoni, G.B., Pievani, M., & Rossi, R. (2019). Whole-brain microstructural white matter alterations in borderline personality disorder patients. *Personality and Mental Health*, *13*. http://dx.doi.org/10.1002/pmh.

Rosanoff, A.J. (1938, reprinted 1947). *Mixed, transitional borderline and miscellaneous groups. In Manual of Psychiatry and Mental Hygiene*, 7th Ed., Hoboken, NJ, US: John Wiley & Sons, Inc., pp. 644-653.

Rosell, D.R. & Siever, L.J. (2015). The neurobiology of aggression and violence. *CNS Spectrums, 20*, 254-279. http://dx.doi.org/10.1017/S109285291500019X.

Ruocco, A.C., Amirthavasagam, S., Choi-Kain, L.W., & McMain, S.F. (2012). Neural correlates of negative emotionality in borderline personality disorder: an activation-likelihood-estimation meta-analysis. *Biological Psychiatry*, *73*(2), 153-160. http://dx.doi.org/10.1016/j.biopsych.2012.07.014.

Ruocco, A.C., Amirthavasagam, S., & Zakzanis, K.K. (2012). Amygdala and hippocampal volume reductions as candidate endophenotypes for borderline personality disorder: a meta-analysis of magnetic resonance imaging studies. *Psychiatry Research: Neuroimaging, 201,* 245-252. http://dx.doi.org/10.1016/j.pscychresns.2012.02.012.

Ruocco, A.C., Rodrigo, A.H., McMain, S.F., Page-Gould, E., Ayaz, H., & Links, P.S. (2016). Predicting treatment outcomes from prefrontal cortex activation for self-harming patients with borderline personality disorder: a preliminary study. *Frontiers in Human Neuroscience, 10*(220). http://dx.doi.org/10.3389/fnhum.2016.00220.

Schmahl, C., Berne, K., Krause, A., Kleindienst, N., Valerius, G., Vermetten, E., & Bohus, M. (2009). Hippocampus and amygdala volumes in patients with borderline personality disorder with or without post traumatic stress disorder. *Journal of Psychiatry Neuroscience, 34*(4), 285-295. PMID 19568480.

Schmahl, C. & Bremner, J.D. (2006). Neuroimaging in borderline personality disorder. *Journal of Psychiatry Research*, 40(5), 419-427. http://dx.doi.org/10.1016/j.jpsychires.2005.08.011.

Schmahl, C.G., Vermetten, E., Elzinga, B.M., & Bremner, J.D. (2003). Magnetic resonance imaging of hippocampal and amygdala volume in women with childhood abuse and borderline personality disorder. *Psychiatry Research: Neuroimaging, 122,* 193-198. http://dx.doi.org/10.1016/S0925-4927(03)00023-4.

Schulze, L., Domes, G., Kruger, A., Berger, C., Fleischer, M., Prehn, K…Herpertz, S.C. (2011). Neuronal correlates of cognitive reappraisal in borderline patients with affective instability. *Biological Psychiatry, 69*(6), 564-573. http://dx.doi.org/10.1016/j.biopsych.2010.10.025.

Sescousse, G., Caldu, X., Segura, B., & Dreher, J.-C. (2013). Processing of primary and secondary rewards: a quantitative meta-analysis and review of human functional neuroimaging studies. *Neuroscience and Biobehavioral Reviews, 37,* 681-696. http://dx.doi.org/10.1016/j.neubiorev.2013.02.002.

Soares, J.C. & Mann, J.J. (1997). The anatomy of mood disorders-review of structural neuroimaging studies. *Biological Psychiatry*, *41*, 86-106. http://dx.doi.org/10.1016/S0006-3223(96)00006-6.

Soloff, P., Nutche, J., Goradia, D., & Diwadkar, V. (2008). Structural brain abnormalities in borderline personality disorder: a voxel-based morphometry study. *Psychiatric Research, 164*(3), 223-236. http://dx.doi.org/10.1016/j.pscychresns.2008.02.003.

Soloff, P., Pruitt, P., Sharma, M., Radwan, J., White, R., & Diwadkar, V.A. (2013). Structural brain abnormalities and suicidal behavior in borderline personality disorder. *Journal of Psychiatric Research*, *46*(4), 516-525. http://dx.doi.org/10.1016/j/jpsychires.2012.01.003.

Sosic-Vasic, Z., Eberhardt, J., Bosch, J.E., Dommes, L., Labek, K., Buchheim, A., & Viviani, R. (2019). Mirror neuron activations in encoding of psychic pain in borderline personality disorder. *NeuroImage: Clinical*, *22*. http://dx.doi.org/10.1016/j.nicl.2019. 101737.

Stanfield, A.C., McIntosh, A.M., Spencer, M.D., Philip, R., Gaur, S., & Lawrie, S.M. (2008). Towards a neuroanatomy of autism: a systematic review and meta-analysis of structural magnetic resonance imaging studies. *European Psychiatry*, *23,* 289-299. http://dx.doi.org/10.1016/j. eurpsy.2007.05.006.

Steele, H. & Siever, L. (2010). An attachment perspective on borderline personality disorder: advances in gene-environment considerations. *Current Psychiatry Reports*, *12*(1), 61-67. http://dx.doi.org/10.1007/ s11920009-0091-0.

Steffens, D.C., Bryum, C.E., McQuoid, D.R., Greenberg, D.L., Payne, M.E., Blitchington, T.F…Krishnan, K.R. (2000). Hippocampal volume in geriatric depression. *Biological Psychiatry*, *48*, 301-309. http://dx.doi.org/10.1016/S0006-3223(00)00829-5.

Stern, A. (1938). Psychoanalytic investigation of and therapy in the borderline group of neuroses. *The Psychoanalytic Quarterly, 7*, 467-489. http://dx.doi.org/10.1080/21674086.1938.11925367.

Vega, D., Ripolles, P., Soto, A., Torrubia, R., Ribas, J., Monreal, J. A…Marco-Pallares, J. (2018). Orbitofrontal overactivation in reward processing in borderline personality disorder: the role of non-suicidal self-injury. *Brain Imaging and Behavior, 12.* http://dx.doi.org/10.1007/s11682-017-9687-x.

Vythilingam, M., Heim, C., Newport, J., Miller, A.H., Anderson, E., Bronen, R…Bremner, J.D. (2002). Childhood trauma associated with smaller hippocampal volume in women with major depression. *American Journal of Psychiatry, 159*, 2072-2080. http://dx.doi.org/10.1176/appi.ajp.159.12.2072.

Wall, P.M. & Messier, C. (2001). The hippocampal formation-orbitomedial prefrontal cortex circuit in the attentional control of active memory. *Behavioral Brain Research, 127*, 99-117. http://dx.doi.org/10.1016/s0166-4328(01)00355-2.

Walter, M., Gunderson, J.G., Zanarini, M.C., Sanislow, C.A., Grilo, C.M., McGlashan, T.H…, Skodol, A.E. (2009). New onset of substance use disorders in borderline personality disorder over 7 years of follow-up: findings from the collaborative longitudinal personality disorders study. *Addiction, 104,* 97-103. http://dx.doi.org/10.1111/j.1360-0443.2008.02413.x.

Williams, J.M.G. & Broadbent, K. (1986). Autobiographical memory in suicide attempters. *Journal of Abnormal Psychology, 95*, 144-149. http://dx.doi.org/10.1037/0021-843X.95.2.144.

Wingenfeld, K., Spitzer, C., Rullkotter, N., & Lowe, B. (2010). Borderline personality disorder: hypothalamus pituitary adrenal axis and finding from neuroimaging studies. *Psychoneuroendocrinology*, *35*(1), 154-170. http://dx.doi.org/10.1016/j.psyneuen.2009.09.014.

Wolf, R.C., Sambataro, F., Vasic, N., Schmid, M., Thomann, P.A., Bienentreu, S.D., & Wolf, N.D. (2011). Aberrant connectivity of resting-state networks in borderline personality disorder. *Journal of Psychiatry and Neuroscience*, *36*(6), 402-411. http://dx.doi.org/10.1503/jpn.100150.

Zeki, S. & Romaya, J.P. (2008). Neural correlates of hate. *PLos ONE*, *3*(10), e355g. http://dx.doi.org/10.1371/journal.pone.0003556.

Zilles, K. (2018). Brodmann: a pioneer of human brain mapping-his impact on concept of cortical organization. *Brain: A Journal of Neurology, 141,* 3261-3278. http://dx.doi.org/10.1093/brain/awy273.

Zutphen, L.V., Siep, N., Jacob, G.A., Domes, G., Sprenger, A., Willenborg, B…Arntz, A. (2019). Impulse control under emotion processing: an fMRI investigation in borderline personality disorder compared to non-patients and cluster-C personality disorder patients. *Brain Imaging and Behavior*. http://dx.doi.org/10.1007/s11682-019-001161-0

In: Borderline Personality Disorder
Editor: Charles M. Lepkowsky
ISBN: 978-1-53618-021-3

Chapter 4

EVIDENCE-BASED MODELS OF TREATMENT FOR BORDERLINE PERSONALITY DISORDER

Chi-Sing Li[1,*], PhD, Robert J. Lugar[2], EdD, Reade Dowda[3], PhD, Diane Smedley[4] and Yu-Fen Lin[5], PhD

[1]Department of Counselor Education, Sam Houston State University, Huntsville, Texas, US
[2]Diversity Counseling Services, Dallas, Texas, US
[3]Advanced Education Programs Department, Fort Hays State University, Hays, Kansas, US
[4]Department of Educational Psychology and Leadership, Texas Tech University, Lubbock, Texas, US
[5]School of Human Services, UNT Dallas, Dallas, Texas, US

ABSTRACT

A brief history of Cognitive Behavioral Therapy (CBT) is followed by discussion of its application in the treatment of Borderline Personality

* Corresponding Author's E-mail: chisingli@shsu.edu.

Disorder (BPD). Research is cited indicating that most evidenced based treatment approaches to BPD stem from CBT, including Dialectical Behavior Therapy (DBT). Inpatient and outpatient treatments are discussed, including the role of psychopharmacology. Research is summarized addressing the most commonly prescribed drug classes for BPD.

Keywords: Cognitive Behavioral Therapy, Dialectical Behavior Therapy, inpatient and outpatient treatment, psychopharmacology

A REVIEW

Borderline Personality Disorder's (BPD's) reputation as a challenging psychiatric diagnosis has led many clinicians to avoid working with BPD clients. Consequently, it is difficult to find psychotherapists who are competent, effective, and willing to work with BPD clients (Choi-Kain, Finch, Masland, Jenkins, and Unruh, 2017). BPD's reputation is based in fact that BPD is a complex diagnosis. Comorbidity is evident in 75% of BPD clients (Sauer-Zavala, Bentley, and Wilner, 2016). Data presented by Dingfelder (2004) suggest that up to 30 percent of those who require mental health services have at least one personality disorder, and of those personality disorders, BPD is the most commonly treated disorder. Dingfelder's data also indicate that clients diagnosed with BPD drop out of treatment 70 percent of the time, ostensibly because BPD is difficult to treat effectively, and ineffective treatment models are often employed. Gunderson et al. (2011) concurred, describing borderline personality disorder (BPD) as difficult to treat, chronic and intractable compared to other personality disorders. This conclusion was drawn from their 10-year longitudinal study comparing the course of BPD psychopathology and social functioning with that of other personality disorders and major depressive disorder (MDD). Results from this study indicated that BPD patients experience significantly more severe and persistent impairment in social functioning than patients diagnosed with other personality disorders or

MDD. The authors suggest that as a consequence, BPD represents a greater public health burden than other personality disorders or MDD.

Outcome research data have been used to identify the more effective treatment models for BPD, which are commonly referred to as evidenced based therapy (EBT) approaches. BPD is now effectively treated by a growing number of evidenced based treatments and through training, by increasingly competent clinicians (Choi-Kain et al., 2017).

Cognitive Behavioral Theory: A Theoretical Foundation

Cognitive Theory posits that psychological difficulties are the consequence of faulty cognitions. Cognitive Behavioral Therapy (CBT) describes a broad spectrum of psychotherapeutic interventions based on Cognitive Theory, initially developed in part by Aaron Beck (1970) and Albert Ellis (1962). Ellis and Beck hypothesized that psychological and emotional problems originating in maladaptive thought processes cause psychological, emotional, and behavioral disorders. According to Beck (1970), maladaptive cognitions form general belief systems, or schemas, about the world, the self, and others that interfere with the client's ability to function in social and interpersonal situations. The basic goal of cognitive behavioral theory is to alter maladaptive thought processes in order to promote symptom reduction while facilitating overall improvement in psycho-social and interpersonal functioning. According to Hofmann (2011), modern CBT refers to a class of interventions that include a variety of cognitive, behavioral, and emotion-focused techniques. McMain, Newman, Segal, and DeRubeis (2015) describe cognitive behavioral therapy as an umbrella term that encompasses and is part of many of the therapeutic treatments utilized today in the treatment of mental illness. Although treatment approaches vary in specific technique, they almost all share and include some aspect of cognitive behavioral therapy (McMain et al., 2015).

Therapeutic use of cognitive behavioral theory is widespread, and has been heavily researched regarding efficacy and value (Hofmann, Asnaani, Vonk, Sawyer, and Fang, 2012). An influential and comprehensive study on the efficacy of cognitive behavioral theory was conducted by Butler, Chapman, Foreman, and Beck (2006), in which meta-analyses of 332 clinical trials was conducted to examine the efficacy of CBT treatment. The authors concluded that the CBT studies they examined were both methodologically sound and appeared to demonstrate improvement in outcome, with CBT as the primary variable. A study conducted by Hofmann et al. (2012), provided a comprehensive survey of meta-analyses examining the efficacy of CBT. The authors identified 269 meta-analytic studies, reviewed a representative sample of 106 meta-analyses, and examined the application of CBT to a variety of psychological problems. The authors concluded that cognitive behavioral therapy has been used for a wide range of psychological problems and that CBT is the most widely studied and utilized form of psychotherapy. They also concluded that the evidence-base of CBT is robust, while stating that there remains a need for additional empirical studies to examine the efficacy of this approach. The authors concluded that regardless of the specific therapeutic approach, almost all evidence-based treatments (EBTs) have a cognitive behavioral component that is integral to treatment (Hofmann, et al., 2012).

In consideration of treatment for BPD, it is important to have a competent understanding of the theoretical causal factors related to BPD, and some familiarity with the historical research in the treatment of this disorder (Linehan, 1993). One's theoretical understanding of BPD pathology generally directs one's treatment approach. A brief summary of some of the more prominent EBTs is discussed below in relation to a cognitive behavioral component followed by a more extensive review of Cognitive Behavioral Therapy as an EBT for BPD.

Mentalization-Based Treatment (MBT)

Mentalization-based treatment (MBT) is another evidenced based treatment (EBT) that was developed at the National Health Services (NHS) in the United Kingdom by Bateman and Fonagy (2010). This treatment approach focuses on the individual's capacity to imagine the thoughts and feelings of others, as well as those in one's own mind, in an attempt to understand interpersonal interactions that occur around them. Psychological disturbance is theorized as arising when a patient stops accurately mentalizing oneself and others. These inaccuracies lead the patient to develop irrational belief systems about other's motives and behaviors. These errant belief systems create pathological constructs surrounding their reality, complicated by a desperate need for proof of feelings through action. Theorists who utilize this approach assume that attachments become over-exaggerated, leading to distress and difficulty coping, rather than providing safety and security. The goal of MBT is to strengthen the patient's ability to accurately mentalize the objects of attachment. The structure of MBT includes weekly individual sessions, weekly group therapy, and a reflecting team that helps support counselors in their work with clients. Bateman and Fonagy look at mentalization as a process that all human beings use to make sense of each other and of oneself. Mental disorders are seen as a direct result of difficulty with mentalization. The authors additionally suggest that those with borderline personality disorder diagnoses consistently show reduced capacities to mentalize, which in turn leads to problems with emotional regulation combined with difficulty managing impulsivity in their ability to manage interpersonal relationships. MBT is considered a brief therapy approach treatment that focuses interventions on the development of mentalizing. MBT requires relatively little additional training (compared to some of the other EBTs) with additional general clinical training.

Mentalization theory is rooted in Bowlby's attachment theory (Bowlby, 1958) and its elaboration by contemporary psychologists (Bateman & Fonagy, 2010). Clinical assumptions revolve around the notion that patients with borderline personality disorder have a history of disorganized attachment, leading to problems with emotional regulation, attention, and self-control. This theory suggests that these problems are mediated through a failure to develop a robust mentalizing capacity. Theoretically, it is one's understanding of others while also being understood by caring, nurturing caregivers that provides for a safe and healthy environment in which to grow. Bateman and Fonagy suggest that interruption in this process through trauma cause impairment in multiple areas, and in particular in the development of social/cognitive capacities necessary for mentalization. Mentalization-based treatment focuses on stabilizing the sense of self and helping the patient maintain an optimal level of arousal in the context of a well-managed (i.e., not too intense and yet not too detached) attachment relationship between the patient and the therapist. As one reviews the description of this approach, it is clear that cognitive processes are an integral part of the etiology of this problem and a necessary component of the treatment approach.

Systems Training for Emotional Predictability and Problem Solving (STEPPS)

Systems Training for Emotional Predictability and Problem Solving (STEPPS) is another Evidenced Based Treatment that has a cognitive behavioral therapy component. It consists of a 20-week manual-based group treatment program for outpatients with borderline personality disorder that combines cognitive behavioral elements and skills training along with a systems component. Blum et al. (2008) have demonstrated the efficacy of this treatment approach in their study of 124 subjects diagnosed with borderline personality disorder that compared STEPPS treatment modality to treatment as usual (TAU) in a randomized controlled trial. Treatment is facilitated by two co-facilitators that lead the groups followed by lesson plans that include three main components; psycho education, emotional management skills training, and behavior management skills. These researchers conclude in their study that STEPPS, as an adjunctive group treatment, can deliver clinically meaningful improvements in borderline personality disorder-related symptoms while also enhancing the patient's ability to function adaptively.

Transference-Focused Psychotherapy (TFP)

Transference-focused psychotherapy (TFP) is based on Otto Kernberg's conceptualization of Borderline Personality which was developed in the 1960s and 1970s (Kernberg, 1970). It is a manualized, psychoanalytically oriented psychotherapy defined by its focus on identity diffusion, primitive defense mechanisms, unstable reality testing, internally and externally expressed aggression, and conflicted internal working models of relationships as key features of personality disorders at the borderline level (Choi-Kain et al., 2017). TFP focus is on the interpersonal dynamics in the patient's life and the resultant intense emotional states. These dynamics emerge in the interpersonal relationship with the therapist in the transference and are jointly examined to resolve the splits between good and bad that drive instabilities in affect and relationships. Change occurs via helping patients achieve more balanced, integrated, and coherent ways of thinking about oneself and others. Structure is two weekly individual therapy sessions, without group therapy and is more compatible for individual therapists not working in teams. The elements of cognitive behavior therapy are not as present in this approach, however there is attention given to cognitions related to how one thinks about oneself.

Structured Clinical Management (SCM) and General Psychiatric Management (GPM)

Structured Clinical Management (SCM) and General Psychiatric Management (GPM) are broad treatment approaches to borderline personality disorder that have been used in psychiatric treatment centers almost since the origin of its diagnosis (Choi-Kain et al., 2017). These approaches emerged as a necessary adjunct to ongoing treatment of this disorder in order to accentuate progress in therapy and help manage BPD symptoms. Both of these approaches are based on a case management model where interventions rely on common sense and are learned easily by generalist clinicians. The focus is on the life outside of therapy. Patients typically meet once per week and the treatment is multimodal while facilitating the use of additional resources such as psychopharmacological interventions, group therapy, family therapy, and coordination across providers. The primary focus is on the interpersonal hypersensitivity symptoms of BPD, understanding that these symptoms are of primary concern while attempting to help the patient understand his or her sensitivities and responses. Given that this approach is an ancillary support to other treatment approaches that treat BPD, cognitive behavioral therapy is incorporated into one if not several of the therapies this model is set up to support.

Schema-Focused Therapy (SFT)

Schema-Focused Therapy (SFT) most closely resembles a traditional cognitive behavioral therapy approach. SFT is considered an integrative cognitive therapy that focuses on generating structural changes to the patient's personality and belief system (Kellogg & Young, 2006). Therapy occurs via individual therapy sessions twice weekly as the therapist utilizes a variety of behavioral, cognitive, and experiential techniques. SFT encourages an attachment between the therapist and the client, a process described as "limited re-parenting" (Kellogg & Young, 2006). According to Geisen-Bloo et al. (2006), the primary goal of SFT is to reorganize the patient's inner structure through limited re-parenting, experiential imagery and dialogue work combined with cognitive restructuring and education, in order to interrupt behavioral patterns. Schema Focused Therapy was initially developed by Jeffrey Young, PhD, while on the faculty with the Department of Psychiatry at Columbia University in the mid-1980s. He is known to have established the first Schema Therapy Institute in the mid-1990s in Manhattan, New York (Geisen-Bloo et al., 2006). SFT was further developed and became more adapted to the study of borderline personality disorder in The Netherlands as Josephine Giesen-Bloo and Arnoud Arntz (2006) conducted a well-controlled outcome study wherein the researchers compared Schema Focused Therapy with Transference Focused

Psychotherapy (TFP) in the treatment of borderline personality disorder. In this study, the researchers were able to demonstrate that SFT provided significant improvement in the symptoms of the borderline personality disorder patient after treatment and functioned significantly better after the first year, with improvement occurring more rapidly in the SFT group. There was continuing improvement in subsequent years. Thus, investigators concluded that both treatments had positive effects, with Schema Therapy being significantly more successful. Schema Therapy is an integrative approach founded on the principles of cognitive-behavioral therapy and then expanded to include techniques and concepts from other psychotherapies. Schema therapists help patients to change their self-defeating patterns using cognitive behavioral, and emotion-focused techniques. The treatment focuses on the relationship with the therapist, daily life outside of therapy, and the traumatic childhood experiences that are common in this disorder. Schema Therapy's effectiveness arises in part from its use of limited re-parenting which is dissimilar to other approaches to BPD. Both Schema Therapy and Transference Focused Psychotherapy focus on deeper personality change, in comparison to other recent treatments that have been limited to the reduction of specific behavioral symptoms. This focus appears to not only reduce symptoms such as self-destructive behaviors and emotional dysregulation but also seems to help resolve issues at a deeper core level (Kellogg & Young, 2006). A primary focus on treatment is directed at changing negative patterns of thinking, feeling and behaving and developing healthier alternatives to replace them in order to repair dysfunctional schemas that essentially control patient's maladaptive behavior and thought processes. This clearly is reflective of a cognitive behavioral approach. Cognitive Behavior Therapy as an effective treatment to borderline personality disorder.

Cognitive-Behavioral Therapy (CBT)

While many of the effective EBTs for BPD include some form or component of Cognitive Behavioral Therapy, CBT alone in and of itself is a proven effective treatment for BPD. Matusiewicz, Hopwood, and Lejuez (2010) investigated research published from 1980 to 2009 which included 45 publications evaluating the outcome of cognitive behavioral interventions for personality disorders. The authors concluded that CBT is an effective treatment approach for reducing symptoms and improving functional outcomes among patients with BPD. The authors also concluded that the use of CBT for treating borderline personality disorders and avoidant personality disorders had the most extensive empirical support, including numerous randomized clinical trials. CBT treatments for BPD have been studied more extensively in randomly controlled studies than treatments for any other diagnosis. Davidson, Tyrer, Norrie, Palmer, and Tyrer (2010) demonstrated that cognitive behavioral therapy significantly reduced the symptoms of borderline personality disorder when compared to treatment as usual (TAU). The authors conducted a randomized clinical study of 106 patients who were diagnosed with BPD and studied follow-up data of the patients over a 6-year period. Although CBT was not seen as demonstrating a significant cost effective advantage to treatment as usual, it was clear that there was significant reduction of BPD symptoms with CBT.

One of the most cited research studies of cognitive behavioral therapy in the treatment of borderline personality disorder is the randomized controlled trial BOSCOT study conducted by Kate Davidson et al. (2006). The goal of this study was to determine whether the addition of cognitive behavioral therapy to treatment as usual (CBT plus TAU) in participants with borderline personality disorder would have an impact on the number of participants with emergency psychiatric visits, accident and emergency room contact, or episodes of self-harm. Treatment was conducted over a twelve-month period followed by twelve months of follow-up. The study was conducted in Glasgow, London and Ayrshire, where TAU was routinely practiced. All participants met criteria for at least 5 items of borderline personality disorder diagnostic criteria, had received either in-patient psychiatric services or an assessment at emergency services or had an episode of deliberate self-harm (either suicidal act or self-mutilation) in the previous 12 months.

In the BOSCOT study, CBT was defined as a structured, time limited, psycho-social intervention wherein patients were encouraged to focus on their beliefs and behavior that impaired their ability to socially and interpersonally function. Each participant was exposed to thirty sessions of CBT over a one-year period, each lasting up to one hour. The objective was to address long-standing problems and to develop new ways of thinking and behaving. Priority was given to behaviors that caused harm to self or others. In addition, participants received the usual treatment they would have received if the trial had not been in place.

Treatment as usual (TAU) was defined as the standard treatment they would have received if the trial had not been in place. Although standard treatment varied depending on the location of the participant, it was assumed that all participants would be engaged with mental health services in their area and would have some contact and access to emergency services for repeated self-harm episodes. The authors concluded that the addition of CBT to usual treatment significantly reduced the frequency and severity of several BPD symptoms, including suicidal behavior, dysfunctional beliefs, and overall perceived psychological distress. Because therapists can be trained in CBT with relative ease compared to some of the more technical treatments for BPD, the authors suggested that CBT can be utilized in many community areas where highly specialized BPD therapy approaches are not available.

Davidson et al. (2010) conducted a 6-year follow-up study of the BOSCOT trial in order to determine whether there was continued reduction in symptoms of the BPD patients that were part of this study. CBT was again compared to TAU for BPD patients. The authors obtained data for 82% of the patients from the BOSCOT trial and determined that over half of the patients who met the criteria for BPD and were treated with CBT continued to experience significant symptom reduction compared to those who were treated with TAU, including reduced rates of admission into hospital or emergency room services.

Cognitive-Behavioral Therapy (CBT) in Group Settings

Research indicates that the use of cognitive behavioral techniques in a group therapy environment is effective in the treatment of BPD. Schilling, Moritz, Kriston, Krieger, and Nagel (2018) studied the efficacy of meta-cognitive training for patients with borderline personality disorder (B-MCT) as an adjunct to standard treatment. They evaluated the effectiveness of this new approach against the control condition of TAU. Seventy-four inpatients with BPD were randomly assigned to metacognitive training for BPD in addition to TAU. The authors concluded that B-MCT was an effective tool that helped reduce symptoms for those who had been diagnosed with BPD.

Nenadic, Lamberth, and Reiss (2017) studied Farrell and Shaw's group schema therapy (GST) (Farrell & Shaw, 2012) in the treatment of BPD. In a pilot study implementing GST in acute psychiatric in-patient settings, Nenadic et al. (2017) suggested that GST is an effective long term treatment for BPD. Van Vreeswiik, Spinhoven, Eurelings-Bontekoe, and Broersen (2014) investigated whether short term schema cognitive behavioral group therapy (SCBT-g) in an outpatient clinic setting was associated with changes in symptom severity. Using 63 psychiatric outpatient participants in a naturalistic pre-treatment post-treatment design, the authors determined that SCBT-g was associated with reduced symptom severity in more than half of the psychiatric outpatients. The authors suggested that SCBT-g might be effective not only for treating BPD, but for other personality disorders as well.

Cognitive-Behavioral Therapy (CBT) and Comorbidity with BPD

Trauma and PTSD are over-represented in the BPD population (Kredlow et al., 2017). Numerous studies have investigated the efficacy of CBT for patients with comorbidity for BPD and PTSD (Kredlow et al., 2017). Holder, Holliday, Pal, and Suris (2017) investigated the effectiveness of Cognitive Processing Therapy (CPT) for twenty-seven BPD female veterans with military sexual trauma-related PTSD. The authors concluded that CPT was effective in reducing PTSD symptoms, and indicated support for the use of CPT in female veterans with PTSD and comorbid BPD. Kredlow et al. (2017) also studied the effects of CBT with BPD patients also diagnosed with PTSD. The authors conducted analyses on data from two randomized controlled trials of a CBT program for PTSD in individuals with severe mental illness (SMI) to examine the feasibility, tolerability, and effectiveness for individuals also diagnosed with BPD. 72 participants in 2 controlled studies were treated with CBT in addition to either TAU or brief therapy. Participants treated with CBT showed significantly greater reduction in PTSD symptoms, depression, and self-reported physical health problems than those who were treated with either brief therapy or TAU.

CBT has been shown to be effective in the treatment of serious mental illness (SMI) with psychosis. Interestingly, 21-54% of patients diagnosed with BPD experience auditory verbal hallucinations. Slotema et al. (2017) used CBT for patients with BPD who also experienced auditory verbal hallucinations (AVH). The authors concluded that CBT is beneficial in the treatment of BPD patients who also meet the diagnostic criteria of SMI with psychosis, regardless of whether or not the patient was taking antipsychotic medication.

Lis and Myhr (2016) concur that (CBT) is an evidence-based treatment approach and that it has been shown to be effective in the treatment for most psychiatric disorders. However, they suggest that there are conflicting data in the literature regarding whether a comorbid personality disorder worsens the prognosis of CBT for depression, anxiety, and other complaints. Lis and Myhr (2016) conducted a pre-test post-test study for patients who were diagnosed with either borderline personality disorder, obsessive compulsive disorder or no personality disorder using cognitive behavioral therapy as the primary intervention. The data indicate that although there was significant improvement in outcome after treatment with obsessive compulsive disorder patients, those diagnosed with borderline personality disorder had a greater response to CBT than the other disorders that were treated.

Pascual et al. (2015) studied the differences between cognitive rehabilitation intervention and psycho-educational interventions, noting that

BPD patients tend to have a higher rate of remission than most other disorders. They conducted a 16 week multicenter, randomized, positive-controlled clinical trial for 70 outpatients with BPD who were randomized to either cognitive rehabilitation or psychoeducational group interventions. A follow up was conducted after 6 months to determine outcomes. The authors concluded that both cognitive rehabilitation and psychoeducational interventions improve overall functioning in daily life in subjects with BPD. However, post-hoc analyses showed that only cognitive rehabilitation significantly increased psychosocial functioning.

Zanarini, Frankenburg, Reich, and Fitzmaurice (2012) examined the commonly-held belief that BPD is more difficult to treat than other personality disorders. In a 16 year follow-up study of 290 inpatients with BPD compared to other Axis II disorders, they found that borderline patients were consistently slower to achieve recovery than those diagnosed with other personality disorders, and that for BPD patients remission and symptom recurrence occurred more rapidly and at a substantially higher rate. The authors suggested that understanding the cognitive processing of BPD and utilizing techniques to alter impaired processing is of paramount importance in the treatment of this disorder. Soloff, White, Omari, Ramaseshan, and Diwadkar (2015) tested this hypothesis, using 16-week cognitive rehabilitation and psychoeducational interventions with BPD patients who were re-evaluated 6 months after treatment. The researchers concluded that both treatments were efficacious for improving daily functioning, with significant symptom reduction.

Dialectical Behavior Therapy (DBT)

Dialectical Behavior Therapy (DBT) was specifically designed to treat extreme suicidal ideation and borderline personality disorder (Chugani, 2017; Neacsiu, Ward-Ciesielski, & Linehan, 2012; Rizvi, Steffle, & Carson-Wong, 2013). DBT is the most researched therapy for borderline personality disorder (Kröger, Harbeck, Armbrust, & Kliem, 2013). A focus of research has been DBT's effectiveness in reducing the frequency and severity of symptoms associated with BPD (Ben-Porath, 2015; Lynch, Chapman, Rosenthal, Kuo, & Linehan, 2006; Navarro-Haro et al., 2018; Neacsiu, Lungu, Harned, Rizvi, & Linehan, 2014). Marsha Linehan was one of the first researchers to conduct a randomized controlled trial (RCT) and publish evidenced based research articles specific to BPD. She demonstrated that DBT was significantly more effective (i.e., yielded more significant reduction in parasuicidal behavior, inpatient psychiatric stays, and treatment drop out) than treatment as usual (TAU). Since then, over 15 manualized therapies have been tested, some of which have been established as evidenced based treatments (EBTs) for BPD (Choi-Kain et al., 2017).

DBT focuses on four main skill sets: mindfulness, emotional regulation, distress tolerance, and interpersonal effectiveness (Lenz & Del Conte, 2018; Linehan, 2015). The DBT treatment process consists of four main fundamental parts including individual therapy, weekly skills training in a group, telephone coaching, and consultation for the therapy team. DBT is being used to treat many different populations and across cultures because of its effectiveness and growing empirical evidence. DBT has proven to be effective with adults (Kröger et al., 2013; Linehan, 2015; Lynch et al., 2006), and is also being used effectively with adolescents (Germán, et al., 2015; Hunnicutt Hollenbaugh & Lenz, 2018; Lenz & Del Conte, 2018). Dialectical Behavior Therapy for adolescents (DBT-A) is advantageous in treating many concerns facing adolescents such as depression, anxiety, and maladaptive behavior (Hunnicutt Hollenbaugh & Lenz, 2018). DBT's flexibility allows culture to be taken into consideration which is one of the reasons it is being used with many cultures and in other countries. Researchers have found it beneficial in working with transgender clients (Sloan, Berke, & Shipherd, 2017), clients in Egypt (Abdelkarim, Nagui, Esmaiel, & Helal, 2016), Latina clients (Germán et al., 2015), Native American and Alaskan Native clients (Beckstead, Lambert, DuBose, & Linehan, 2015), and deaf clients (O'Hearn & Pollard, 2008).

Marsha Linehan found that focusing on change alone resulted in clients feeling invalidated, while a focus on acceptance alone was perceived as dismissive to problem severity. For that reason, she began to focus on finding a balance between acceptance and change. DBT does not merely focus on the disorder.Rather, the presenting issue, emotional concerns, and environmental factors are all addressed in a holistic approach to improving the client's well-being (Lynch et al., 2006). DBT is flexible and includes a team where concerns are discussed and treatment is collaborative, which fits well when working with complicated diagnoses (Linehan & Wilks, 2015). Another reason DBT is effective is the length of time clients spend in therapy. Spending more time in therapy allows clients to address issues with therapists and other group members, and work through conflict resolution instead of terminating relationships as they might in their personal lives (Linehan, 2015). This builds hope and the expectation that a client can maintain interpersonal relationships by working through issues that arise.

Borderline Personality Disorder and Hospital Treatment

In general, personality disorders are diagnosed when a patients' behavior is outside of cultural and societal expectations, is pervasive and inflexible, has an onset during early adulthood, and leads to distress and/or impairment (APA, 2013). According to the *Diagnostic and Statistical Manual of Mental Disorders, Fifteh edition (DSM-5)* (APA, 2013), BPD is a specific type of personality disorder that is marked by erratic and unstable behavior patterns in interpersonal relationship difficulties, self-image, and increased impulsivity. Due to the cluster of symptoms associated with BPD, these patients are often admitted for hospitalization due to safety concerns. The unique symptoms of BPD that lead to increased hospitalization rates, the specifics of hospital treatment, and what evidence-based treatments are currently used for BPD in psychiatric hospital settings will be discussed.

BPD Symptomology and Hospital Treatment

BPD diagnostic criteria include unstable patterns of interpersonal relationships, erratic and impulsive behavior, and unstable self-image (APA, 2013). The unstable patterns of interpersonal relationships are often expressed in a "hot and cold" intense approach to relationships. When a relationship appears to be ending, or there is a chance of experiencing any form of rejection, a patient with BPD often becomes desperate to avoid abandonment by others. The abandonment is internalized, and the patient is likely to label themselves as "bad" or "worthless" (Axelrod, Perepletchikova, Holtzman, & Sinha, 2011). This is often when impulsive behaviors are displayed in order to mitigate the painful feelings, and there is a greater likelihood of non-suicidal self-injury (NSSI) and/or suicidal thoughts and behavior (Bloom, Woodward, Susmaras, & Pantalone, 2012).

Patients with BPD have higher rates of NSSI and a completed suicide rate 50 times greater than the general population (APA, 2001). Mental health practitioners working outside of the acute psychiatric hospital setting have an obligation to ensure the safety of their patients. It is difficult for practitioners to ensure safety when patients report a desire to participate in self-harming behaviors. Due to the high rates of self-harm behaviors reported by patients with BPD, NSSI or suicidal behaviors are the primary reason for hospitalization of this population (Gunderson, 2009). This lability of symptoms and impulsivity combined with heightened rates of self-harm often leaves practitioners uncomfortable managing these symptoms outside of a hospital setting (Hörz, Zanarini, Frankenburg, Reich, & Fitzmaurice, 2010).

Mental health practitioners can provide services to patients in a variety of treatment settings. During times of crisis, patients can be admitted to psychiatric hospitals for both stabilization and safety (National Alliance on Mental Illness, 2019). Admission to an inpatient hospital unit typically requires that the patient is either likely to cause harm to self or others (e.g., suicidal or homicidal behaviors) or is acting in an erratic manner due to the effects of a psychiatric symptom (e.g., psychosis or mania). On rarer occasions, admission to an inpatient unit may be due to the desire of a psychiatrist to monitor medication adjustments or monitor electroconvulsive therapy.

Psychiatric hospitals often also offer day programs called partial hospitalization programming (PHP) and/or intensive outpatient programming (IOP). PHP typically requires attendance five to seven days a week for upwards to ten hours a day. IOP attendance is considered a less acute level of treatment, usually two to five days a week, and for fewer hours, around four hours per day of programming. Both programming types allow patients to go home at night. Often PHP and IOP are used to transition patients from inpatient care to daily life after a mental health crisis. Sometimes mental health practitioners and psychiatrists will recommend PHP/IOP treatment when inpatient treatment is inappropriate or unfeasible. For patients with BPD, neither inpatient treatment nor PHP/IOP treatment are a panacea. However, both have demonstrated efficacy with evidence-based treatments to reduce symptomology and lower hospitalization rates.

Inpatient Treatment for BPD

Almost 75% of people who meet the diagnostic criteria for BPD will have at least one lifetime hospitalization, while subsequent hospitalizations are more likely with BPD than with any other mental health disorder (Widiger & Weissman, 1991). Paradoxically, there is relatively little research regarding effective treatments within the inpatient treatment setting. At this time, dialectical behavior therapy (DBT) appears to be the most popular and well researched modality used with patients who have BPD and seek inpatient treatment (Bloom, Woodward, Susmaras, & Pantalone, 2012; Kröger et al., 2013).

Bloom et al. (2012) conducted a review of published studies where researchers made modifications to standardized DBT treatment for inpatient hospital implementation. From their review, the authors found that when DBT was adapted to fit the treatment setting, patients experienced a reduction in symptoms of borderline personality disorder. According the Bloom et al., the reduced symptoms included “self-harm behaviors, depressive symptoms, anxiety symptoms, and dissociative experiences" (p. 885). There is also some evidence that inpatient DBT treatment can lead to reduction in hostility, anger, and suicidal ideation. The authors found that not only were gains made during treatment, but much of the reduction in symptoms was maintained post treatment. One study that Bloom et al. reviewed found treatment improvements lasting nearly two years post treatment.

Kröger et al. (2013) conducted a study on 1,423 patients of mixed gender with BPD who received three months of inpatient treatment. This study was unique due to both its large sample size and studying both men and women. Participants reported a significant decrease in BPD symptoms during treatment. 45% of participants experienced an improvement in symptoms and 14.8% experienced symptoms at a rate that is similar to the general population. This study included data regarding participants with comorbidities. The results indicate that there is a higher likelihood of complications to treatment compliance when a patient has an additional psychiatric disorder, especially including a substance use disorder.

Outside of DBT, there is scarce research showing inpatient treatment efficacy with BPD and any other therapeutic modality. Strauss, Mestel, and Kirchmann (2011) studied the change in attachment status of patients with BPD seeking inpatient treatment. The authors hypothesized that a change in attachment status would be associated with positive psychological outcomes. Strauss et al. expected that a significant proportion of the 40 participants would move from an insecure to a secure attachment style. Using a combination of psychodynamic and person-centered orientations, the participants received a variety of group therapies for an average of 12 weeks. The authors reported that their hypothesis of participants moving from insecure to secure attachment was not supported. However, a large portion of the participants did change from ambivalent attachment to an avoidant attachment. This move from ambivalent to avoidant was described by the authors as "deactivating the attachment system" (p. 281), and that this deactivation was associated with positive outcomes. Additional research is needed on the effects of changing attachment status on BPD symptoms.

Anecdotally, many hospitals employ cognitive behavioral therapy due to its longstanding position as an evidence-based modality.

Inpatient treatment is currently considered by many to be the best treatment for clients in crisis; however, it comes with risks and concerns. A major concern is the cost of inpatient treatment. With little evidence-based research to back up the efficacy of inpatient treatment, it is difficult to justify the large cost of hospitalization. Costing at least $8,000 and increasing the involvement of managed health care systems, the availability of data to justify inpatient treatment has become increasing important (Bales et al., 2012; Bateman & Fonagy, 2003). The high rates of BPD hospitalization make it increasingly important to conduct research on patients with BPD seeking inpatient hospital treatment (Leichsenring, Leibing, Kruse, New, & Leweke, 2011).

Inpatient hospitalization might also involve some risks, including the reinforcement of undesirable symptoms in patients with BPD. Bloom et al. refer to concern about suicidal behavior having a "contagion" effect among an inpatient treatment setting for patients with BPD. Depending on the reasoning behind the patient's behaviors, inpatient hospitalization might reinforce undesirable behaviors in the BPD population. (Linehan, 2018). If suicidal behavior is an act of avoidance, then placing the patient in inpatient care unintentionally allows for the avoidance to occur. It appears that the BPD individual is more likely to engage in suicidal behavior in the future as an avoidance tool (Bloom et al., 2012), eventuating in systematic drains on community resources and an intensification of patient symptoms.

Finally, comorbidities are common in patients with BPD. Common occurring comorbidities include depression, anxiety, and substance use disorders. As seen in the study conducted by Kröger et al. (2013), comorbidities can complicate treatment compliance. Kröger et al. found that when a patient with BPD had a comorbidity, the patient was less likely to maintain regular treatment attendance. Since comorbidities with BPD are common, it is important that inpatient treatment includes interventions that assistance patients with both BPD and other mental health disorders. Kröger et al. also noted that addressing social enviroments and including family interventions may increase the effectiveness of inpatient treatment for this population. Sometimes inpatient treatment is not appropriate for a patient with BPD, but the patient might still need a higher level of intervention than weekly outpatient psychotherapy. In this situation, PHP/IOP programming plays a vital role in sypmtom management for patients with BPD.

Day Hospitalization Treatment for BPD

PHP and IOP treatment settings provide patients with the ability to participate in daily life while receiving intensive treatment for BPD. Similar to inpatient treatment, there is relatively scare research evaluating the efficacy of evidence-based treatment for this treatment setting. Bales et al. (2012) studied the use of a manualized approach, mentalization-based treatment (MBT), as a therapeutic modality with 45 patients with BPD in a day hospital program. Researchers checked in with participants at the beginning of treatment and then at six months, twelve months, and eighteen months from the initiation of treatment. Patients experienced significant reduction in suicide attempts, self-harm, and inpatient hospitalizations during treatment. Attendance rates were favorable and BPD symptoms improved over the course of treatment.

An additional study using MBT with a day hospitalization program was conducted to look at long term efficacy (Bales et al., 2015). Using a matched control study, researchers compared the outcomes of patients with BPD receiving MBT day hospital treatment to those receiving other specialized psychotherapeutic treatment (OPT). Data were collected at baseline, 18 months into treatment, and 36 months into treatment. While both groups saw improvement in BPD symptomology, those receiving MBT saw greater improvements with large effect sizes. These improvements included better emotion regulation, increased stability of self-image, improved frustration tolerance, improved responsibility, and increased intimacy and relationship tolerance. In addition to MBT, DBT is also noted an as effective treatment modality in both PHP and IOP treatment settings (Axelrod, Perepletchikova, Holtzman, & Sinha, 2011; Bloom et al., 2012).

PHP and IOP provides patients with BPD the opportunity to transition les abruptly from inpatient treatment to the stressors of daily life. Day hospital treatment also allows for patients to continue working, manage childcare, and participate in the stressors that often resulted in the need for inpatient treatment. As mentioned earlier, inpatient treatment can be used to avoid stressors in life. PHP and IOP program circumvent this by providing consistent and intense treatment while the patient participates in their own lives including stressors. While this seems to be in the patient's best interest, what it does not address is concerns for safety.

Inpatient hospitalization typically occurs in a controlled environment where patients are not free to come and go due to safety risks. The same is not true for day hospitalization. Mental health practitioners must be cognizant of who they recommend as appropriate for this level of care. Stability should be reached along with a cessation of self-harming behavior. It is important to establish the patient's support system and safety planning at the initiation of treatment as an added protective factor when there is documented risk of suicide.

Psychopharmacological Treatment for BPD

Borderline personality disorder (BPD) has a population prevalence of 1.9% to 5.9% (APA, 2013). BPD is often marked by a pervasive pattern of unstable personal relationships, affect instability, impulsivity, and increased rates of non-suicidal self-injury (NSSI) and/or suicidality. According to Limandri (2018), BPD was initially recognized as a disorder of psychological origination due to environmental factors such as childhood sexual abuse or childhood neglect. This perspective created a gap in treatment between personality disorders and disorders such as schizophrenia and bipolar disorder that were deemed biological in nature (Gabbard & Ball, 2009). With the advent of new technologies that allow for improved understanding of the complexities of brain function, genetics, environmental factors, and the interactions of each component, there is increased potential in treating BPD biologically with targeted psychopharmacology (Gabbard

& Ball, 2009; Limandri, 2018). Prior to beginning psychopharmacological treatment with a patient who has BPD, there are key steps mental health care providers can take that are likely to improve outcomes for this population.

The patient and clinician both benefit when treatment begins focused on the patient-clinician relationship. Treatment should be driven by what is best for the patient, ideally not increasing patient symptoms through an unstructured and unclear treatment protocol. Patients with BPD benefit from clear boundaries and structure as part of their treatment protocol. Clinicians should have a structured treatment protocol for this population that includes clear expectations of both clinician and patient (Limandri, 2018). The goal is to affirm understanding at the outset of treatment as a proactive measure to avoid feelings of rejection by the patient during the course of treatment (Silk, 2011).

Treatment should also include a multidisciplinary approach prior to introducing psychopharmacology. Patients with BPD often have a treatment team that may consist of counselors, case managers, educators, and family/social supports that play a vital role in the patients' treatment outcome. According to Silk (2011), collaboration is key in treating patients with BPD. Silk mentions that these collaborations are important due to the intense effect interpersonal relationships have on these patients' symptoms. Silk goes on to explain that these patients tend to report symptomology based on the patients' current affective state, which can be heavily influenced by externalization, denial, and projection. This creates a safety concern, because BPD symptomology often includes episodes of NSSI and suicidality. In addition to safety concerns, patients with BPD struggle with medication compliance and maintenance. There are many reasons patients may become treatment resistant. Symptom reduction is often more easily achieved than re-engaging in vocational activities and relationships, which can discourage patients regarding treatment effectiveness (Choi-Kain, Glasserman, & Finch, 2017; Tohen, 2014). Due to the specific components of BPD, patients benefit when mental health professionals keep an open dialogue with all members of the patients' treatment team.

Once the structure of treatment is established, treating providers must consider current medication treatment guidelines in conjunction with the often highly individualized needs of patients with BPD (Stephan, Krawitz, & Jackson, 2007). Both the APA and the UK National Institute for Clinical Excellence (NICE) recommend psychotherapy as the first line of treatment for BPD (Broadbear et al., 2016; Martín-Blanco et al., 2017; Stephan et al., 2007). Psychotherapy modalities such as dialectical behavior therapy, mentalization based therapy, and cognitive behavioral therapy have all shown efficacy in the reduction of BPD symptoms. According to Martín-Blanco et al. (2017), there is some differentiation between the APA and NICE in pharmacological treatment recommendations. The APA recommends symptom targeted treatment, and NICE recommends using medication only where there are clear comorbidities. However, there is a clear consensus against the use of polypharmacy in the treatment of BPD. Polypharmacy is defined as the use of multiple medications to treat a single disorder. This practice is not recommended for patients with BPD (Martín-Blanco et al., 2017; Paolini, Mezzetti, Pierri, & Moretti, 2017).

While guidelines for medication management of BPD clearly state that medication should only be used when targeted towards specific symptoms and polypharmacy should be avoided, treating clinicians often do not follow these guidelines in actual practice. In a study performed by Haw and Stubbs (2011), the authors found that of their 79 participants with a BPD diagnosis, 80% were receiving at least one medication for BPD and 48% were receiving two or more medications for BPD. The authors stated that this finding mirrored a recent UK community survey of outpatients with BPD, in which 79% were receiving at least one medication targeted to BPD and 40% were receiving two or more medications for BPD. The study conducted by Martín-Blanco et al. (2017) had similar single medication (over 80%) and polypharmacy (42%) results. The reasons doctors prescribe against the guidelines are not well understood, and may include lack of access to specialized psychotherapy, patient comorbidity and symptoms, and physician empathy to resolve patient pain and suffering (Martín-Blanco et al., 2017; Silk, 2011).

As Paolini et al. (2017) mention, there is a paucity of research regarding medication efficacy with BPD. At this time, there is no psychotropic medication that is targeted for BPD or has received approval as a treatment protocol (Stoffers & Lieb, 2015; Tohen, 2014). When clinicians opt to use psychotropic medications to treat BPD, there are complexities that should be considered in order to provide optimal treatment outcomes. First, comorbidities are prevalent in this patient population. In the study by Martín-Blanco et al. (2017), almost three quarters of the participants presented with comorbid disorders. Similar prevalence was found in additional studies (Haw & Stubbs, 2011; Paolini et al., 2017). Comorbidities often present as psychiatric disorders such as bipolar disorder or major depressive disorder, eating disorders, and substance/alcohol use disorders (Gianoli, Jane, O'Brien, & Ralevski, 2012; Limandri, 2018). Determining the efficacy of treatment protocols is often complicated by the prevalence of comorbidities associated with BPD (Broadbear et al., 2016). In the less prevalent case of no comorbidity, treatment guidelines state that patients with BPD should not receive medication and instead be treated through the use of psychotherapy only (Martín-Blanco et al., 2017).

According to Stephan et al. (2007), clinicians should include patients in making treatment decisions. Stephan provides three decision making models that are regularly used in healthcare: the perfect agent model, the shared decision-making model, and the informed decision-making model. The perfect agent model and informed decision-making model sit on opposite sides of this decision-making continuum, with the former having the doctor in complete control and the later having the patient in complete control. Given the symptoms related to BPD, there are safety concerns with providing patients with full autonomy over their healthcare decisions. Stephan et al. cautions that clinicians should use their clinical judgement and keep patient safety at the forefront of treatment decision making. Clinicians treating patients with BPD should strive to participate in a patient-centered decision-making model. This allows for the clinician to create the previously mentioned structure and the patient to exercise their own autonomy and self-efficacy in treatment decision making, which mirrors the psychotherapy goals often set for patients with BPD.

The Four Most Common Prescriptions for BPD

There are four classes of medications that are often administered to patients with BPD. These include antidepressants, mood stabilizers, antipsychotics, and anxiolytic (anti-anxiety) medications. There is a lack of consensus both in research and in clinical practice over the efficacy of any drug class in the treatment of BPD. In addition to current medications used, there is an increase in alternative treatments in an effort to provide relief to patients with BPD.

Antidepressants

Antidepressants are medications used to treat symptoms of depression and more recently some are used in treatment of anxiety. There is a lack of agreement in existing research regarding the efficacy of antidepressants in the treatment of BPD. In research studies noted by Francois, Roth, and Klingman (2015), first generation antidepressants like tricyclic antidepressants (TCA) and monoamine oxidase inhibitors (MAOIs) have some efficacy in treating symptoms. Limandri's (2018) review of the literature showed mixed results, indicating some effectiveness using MAOIs, but citing TCAs as not only ineffective, but at times, harmful. Second generation antidepressants like selective serotine reuptake inhibitors (SSRIs) and serotonin-norepinephrine reuptake inhibitors (SNRIs) are commonly prescribed medications for patients with BPD. SSRIs have been shown to be effective in reducing anger dysregulation, dysphoria, and anxiety in BPD patients (Gabbard & Ball, 2009). While antidepressants are a longstanding medication of choice in the treatment of BPD, there is a recent reduction in the frequency of use by clinicians. This may be due to the lack of research based evidence justifying the use of anti-depressants in treatment of BPD (Paolini et al., 2017).

Mood Stabilizers

Mood stabilizers are another class of medications that are prescribed to patients with BPD. This drug class is typically prescribed to patients with bipolar disorder to stabilize high (mania) and low (depression) mood changes. Short term studies with small sample sizes of Topiramate, Divalproex Sodium, and Lamotrigine show some improvement in patients' anger dysregulation (Francois et al., 2015). However, a year-long study conducted with 276 participants demonstrated no greater symptom improvement with lamotrigine than with placebo (Crawford et al., 2018). Carbamazepine provided no statistically significant improvements in small, double-blind, parallel, placebo controlled study (Francois et al., 2015). There are some concerns regarding the use of mood stabilizers with the BPD population. Due to the toxicity of some mood stabilizers such as Lithium Carbonate, clinicians should consider the patient's history of NSSI and suicidality when assessing for safety in medication decisions. Also, a majority of patients with BPD are women in their reproductive years. Certain mood stabilizers like divalproex sodium have demonstrated increased likelihood of birth defects. Patients with BPD often report difficulty with impulsive behaviors such as unplanned and unprotected sexual activity (Crawford et al., 2018). Since impulsivity puts female patients at a higher risk for pregnancy, clinicians should consider contraception use during treatment decision making. Historically, prescription of mood stabilizers for symptom relief with BPD has been infrequent; however, there has been an increase in prescribing frequency over the last five years (Paolini et al., 2017). Therefore, clinicians should be cognizant of potential unintended consequences of using this drug class with patients with BPD.

Antipsychotics

Antipsychotics are typically prescribed to manage psychosis in patients with disorders such as schizophrenia and bipolar disorder. There are two types of antipsychotics, typical and atypical. Typical antipsychotics are the first generation of antipsychotics and are known to have severe side effects that affect motor control. Atypical antipsychotics are second generation antipsychotics that do not have the same severe side effects as typical antipsychotics. However, atypical antipsychotics can have side effects that interfere with quality of life such as weight gain and decrease in libido. Existing research points to moderate efficacy in the use of both typical and atypical antipsychotics in treating patients with BPD (Francois et al., 2015; Haw & Stubbs, 2011; Martín-Blanco et al., 2017). This drug class appears to assist patients with not only mood stability but also reduction in paranoia, impulsivity, suicidality, anxiety, and interpersonal relationship conflict (Francois et al., 2015). However, there is a concern with compliance in this drug class due to side effects. Typical antipsychotics come with a host of unpleasant side effects including some that affect motor control (e.g., tardive dyskinesia) and therefore quality of life. For patients with comorbid eating disorders, the side effect of weight gain with atypical antipsychotics can deter medication compliance (Limandri, 2018). Despite these concerns, the frequency of prescribing antipsychotics for symptoms of BPD is steadily increasing (Paolini et al., 2017).

Anxiolytics

Anxiolytic medications are typically used to reduce or eliminate symptoms related to anxiety. It is not uncommon for clinicians to prescribe anxiety reducing medications for patients with BPD. Because there is often a history of trauma in patients with BPD, it is not uncommon for patients to have comorbid anxiety disorders such as posttraumatic stress disorder. Caution must be used when prescribing benzodiazepines to patients with BPD. Due to the association of BPD with high rates of suicidal behavior, Limandri (2018) mentions that it is important that clinicians prescribe safe medications that have lower rates of potential overdose. The author goes on to explain that fast-acting anxiolytic medications such as benzodiazepines can be counterproductive to psychotherapy goals. Patients with BPD work on skills such as distress tolerance, self-regulation, and self-control in counseling. Limandri posits that the use of fast-acting anxiolytic medication might behaviorally reinforce the patients' belief that they are unable to manage these feelings. As a result, the preference is to use either an antidepressant that is indicated to reduce anxiety, or a non-sedating anxiolytic medication such as Buspirone.

Future Considerations for the Use of Prescriptions for BPD

With no targeted medication for relief from the symptoms of BPD, clinicians are investigating alternative approaches for helping patients improve their quality of life. These alternative approaches include the use of omega-3 fatty acids, opioid antagonists, adrenergic agonists, hormone focused therapies like oxytocin, and imaging equipment such as fMRIs to better understand brain function in patients with BPD (Gabbard & Ball, 2009; Limandri, 2018; Stoffers & Lieb, 2015). Further research is needed exploring alternative approaches for both efficacy and safety. With ongoing advancements in psychopharmacology, there is hope that in the future, patients with BPD will have access to medications targeted at providing symptom relief.

Summary and Conclusion

Based on decades of outcome research, BPD has a reputation as one of the most difficult psychopathologies to address in treatment. Among the various models of treatment, approaches based on Cognitive Behavioral Theory have the strongest record of research demonstrating efficacy with BPD. Of these, DBT has been studied most extensively, with the most consistent record of good outcome as an effective treatment for BPD, as well as other psychological disorders. Because Cognitive Behavioral Therapy is cost effective and can be administered without the specialized training required for many other evidenced based treatment approaches, CBT might be considered the treatment of choice for BPD, as well as a variety of other psychological disorders. DBT outcome data (Linehan, 2015) indicate that spending more time in therapy renders the best outcomes for BPD when the duration of treatment is at least twelve months. Time-limited models of brief psychotherapy favored by third party payers are not supported by outcome research on BPD, suggesting that fiscally-driven models of care might not yield the best patient care or clinical outcomes. The relative cost effectiveness of extended treatment over less effective time-limited treatment might be evaluated over a more extended time frame using longitudinal research, which is recommended to help clarify this issue.

REFERENCES

Abdelkarim, A., Rizk, D. N., Esmaiel, M., & Helal, H. (2016). Impact of dialectical behavior therapy on incidence of suicidal attempts and non-suicidal self-injury among a sample of Egyptian borderline personality disorder patients. *European Psychiatry, 33*, S323. https://doi.org/10.1016/j.eurpsy.2016.01.709

American Psychiatric Association. (2013). *Diagnostic and statistical manual of mental disorders* (5th ed.). Arlington, VA: Author.

American Psychiatric Association. (2001). *Practice guideline for the treatment of patients with borderline personality disorder*. Washington, D.C.: American Psychiatric Pub.

Axelrod, S. R., Perepletchikova, F., Holtzman, K., & Sinha, R. (2011). Emotion regulation and substance use frequency in women with substance dependence and borderline personality disorder receiving dialectical behavior therapy. *The American Journal of Drug and Alcohol Abuse, 37*(1), 37-42. https://doi.org/10.3109/00952990.2010.535582

Bales, D., Timman, R., Andrea, H., Busschbach, J. J., Verheul, R., & Kamphuis, J. H. (2015). Effectiveness of day hospital mentalization-based treatment for patients with severe borderline personality disorder: A matched control study. *Clinical Psychology & Psychotherapy, 22*(5), 409-417. https://doi.org/10.1002/cpp.1914

Bales, D., van Beek, N., Smits, M., Willemsen, S., Busschbach, J. J., Verheul, R., & Andrea, H. (2012). Treatment outcome of 18-month, day hospital mentalization-based treatment (MBT) in patients with severe borderline personality disorder in the Netherlands. *Journal of Personality Disorders, 26*(4), 568-582. https://doi.org/10.1521/pedi.2012.26.4.568

Bateman, A. & Fonagy, P. (2003). Health service utilization costs for borderline personality disorder patients treated with psychoanalytically oriented partial hospitalization versus general psychiatric care. *American Journal of Psychiatry, 160*(1), 169-171. https://doi.org/10.1176/appi.ajp.160.1.169

Bateman, A. & Fonagy, P. (2010). Mentalization based treatment for borderline personality disorder. *World Psychiatry, 9*(1), 11-15. Retrieved from https://www.ncbi.nlm.nih.gov/pmc/articles/PMC2816926/

Beck, A. T. (1970). Cognitive therapy: Nature and relation to behavior. *Behavior Therapy, 1*(2), 184-200. https://doi.org/10.1016/s0005-7894(70)80030-2

Beckstead, J. D., Lambert, M. J., DuBose, A. P., & Linehan, M. (2015). Dialectical behavior therapy with American Indian/Alaska Native adolescents diagnosed with substance use disorders: Combining an evidence-based treatment with cultural, traditional, and spiritual beliefs. *Addictive Behaviors, 51*, 84. https://doi.org/10.1016/j.addbeh.2015.07.018

Ben-Porath, D. D. (2015). Orienting clients to telephone coaching in dialectical behavior therapy. *Cognitive and Behavioral Practice, 22*(4), 407-414. https://doi.org/10.1016/j.cbpra.2014.02.004

Ben-Porath, D. D. & Koons, C. R. (2005). Telephone coaching in dialectical behavior therapy: A decision-tree model for managing inter-session contact with clients. *Cognitive and Behavioral Practice, 12*(4), 448-460. https://doi.org/10.1016/s1077-7229(05)80072-0

Bloom, J. M., Woodward, E. N., Susmaras, T., & Pantalone, D. W. (2012). Use of dialectical behavior therapy in inpatient treatment of borderline personality disorder: A systematic review. *Psychiatric Services, 63*(9), 881-888. https://doi.org/10.1176/appi.ps.201100311

Blum, N., St. John, D., Pfohl, B., Stuart, S., McCormick, B., Allen, J., Arndt, S., & Black, D. W. (2008). Systems training for emotional predictability and problem solving (STEPPS) for outpatients with borderline personality disorder: A randomized controlled trial and 1-year follow-up. *American Journal of Psychiatry, 165*(4), 468-478. https://doi.org/10.1176/appi.ajp.2007.07071079

Bowlby, J. (1958). The nature of the child's tie to his mother. *International Journal of Psychoanalysis, 39*, 350-371. Retrieved from: https://www.pep-web.org/document.php?id=ijp.039.0350a

Broadbear, J. H., Nesci, J., Thomas, R., Thompson, K., Beatson, J., & Rao, S. (2016). Evaluation of changes in prescription medication use after a residential treatment programme for borderline personality disorder. *Australasian Psychiatry, 24*(6), 583-588. https://doi.org/10.1177/1039856216654391

Butler, A. C., Chapman, J. E., Foreman, E. M., & Beck, A. T. (2006). The empirical status of cognitive-behavioral therapy: A review of meta-analyses. *Clinical Psychology Review, 26*(1), 17-31. https://doi.org/10.1016/j.cpr.2005.07.003

Chapman, A. L. (2006). Dialectical behavior therapy: Current indications and unique elements. *Psychiatry (Edgmont), 3*(9), 62-68. Retrieved from: https://www.ncbi.nlm.nih.gov/pmc/articles/PMC2963469/

Chapman, A. L., Rosenthal, M. Z., Dixon-Gordon, K., Turner, B. J., & Kuppens, P. (2017). Borderline personality disorder and the effects of instructed emotional avoidance or acceptance in daily life. *Journal of Personality Disorders, 31*(4), 483-502. https://doi.org/10.1521/pedi_2016_30_264

Choi-Kain, L. W., Finch, E. F., Masland, S. R., Jenkins, J. A., & Unruh, B. T. (2017). What works with the treatment of borderline personality disorder. *Current Behavioral Neuroscience Reports, 4*(1), 21-30. https://doi.org/10.1007/s40473-017-0103-z

Choi-Kain, L. W., Glasserman, E. I., & Finch, E. F. (2017, November). Borderline personality disorder: Treatment resistance reconsidered. *Psychiatric Times. (34)*11. Retrieved from https://www.psychiatrictimes.com/special-reports/borderline-personality-disorder-treatment-resistance-reconsidered

Chugani, C. D. (2017). Adapting dialectical behavior therapy for college counseling centers. *Journal of College Counseling, 20*(1), 67-80. https://doi.org/10.1002/jocc.12059

Crawford, M. J., Sanatinia, R., Barrett, B., Cunningham, G., Dale, O., Ganguli, P., . . . Lykomitrou-Matthews, G. (2018). Lamotrigine for people with borderline personality disorder: A RCT. *Health Technology Assessment, 22*(17). https://doi.org/10.3310/hta22170

Davidson, K., Norrie, J., Tyrer, P., Gumley, A., Tata, P., Murray, H., & Palmer, S. (2006). The effectiveness of cognitive behavior therapy for borderline personality disorder: Results from the borderline personality disorder study of cognitive therapy (BOSCOT) trial. *Journal of Personality Disorders, 20*(5), 450-465. https://doi.org/10.1521/pedi.2006.20.5.450

Davidson, K., Tyrer, P., Norrie, J., Palmer, S.J. & Tyrer, H. (2010). Cognitive therapy verses usual treatment for borderline personality disorder: Prospective 6 year follow up. *The British Journal of Psychiatry, 197*(6): 456-462. https://doi.org/10.1192/bjp.bp.109.074286

Dingfelder, S. F. (2004). Treatment for the untreatable. *Monitor on Psychology, 35*(3), 46. https://www.apa.org/monitor/mar04/treatment.html

Ellis, A. (1962). *Reason and emotion in psychotherapy.* New York: Stuart.

Farrell, J. M. & Shaw, I. A. (2012). *Group schema therapy for borderline personality disorder: A step-by-step treatment manual with patient workbook.* West Sussex, UK: Wiley-Blackwell.

Francois, D., Roth, S. D., & Klingman, D. (2015). The efficacy of pharmacotherapy for borderline personality disorder: A review of the available randomized controlled trials. *Psychiatric Annals, 45*(8), 431-437. https://doi.org/10.3928/00485713-20150803-09

Gabbard, G. O. & Ball, V. L. (2009). Physical and medical dimensions of borderline personality disorder and the effect of treatment. *Psychiatric Annals, 39*(12), 997-1003. https://doi.org/10.3928/00485718-2009 1123-01

Germán, M., Smith, H., Rivera-Morales, C., González, G., Haliczer, L., Haaz, C., & Miller, A. (2015). Dialectical behavior therapy for suicidal Latina adolescents: Supplemental dialectical corollaries and treatment targets. *American Journal of Psychotherapy, 69*(2), 179-97. https://doi.org/10.1176/appi.psychotherapy.2015.69.2.179

Gianoli, M. O., Jane, J. S., O'Brien, E., & Ralevski, E. (2012). Treatment for comorbid borderline personality disorder and alcohol use disorders: A review of the evidence and future recommendations. *Experimental and Clinical Psychopharmacology, 20*(4), 333. https://doi.org/10.1037/a0027999

Giesen-Bloo, J., van Dyck, R., Spinhoven, P., van Tilburg, W., Dirksen, C., van Asselt, T., … Arntz, A. (2006). Outpatient psychotherapy for borderline personality disorder: A randomized trial of schema focused therapy versus transference focused therapy. *Archives of General Psychiatry, 63*(6), 649-658. https://doi.org/10.1001/archpsyc.63.6.649

Gunderson, J. G. (2009). *Borderline personality disorder: A clinical guide* (2nd ed.). Arlington, VA: American Psychiatric Pub.

Gunderson, J. G., Stout, R. L., McGlashan, T. H., Shea, M. T., Morey, L. C., Grilo, C. M., … Skodol, A. E. (2011). Ten-year course of borderline personality disorder: Psychopathology and function from the collaborative longitudinal personality disorders study. *Archives of General Psychiatry, 68*(8), 827-837. https://doi.org/10.1001/archgenpsychiatry.2011.37

Haw, C. & Stubbs, J. (2011). Medication for borderline personality disorder: A survey at a secure hospital. *International Journal of Psychiatry in Clinical Practice, 15*(4), 270-274. https://doi.org/10.3109/13651501.2011.590211

Hofmann, S. G. (2011). *An introduction to modern CBT: Psychological solutions to mental health problems.* Oxford, UK: WileyBlackwell.

Hofmann, S. G., Asnaani, A., Vonk, I. J., Sawyer, A. T. & Fang, A. (2012). The efficacy of cognitive behavioral therapy: A review of meta-analyses. *Cognitive Therapy Research, 36*, 427–440. https://doi.org/10.1007/s10608-013-9595-3

Holder, N., Holliday, R., Pal, A., & Suris, A. (2017). Role of borderline personality disorder in the treatment of military sexual trauma-related posttraumatic stress disorder with cognitive processing therapy. *Behavior Medicine, 43*(3), 184-190. https://doi.org/10.1080/08964289.2016.1276430

Hörz, S., Zanarini, M. C., Frankenburg, F. R., Reich, D. B., & Fitzmaurice, G. (2010). Ten-year use of mental health services by patients with borderline personality disorder and with other axis II disorders. *Psychiatric Services, 61*(6), 612-616. https://doi.org/10.1176/ps.2010.61.6.612

Hunnicutt Hollenbaugh, K. M. & Lenz, A. (2018). Preliminary evidence for the effectiveness of dialectical behavior therapy for adolescents. *Journal of Counseling & Development, 96*(2), 119-131. https://doi.org/10.1002/jcad.12186

Kellogg, S. H. & Young, J. E. (2006). Schema therapy for borderline personality disorder. *Journal of Clinical Psychology, 62*, 445-58. https://doi.org/10.1002/jclp.20240

Kernberg O. F. (1970). A psychoanalytic classification of character pathology. *Journal of the American Psychoanalytic Association, 18*, 800–822. https://doi.org/10.1177/000306517001800403

Klein, M. (1946). Notes on some schizoid mechanisms. *The Journal of Psychotherapy Practice and Research, 5*(2), 160-179. Retrieved from https://www.ncbi.nlm.nih.gov/pmc/articles/PMC3330415/

Koons, C. R. (2011). The role of the team in managing telephone consultation in dialectical behavior therapy: Three case examples. *Cognitive and Behavioral Practice, 18*(2), 168-177. https://doi.org/10.1016/j.cbpra.2009.10.008

Kredlow M. A., Szuhany K. L., Lo, S., Xie, H., Gottlieb J. D., Rosenberg S. D., & Mueser, K. T. (2017). Cognitive behavioral therapy for posttraumatic stress disorder in individuals with severe mental illness and borderline personality disorder. *Psychiatry Research. 249*, 86-93. https://doi.org/10.1016/j.psychres.2016.12.045

Kröger, C., Harbeck, S., Armbrust, M., & Kliem, S. (2013). Effectiveness, response, and dropout of dialectical behavior therapy for borderline personality disorder in an inpatient setting. *Behaviour Research and Therapy, 51*(8), 411-416. https://doi.org/10.1016/j.brat.2013.04.008

Leichsenring, F., Leibing, E., Kruse, J., New, A. S., & Leweke, F. (2011). Borderline personality disorder. *The Lancet, 377*(9759), 74-84. https://doi.org/10.1016/s0140-6736(10)61422-5

Lenz, A., & Del Conte, G. (2018). Efficacy of dialectical behavior therapy for adolescents in a partial hospitalization program. *Journal of Counseling & Development, 96*(1), 15-26. https://doi.org/10.1002/jcad.12174

Limandri, B. J. (2018). Psychopharmacology for borderline personality disorder. *Journal of Psychosocial Nursing and Mental Health Services, 56*(4), 8-11. https://doi.org/10.3928/02793695-20180319-01

Linehan, M. M. (2018). *Cognitive-behavioral treatment of borderline personality disorder*. New York, NY: Guilford Publications.

Linehan, M. M. (1993). *Cognitive-behavioral treatment of borderline personality Disorder* (1st ed.). New York, NY: Guilford Press.

Linehan, M. M. (2015). *DBT skills training manual* (2nd ed.). New York, NY: The Guilford Press.

Linehan, M. M. (2011). Dialectical behavior therapy and telephone coaching. *Cognitive and Behavioral Practice, 18*(2), 207-208. https://doi.org/10.1016/j.cbpra.2010.06.003

Linehan, M. M., Armstrong H. E., & Suarez, A. (1991). Cognitive-behavioral treatment of chronically suicidal borderline patients. *Archives of General Psychiatry, 48*(12), 1060–1064. https://doi.org/10.1001/archpsyc.1991.01810360024003

Linehan, M. M. & Wilks, C. (2015). The course and evolution of dialectical behavior therapy. *American Journal of Psychotherapy, 69*(2), 97-110. https://doi.org/10.1176/appi.psychotherapy.2015.69.2.97

Lis, E. & Myhr, G. J. (2016). The effect of borderline personality pathology on outcome of cognitive behavior therapy. *Psychiatry Practice, 22*(4), 270-282. https://doi.org/10.1097/pra.0000000000000167

Lynch, T. R., Chapman, A. L., Rosenthal, M. Z., Kuo, J. R. and Linehan, M. M. (2006). Mechanisms of change in dialectical behavior therapy: Theoretical and empirical observations. *Journal of Clinical Psychology, 62*(4), 459-480. https://doi.org/10.1002/jclp.20243

Martín-Blanco, A., Ancochea, A., Soler, J., Elices, M., Carmona, C., & Pascual, J. (2017). Changes over the last 15 years in the psychopharmacological management of persons with borderline personality disorder. *Acta Psychiatrica Scandinavica, 136*(3), 323-331. https://doi.org/10.1111/acps.12767

Matusiewicz, A. K., Hopwood, C. J. & Lejuez, C. W. (2010). The effectiveness of cognitive behavioral therapy for personality disorders. *Psychiatric Clinics of North America, 33*(3), 657-685. https://doi.org/10.1016/j.psc.2010.04.007

McMain, S., Newman, M. G., Segal, Z. V., & DeRubeis, R. J. (2015). Cognitive behavioral therapy: Current status and future research directions. *Psychotherapy Research, 25*(3), 321-329. https://doi.org/10.1080/10503307.2014.1002440

National Alliance on Mental Illness. (2019). *Getting treatment during a crisis*. Retrieved from https://www.nami.org/Learn-More/Treatment/Getting-Treatment-During-a-Crisis

Navarro-Haro, M., Botella, V., Guillen, C., Moliner, V., Marco, R., Jorquera, H., . . . Garcia-Palacios, R. (2018). Dialectical behavior therapy in the treatment of borderline personality disorder and eating disorders comorbidity: A pilot study in a naturalistic setting. *Cognitive Therapy and Research, 42*(5), 636-649. https://doi.org/10.1007/s10608-018-9906-9

Neacsiu, A. D., Lungu, A., Harned, M. S., Rizvi, S. L., & Linehan, M. M. (2014). Impact of dialectical behavior therapy versus community treatment by experts on emotional experience, expression, and acceptance in borderline personality disorder. *Behaviour Research and Therapy, 53*(1), 47-54. https://doi.org/10.1016/j.brat.2013.12.004

Neacsiu, A. D., Ward-Ciesielski, E. F., & Linehan, M. M. (2012). Emerging approaches to counseling intervention: Dialectical behavior therapy. *Counseling Psychologist, 40*(7), 1003-1032. https://doi.org/10.1177/0011000011421023

Nenadić I., Lamberth S., & Reiss N. (2017). Group schema therapy for personality disorders: A pilot study for implementation in acute psychiatric in-patient settings. *Psychiatry Research, 253*, 9-12. https://doi.org/10.1016/j.psychres.2017.01.093

Noll, L., Lewis, J., Zalewski, M., Martin, C., Roos, L., Musser, N., & Reinhardt, K. (2019). Initiating a DBT consultation team: Conceptual and practical considerations for training clinics. *Training and Education in Professional Psychology.* https://doi.org/10.1037/tep0000252

O'hearn, A., & Pollard, R. Q. (2008). Modifying dialectical behavior therapy for deaf individuals. *Cognitive and Behavioral Practice, 15*(4), 400-414. https://doi.org/10.1016/j.cbpra.2008.02.007

Paolini, E., Mezzetti, F. A. F., Pierri, F., & Moretti, P. (2017). Pharmacological treatment of borderline personality disorder: A retrospective observational study at inpatient unit in Italy. *International Journal of Psychiatry in Clinical Practice, 21*(1), 75-79. https://doi.org/10.1080/13651501.2016.1235202

Pascual, J. C., Palomares, N., Ibáñez, Á., Portella, M. J., Arza, R., Reyes, R., … Carrasco, J.L. (2015). Efficacy of cognitive rehabilitation on psychosocial functioning in borderline personality disorder: A randomized controlled trial. *BMC Psychiatry, 16*(5), 298-307. https://doi.org/10.1186/s12888-015-0640-5

Rizvi, S., Steffel, L., & Carson-Wong, A. (2013). An overview of dialectical behavior therapy for professional psychologists. *Professional Psychology: Research and Practice, 44*(2), 73-80. https://doi.org/10.1037/a0029808

Sauer-Zavala, K. H., Bentley, K. H., & Wilner, J. G. (2016). Transdiagnostic treatment of borderline personality and comorbid disorders: A clinical replication series. *Journal of Personality Disorders, 30*(1), 35-51. https://doi.org/10.1521/pedi_2015_29_179

Schilling, L., Moritz, S., Kriston, L., Krieger, M., & Nagel, M. (2018). Efficacy of metacognitive training for patients with borderline personality disorder: Preliminary results. *Psychiatry Research*, *262*,459-464. https://doi.org/10.1016/j.psychres.2017.09.024

Silk, K. R. (2011). The process of managing medications in patients with borderline personality disorder. *Journal of Psychiatric Practice, 17*(5), 311-319. https://doi.org/10.1097/01.pra.0000405361.88257.4a

Sloan, C., Berke, D., & Shipherd, J. (2017). Utilizing a dialectical framework to inform conceptualization and treatment of clinical distress in transgender individuals. *Professional Psychology: Research and Practice, 48*(5), 301-309. https://doi.org/10.1037/pro0000146

Slotema, C. W., Blom, J. D., Deen, M., Niemantsverdriet, M., van der Gaag, M., Hoek, H. W., & Sommer, I. E. (2017). Negative beliefs about voices in patients with borderline personality disorder are associated with distress: A plea for cognitive-behavioural therapy? *Psychopathology, 50*(4), 255-261. https://doi.org/10.1159/000477669

Soloff, P. H., White, R., Omari, A., Ramaseshan, K., & Diwadkar, V. A. (2015). Affective context interferes with brain responses during cognitive processing in borderline personality disorder: fMRI evidence. *Psychiatric Research: Neuroimaging. 233*(1), 23–35. https://doi.org/10.1016/j.pscychresns.2015.04.006

Stephan, A., Krawitz, R., & Jackson, W. (2007). Medication decision-making by adults with borderline personality disorder. *Australasian Psychiatry, 15*(5), 385-389. https://doi.org/10.1080/10398560701439673

Stern A. (1938). Psychoanalytic investigation of and therapy in the borderline group of neuroses. *Psychoanalytic Quarterly, 7*, 467–489. https://doi.org/10.1080/21674086.1938.11925367

Stoffers, J. M., & Lieb, K. (2015). Pharmacotherapy for borderline personality disorder—current evidence and recent trends. *Current Psychiatry Reports, 17*(1), 534. https://doi.org/10.1007/s11920-014-0534-0

Strauss, B. M., Mestel, R., & Kirchmann, H. A. (2011). Changes of attachment status among women with personality disorders undergoing inpatient treatment. *Counselling and Psychotherapy Research, 11*(4), 275-283. https://doi.org/10.1080/14733145.2010.548563

Tohen, M. (2014). Pharmacologic treatments for borderline personality disorder. *The American Journal of Psychiatry, 171*(11), 1139-1141. https://doi.org/10.1176/appi.ajp.2014.14081008

Valentine, S., Bankoff, S., Poulin, R., Reidler, E., & Pantalone, D. (2015). The use of dialectical behavior therapy skills training as stand-alone treatment: A systematic review of the treatment outcome literature. *Journal of Clinical Psychology, 71*(1), 1-20. https://doi.org/10.1002/jclp.22114

Van Vreeswijk, M. F., Spinhoven, P., Eurelings-Bontekoe, E. H., & Broersen J. (2014). Changes in symptom severity, schemas and modes in heterogeneous psychiatric patient groups following short-term schema cognitive-behavioural group therapy: A naturalistic pre-treatment and post-treatment design in an outpatient clinic. *Clinical Psychology & Psychotherapy, 21*(1), 29-38. https://doi.org/10.1002/cpp.1813

Walsh, C., Ryan, P., & Flynn, D. (2018). Exploring dialectical behaviour therapy clinicians' experiences of team consultation meetings. *Borderline Personality Disorder and Emotion Dysregulation, 5*(1), 1-11. https://doi.org/10.1186/s40479-018-0080-1

Widiger, T. A., & Weissman, M. M. (1991). Epidemiology of borderline personality disorder. *Psychiatric Services, 42*(10), 1015-1021. https://doi.org/10.1176/ps.42.10.1015

Zanarini, M. C., Frankenburg, F. R., Reich, D. B., & Fitzmaurice, G. (2012). Attainment and stability of sustained symptomatic remission and recovery among patients with borderline personality disorder and axis II comparison subjects: A 16-year prospective follow-up study. *American Journal of Psychiatry, 169*(5), 476-483. https://doi.org/10.1176/appi.ajp.2011.11101550

In: Borderline Personality Disorder
Editor: Charles M. Lepkowsky ISBN: 978-1-53618-021-3

Chapter 5

OBJECT RELATIONS THEORY AND BORDERLINE PERSONALITY DISORDER

Erik G. Jul*[*], *PsyD
Hawai'i School of Professional Psychology,
Argosy University Honolulu, Hawai'i

ABSTRACT

Classical psychoanalytic thought has advanced in depth and scope. Contemporary psychoanalytic theory can be applied to conceptualization and treatment of Borderline Personality Disorder (BPD). Specifically, the field of Object Relations Theory allows a penetrating look into the organization of the intra- and interpersonal experience of people with BPD. An introduction to Object Relations Theory including key terms and concepts is presented as the foundation for a basic framework for treatment.

Keywords: object relations theory, Klein, Fairbairn, Winnicott, Kernberg

[*] Corresponding Author's E-mail: erikjul.psyd@gmail.com.

Introduction

Borderline personality disorder (BPD) is a complex array of interpersonal patterns and intrapersonal dynamics. From a psychodynamic perspective, object relations theory provides a conceptual framework for understanding the psychodynamic processes within the person with BPD, and describing the manner in which they interact with others. The origins, key conepts and applications of object relations theory will be discussed, with specific attention to its historical role in understaning and treating BPD.

Origins of Object Relations Theory

Object relations theory emerged in the early to mid-20th century as an extension of, reaction to, and evolution of Sigmund Freud's psychoanalytic theory (McWilliams, 2011). The application of object relations theory in psychotherapy is to support an individual's awareness and understanding of early childhood experiences, and consequent development of mental maps and images. Object relations theory deviates from Freud's belief that sexual and aggressive drives are primarily responsible for the formation of the human psyche, and instead places emphasis on the need for relational contact with others as the driving force in the creation and development of the person. By uncovering early relational maps and images, the person in treatment can readjust relationships and improve interpersonal functioning. Freud's early theories of the psyche were used as a foundation upon which object relations theorists expounded. His initial models of the psyche were extended upon to create the field of ego psychology. To better understand object relations theory, it is helpful to review the key concepts developed by Freud and their evolution and application in the fields of ego psychology and object relations theory.

Freud's Contributions and Foundational Theory

Freudian theory ushered in a new era of understanding of the human psyche (McWilliams, 2011). He developed several models that were synthesized to create the Structural Model of the mind and focused on the dynamic interplay of conscious and unconscious experience. This advancement in theory provides contemporary theorists and clinicians useful tools for understanding and treating Borderline Personality Disorder. In addition to the Structural Model, Freud's Topographic Model, Adaptive Model and Genetic Model will be included in an overview of the foundations of contemporary psychoanalytic theory.

Structural Model

The Structural Theory of Mind posits that the mind has three components: the Id, the Ego, and the Superego (Freud, 1964/1933). Freud saw the Id as a primitive and instinctual part of the mind that operates on the pleasure principle, seeking immediate gratification of need, which is described as drive. The Id was described as unreasonable or "prerational," locked into primitive understandings of desire and fear, outside the awareness of the conscious mind.

Freud saw the Ego as a necessary adaptation to the Id, providing the ability to bring order to chaos. The Ego operates on developed logic in tune with the reality principle (Freud, 1964/1933). The main function of the Ego was seen as managing and organizing strong urges and desires from the unconscious Id. The Ego, while overwhelmed initially in the human lifespan, develops in strength and ability over time to tame the Id to some degree. The Ego makes use of various defense mechanisms (against chaos and anxiety) to influence the Id. Some defense mechanisms are learned and implemented early in infancy at the preverbal level, while others arise and evolve at later chapters of development. The Ego is what people use to describe their sense of "me" or "I."

Ego psychology views personality as a dynamic interaction between ego defense mechanisms whose interplay defines a person's tolerance for distress and interactions with others. Ego psychology developed terminology to describe the "observing ego," the self-reflective function of humanity (Ormont, Hunt, & Corman, 1964). Specifically, we can be aware of elements of our experience as being "me" or "not me."

The term "Superego" was developed by Freud to describe the socializing element of society, the morality principle and conscience (Freud, 1964/1933). The task of the Superego is to exert influence and pressure on the ego to conform to society's demands, preventing the Id from acting out unconscious drives to minimize the risk of consequences for poorly managed behavior.

The Id, Ego, and Superego translate into "it," "me," and "above me," indicating their relationships with one another (Freud, 1964/1933). In psychoanalysis, people diagnosed with mental illness were categorized around the structures of ego psychology, and were treated for having too much or not enough Id, Ego, or Superego in their personality structure. The dynamic that arose from the interaction of the mind's parts allowed clinicians to understand where underdevelopment or maladjustment may be located, and how to support healthier organization. Ego psychology was successful in creating a general matrix of character diagnosis based on the types of defense mechanisms and manner of organization of the individual's mind. Mental illness was seen as a function of maladaptive defenses, and the focus of treatment was placed on creating a stable enough mind to tolerate seemingly intolerable unconscious experiences.

Topographic Model

The topographic model of the mind was created by Freud as a map of the psyche and the three levels of consciousness: the unconscious, preconscious, and conscious elements of mind (Freud, 1933, 1964). These "systems of consciousness" were seen as separate yet interrelated elements.

The unconscious was defined primarily as material inaccessibility to conscious awareness (Freud, 1964/1933 ibid). The preverbal ideas, wishes, and affective states of the unconscious powerfully shape the tone of the conscious mind, and have been described at times as "unthought known," unperceived yet graspable at an intuitive or sensate level.

The preconscious system was defined as the route to which unconscious material was made conscious through thought patterns (Freud, 1964/1933). A primary role of the preconscious was to connect unconscious material to logical-linguistic processes of the conscious mind.

The conscious mind was seen to be the organizer of attention and awareness, and was attributed with higher level thinking processes such as reasoning and decision-making (Freud, 1964/1933 ibid). The conscious mind allows a person to explore and analyze cognitive and affective experiences.

The interplay between the three components of the mind was thought to allow the human experience to filter mental content into conscious awareness from unconscious sources (Freud, 1964/1933 ibid). Experiences that are appraised as too disruptive may be transformed into less direct expression that is manageable or more acceptable to the conscious mind. For example, a person with BPD may act out disturbed relationship patterns by projecting inner pain onto others, rather than confronting the tension more directly within themselves.

Adaptive Model

The adaptive model focuses on the perspective of Ego as an adaptive, dynamic process (Freud, 1964/1933 ibid). Hartmann (1958) dichotomized the processes into autoplastic and alloplastic types, wherein people either have the capacity to adapt themselves to the environment (autoplastic) or the environment to themselves (alloplastic). The Ego is seen as responsible for these dynamic processes of organization. In order to accomplish the task of adaption, the Ego was seen to create internal models or representations of reality and the others/objects within it.

The internal models include elements from memory learning, language, intelligent multisensory processing, etc. Mental representations allow people to reflect on past/present experiences, explore emotional meaning, and generally guide how a person interacts with his or her environment in the present moment. The Ego's adaptive ability to organize reality plays a pivotal role in the lives of people with Borderline Personality Disorder, and affects the manner in which they manage and engage in their relationships with self and others/objects. To accommodate developmental arrest and relationship injury, they are thought to unconsciously distort their internal maps to create greater stability.

Genetic Model

Freud's genetic model contributed to the understanding of the mind as unfolding and developing in relative stages (Freud, 1964/1933ibid). He emphasized the necessity of interpersonal contact for the developing mind, and predicted negative behavioral consequences when an infant's needs are unmet. The genetic model focused on psychosexual stages, and Freud placed importance on sexuality across development as a primary motivator to connect.

According to the genetic model, the developing psyche is grounded in a physical body and connects to caregivers through meaningful bodily zones. Freud focused on specific areas of anatomy that serve as triggers for excitation and discharge of energy (Freud, 1964/1933ibid). On the path toward adulthood, Freud described the developing person as going through oral, anal, urethral, phallic, latency, and genital phases.

Each stage carries a set of tasks and challenges to navigate in the self and other/object dyad. Earlier interactions were thought to be more foundational to personality organization, so that unmet needs or injury to the psyche in early life carry heavier consequences. Through the lens of this model, people with borderline personality organization struggle with themes related to early phases of development (McWilliams, 2011).

According to this model, people with borderline personality organization often demonstrate relationship and behavior patterns linked to the anal stage of psychosexual development (McWilliams, 2011). This phase is typically occurs between 18 months and three years of life. The developing person begins to put thoughts into words, notably "no, me, and mine." The site of the anus and mastery over defecation brings into greater focus themes around mastery and control, and the holding on versus letting go of material, physical, and mental. The young child works to master their environment and social power increases with the development of language. Importantly, the child has begun to have willful control over the body, some mastery over the environment (others/objects), and initial awareness of difference between biological differences between self and others.

In summary; Freud's contributions to the understanding of the structure and dynamic of the psyche led to Neofreudian theorists and contemporary psychoanalysis as a field to shift into advanced knowledge and understanding of Borderline Personality Disorder phenomenon. Object relations theory was built upon the ideas of Freud, or in reaction to them, leading to a more comprehensive theory of pathology and treatment.

Object Relations Theory: Key Terms and Primary Contributors

The developments of object relations theory reflect the original ideas of Freud, with notable shifts of focus. While not exhaustive, the following section demonstrates key concepts and terms of object relations theory, as linked to the theorists that developed them.

Key Concepts

Self

The self is the internal image, both conscious and unconscious, a person creates for themselves.

Other/Object

Other/object is used as a joint term in this chapter to describe the relation between the self and real or imagined people, objects, and ideas in a person's life. For example, the other/object could be different images of the mother figure. It could be mother of the present, mother of the past, or imagined mother image. There is no *absolute* image of mother, only the multi-faceted image that is created and evolves over time. The other/object can also represent objects such as a blanket (image of safety), shoe (image of sexuality), the American flag (image of relative kinship/community) or America as a country.

Representation

Representation describes the way the self possesses the image of the other/object or self. Object relations describes the mental representation of other/object and self.

External Other/Object

An actual other person or object that has been invested with emotional energy.

Internal Other/Object

The internal representation of another person or object that has been invested with emotional energy.

Self-Representation

The representation of identity created by a person, in relation to other/objects.

Self-Other/Object Confusion

The blurring or loss of boundaries between the person's self and the other/object. This is a hallmark experience of people with BPD.

Part Other/Object

An incomplete, underdeveloped, and often maladaptive image of the other/object.

Whole Other/Object

A more complete understanding of the other/object, with intact and accurate self and other/object boundaries and appreciation for the autonomy of existence of the other/object.

PRIMARY CONTRIBUTORS AND CONCEPTS

Melanie Klein

Melanie Klein (1964) is often credited as the founder of object relations theory. She emphasized infant interactions with caregivers and focused her research on the preverbal, prerational processes that are abound in the parent-infant dyad. Klein viewed her work as an extension of Freud's and based much of her work on the psychosexual model of development, yet de-emphasized the management of sexual urges as primary (Klein, 1964). Her contribution to psychoanalysis derived from her clinical work with children, and her therapeutic work helping the child work through conflicts and relationships. Where Freud focused on the development of the psyche in the first few years of life, Klein focused on the first months of caregiver-child interaction.

W.R.D. Fairbairn

W.R.D Fairbairn (1952) saw the person as primarily seeking relationships. The emphasis is placed on how the other/object had related to the person, and the gradual shift from complete dependency towards interdependence. He focused specifically on how the infant had been treated and what internal representations or models they created to manage relationships with caregivers. He studied and described ways in which early internal models continued to affect the person unconsciously in adulthood. Object relations theory focuses less on the previous Freudian models of development, and instead emphasizes themes related to safety, autonomy, and the challenges of separation and individuation (Fairbairn, 1952).

D.W. Winnicott

Winnicott began his career as a pediatrician; through observation of caregiver-infant dyads he theorized about "good enough" care. He described a holding phase, wherein the infant and mother began physical bonding; the emergence of the mother-infant dyad; and eventual mother-father-infant bonding. While his theory was biased in its use of the nuclear family type as a model, he further developed the concept of "good enough parenting."

Margaret Mahler

Margaret Mahler furthered the field with her research on separation-individuation dynamics and the adaptive psychological and physical holding space. She described "psychological birth" as a developmental event. Her separation-individuation theory has four stages: differentiation and development of body awareness; practicing phase and development of physical mobility; rapprochement phase and development of autonomy; and the object constancy phase and development of internal, stable images of early caregivers.

Otto Kernberg

Kernberg brought focus to Borderline Personality Disorder as the result of early caregivers relating in ways that provoke intense hurt/anger and aggression in the child's life (Kernberg, 1975). He saw caregivers who were perceived as dangerous or threatening and consistently hated and feared as creating conditions for BPD to emerge. Kernberg was the first to elaborate on the specific application of object relations theory for the treatment of BPD (Kernberg, 1976).

James Masterson

Masterson provided a clear definition of BPD, its etiology and treatment (Masterson, 1976). His writings provide detailed case studies that illustrate variants of borderline pathology and how the therapist might address specific behaviors that arise during progressive stages of psychotherapy.

Heinz Kohut

Kohut viewed the self as a composite of internalized objects (Kohut, 1977). He described personality disorders as the consequence of unintegrated part-self units (Kohut, 1984a). His descriptions of the process of psychoanalysis provde a foundation for understanding borderline personality pathology and a method for its treatment Kohut, 1984b).

Object Relations Theory: Further Concepts

As object relations theory progressed, there was a strong similarity with the work being done by theorists in the United States such as Karen Horney, Frieda Fromm-Reichmann, Harry Stack Sullivan, and Erich Fromm, amongst others, who identified as "Interpersonal Psychoanalysts." (McWilliams, 2011).

Both object relations theorists and interpersonal theorists deemphasized the person being treated as an object and focused on the experience of the relationship between the therapist and the patient. Interpersonal theorists further placed less emphasis on the infantile, unconscious models of the past and instead focused on the creation of a healthy, connected relationship in the present moment (McWilliams, 2011).

Object relations theorists departed from more traditional Freudian interpretations of the mind, and found less use in separating the mind into the Id, Ego, and Superego. They observed the mind had unintegrated "Ego states" that could function differently and at times seem out of awareness of one another (Hamilton, 1988). When experiencing strong and unintegrated ego states, a person could think, feel, and act in a manner with limited to no grasp on the reality of their situation. Simply put, the "then and there" of the past or a distorted internal model was eclipsing the more objective reality of the "here and now."

The emergence of the object relations perspective shifted the nature of treatment from the analysis of the person (with a higher potential to objectify and reduce them to a set of instincts, drives, and elements) towards a mutual experience between a helping other and a person in need. Theorists and clinicians learned treatment efficacy increased when they attended to the relational space in-between the person and themselves (Mitchell, 1988). During interactions they sought to identify the image of the maladaptive caregiver or early internalized object that was activated.

Object relations clinicians attended to defense mechanisms that arose to manage the *here and now* relationship while the person was activated, and sought to provide healthier ways of interacting and to encourage healthier defenses. Essentially, their aim was to trend towards greater states of organization when activated, using awareness and accurate empathy as the cornerstones of the therapeutic relationship.

Fromm-Reichman (1950) captured the sentiment in saying, "The patient needs an experience, not an explanation." Whereas classic psychoanalysis had sought to make the unconscious more conscious and give insight to a receiving other, contemporary psychoanalysis sought to create an emotionally corrective experience within the relational field.

With object relations theory, the clinician could listen for poorly integrated "ego states," and identify shifts in thinking, feeling, and behavior as signs that an "introjected" internal other was activated (Bromberg, 1991,

1998). Introjection is the unconscious adoption of adaptive or maladaptive elements from another other/object. Examples could be critical attitudes and beliefs heard as one's own voice or the internal experience of another's voice in the psyche.

The clinician could understand the person as needing healthy psychological separation and individuation and better mental representations. This could increase in general psychological organization (affect tolerance, capacity to self-soothe, higher order thinking and decision-making processes, etc.).

Object relations theorists and clinicians were able to comprehend the instability of people with BPD as identifiable patterns from past and present (McWilliams, 2011). The patterns could be seen as a strategy to recreate previous relationships, and the person pulling for the supportive other to behave like caregivers or other/objects from earlier childhood. The clinician could lend a more developed ego and observing ego as "ego strength" to the person, and assist in identifying and integrating chaotic ego states.

This method of treatment allowed clinicians to take greater ownership of their own subjective experience of the person with borderline states of organization. There was an emergence of clinicians and theorists openly sharing their own reactions with the person in need of help; they saw this as valuable treatment information rather than evidence of incomplete understanding from an "expert" (Winnicott, 1949). Transference and Countertransference refer to the unconscious experience that is acted out on the clinician (transference) and then received and acted out again on the patient by the clinician (countertransference).

Henirich Racker (1968) developed a useful framework for understanding of the transference-countertransference relationship, stating that the clinician experiences "concordant" and "complementary" states of countertransference. Concordant experiences were defined as the clinician feeling as the patient had when a child, whereas complementary countertransference experiences were defined as feeling how the patient's other/object had felt around the patient as a child. One may feel like the shamed child (concordant) or the shaming parent (complimentary). This identification allows the clinician to become more self-aware when in a chaotic relationship exchange a patient with BPD.

Borderline Personality Disorder as Level of Organization

To further assist the helping field with accurate diagnosis and treatment, object relations theorists found utility in identifying a patient's level of organization along a spectrum, and the person's general character type (McWilliams, 2011). The following describes the Neurotic-Borderline-Psychotic (NBP) levels of organization and common defense mechanisms that cluster around the Borderline level of organization (and inform character).

Origin of the Organizational Spectrum

Early 20th century descriptions of how human personality develops and functions centered around a dichotomy popularized by Emil Kraepelin (Jablensky, 2007). There existed a need to understand various psychopathologies and to develop a taxonomic system.

Kraepelin can be viewed as the father of contemporary diagnostic classification (Jablensky, 2007). He worked to identify syndromes with common characteristics, and to develop theories related to etiology. In the early 20th century, analytically-oriented therapists often followed the trend to identify people along a neurotic and psychotic continuum of organization, the main distinctions being that people who were neurotically organized were in touch with reality and those with psychotic levels of organization were not (McWilliams, 2011). Upon the development of the structural model of the mind by Freud, people were diagnosed in relation to their psychological infrastructure. People organized as neurotic were seen as suffering because the psyche and its defenses had become too rigid and broadly applied, and thus cut off from vital energetic resources. People organized at a psychotic level were seen to suffer because their ego defenses had become consistently overwhelmed by powerful primitive urge and energy from the id.

The neurotic-psychotic continuum allowed movement along these lines of development (McWilliams, 2011). At times, patients may be more or less organized, and the psyche could have a range within this continuum on which the psyche constitutionally existed. This promoted the belief that treatment could allow patients to organize upward and trend towards healthier states of being. As defenses were strengthened, patients would potentially manage their inner space in more adaptive ways.

The delineation of Borderline level of organization was in its infancy, even in the late 19th century as some psychiatrists were identifying people who did not fit into the neurotic or psychotic categories. Earlier psychiatrists observed patients who appeared to be in a psychological borderland within the continuum (Rosse, 1890).

Hoch and Polatin (1949) described the psychological borderland as a "pseudoneurotic schizophrenia," and were attempting to classify people who appeared to be too organized to be out of touch with reality, and too disturbed to be described as neurotically organized. By the mid-20th century, theorists and practitioners increasingly became aware of the limitations of the Neurotic-Psychotic continuum, and the conversation shifted to describing and treating patients who appeared to be character disordered and manifesting chaotic emotional and cognitive patterns. In the absence of hallucinations or delusions, these people were not psychotic, yet were chaotic enough to be less organized than neurotic.

A 1968 study formally delineated a "borderline syndrome" to fit within the lower range of neurotic organization and the upper range of psychotic organization (Grinker, Werble, & Drye, 1968). Noting that their patients with this syndrome could see significant movement along the continuum depending on a variety of influential factors. Influx of further research and clinical anecdote, and the writings of personality theorists such as Otto Kernberg, James F. Masterson, and others allowed the borderline syndrome concept to get a foothold and foundation within the psychoanalytic community.

With the publication of the Diagnostic and Statistical Manual, 3rd Edition (American Psychiatric Association, 1980) the borderline level of organization as a concept was categorized as "borderline personality disorder." The DSM-III defined borderline personality disorder in a more simplistic way than it was often written about; this allowed for greater researchability. This attempt for parsimony has had both benefits and drawbacks. Borderline personality disorder has received a greater research focus. However, arguably the theoretical shift from classifying borderline personality phenomenon as a discrete category of personality disorder appears to have decreased clinical utility and theoretical accuracy (McWilliams, 2011).

Overview of the Neurotic-Borderline-Psychotic (NBP) Structure

In McWilliam's (2011) manual of psychoanalytic diagnosis, she classifies the psychotic-, borderline-, and neurotic- levels of organization as being comprised of favored defenses level of identity integration capacity for reality testing awareness of one's own psychopathology quality and nature of primary and early conflict and pattern of transference and complementary countertransference. She finds evidence for these elements in behavioral observations and patterns of communication within initial sessions and beyond.

Neurotic

Freud originally used the neurotic level of organization to describe people with intact reality testing; experiencing pathology of a nonorganic nature; and absent psychotic features, psychopathic features, and bipolar features. People organized at a neurotic level often have emotional distress, but are well enough organized that they are not severely emotional chaotic nor experiencing psychosis (McWilliams, 2011).

People organized at a neurotic level have developed mature defenses that remain in touch with reality. The array of defenses are more flexibly applied, however certain emotionally resonant patterns will create personality rigidity (McWilliams, 2011). Oftentimes, repression and suppression are the defenses of choice, creating tension within the psyche as they intentionally "look away" from emotionally distressing psychic conflict. Notably, more basic and primitive defenses such as denial, splitting, projective identification, and departures from reality are less prominent.

People who are more well-organized at the neurotic level have more cohesive sense of who they are and have had good enough identity development (Erikson, 1968). The ability for more mature processing of distressing psychic material allows the person to integrate complex, painful experiences. This is evidence that the organizing ego has sufficient strength to hold the elements in awareness and organize. Additionally, the person is behaviorally consistent and experiences general continuity of self. They have capacity for an observing ego with which they can become aware of and critique their own experience (Sterba, 1934).

Psychotic

In Freud's conceptualization, the patient at the psychotic end of the continuum will present as disorganized in identity, emotional experience, sensory and perceptual experience, and cognitively. People primarily organized at the psychotic level evidence strong, primitive defense mechanisms such as denial, primitive idealization and devaluation, primitive projection and introjection, omnipotent control, splitting, dissociation, acting out, and somatization (McWilliams, 2011).

The painful and disturbed experience of the person with psychotic personality organization is often at a preverbal level and mostly unconscious. The chronically distressed ego struggles to maintain a coherent, integrated sense of identity and is consistently in peril of losing contact with what most would call reality. The capacity for reflective awareness is thin and severely underdeveloped. This often creates tension between the patient and the clinician, who may be seen as threatening. Strong primitive, emotional experience has overtaxed psychic mechanisms for stability. Some people are chronically in this state, while others may organize at higher levels and drop into more psychotic states when stressed and regressed.

Borderline

In the Freudian model, a defining feature of personalities organized at the borderline level is the primitive defense mechanisms they use to regulate their relation to self and other/objects (McWilliams, 2011). Defense mechanisms used to control inner experience are characteristically: splitting, projective identification, denial. There is significant overlap with primitive defenses used by patients in a psychotic state. Patients with borderline tendencies may regress into transient psychotic organization when stressed.

Notably, high levels of emotional dysregulation are a part of the patient's attempt to make contact with their reality, and often the patient may split themselves or others/objects into "all good, all bad" perceptions. This is an attempt at understanding the complicated nature of their attachments, and a still developing attempt at integration of complex and emotional experience. Splitting is a defense mechanism where the patient experiences black and white, all good/all bad thinking. This is an interplay of primitive idealization and devaluation.

Patients with BPD often struggle to develop a cohesive sense of identity. Underdeveloped identity integration may leave the patient at a loss when asked to describe themselves (McWilliams, 2011). Their overstressed ego has difficulty finding solid foundation with which to construct the psyche, and they may have difficulty in describing themselves, or may often change their perception of themselves as a reflection of the splitting mechanism.

The patient's ability to self-reflect will be hindered, and their observing ego will struggle to maintain accurate perceptions. This indicates the patient has had, and may still have, difficulty finding accurate mirroring from supportive others. Mirroring is the process through which we develop stable identity. Mirroring allows us to see ourselves through the eyes of others, giving important information about how we are perceived by others. Accurate mirroring allows stable self-representations, while inaccurate mirroring creates identity confusion and poor integration.

Internal and external stressors may cause a person with borderline phenomena to organize upwardly or downwardly in the continuum. At times the patient may present well enough to seem nearly neurotically organized. Patients with BPD are characteristically prone to rapid and drastic shifts in presentation, often prompted by unmet emotional/relational needs.

TREATMENT: NEED TO INTEGRATE PART SELF AND PART OBJECT RELATIONS

Treatment for patients with BPD is multifaceted, and attends to the person as a whole within their environment. The patient often responds best to a multi-disciplinary team that attends to their biopsychosocial needs. This chapter describes a treatment method that embraces both general principles of effective psychotherapy, and addresses treatment and methods specific to object relations theory.

Empirically Supported Principles of Psychotherapy

Although there are different approaches to psychotherapy, and Object Relations is one of them, there are undergirding principles of change that support the therapeutic space. Due to the strong focus placed on the relationship between the patient with BPD and the clinician, these empirically supported principles of change are even more vitally important.

The following principles of change can be understood to be common to most forms of psychotherapy (Goldfried, 1980/1982)

- Promoting hope for change and attending to the patient's expectation and motivation to change:
  Promotion of hope and expectation was present as early as Freud's work in psychoanalysis, where he encouraged patient's to anticipate success in "talk therapy" (Gay, 1985). A patient who has engaged in dialogue about expectation and motivation to change, and who has shifted from precontemplation to a contemplation stage, is more likely to find success in treatment (Prochaska, Norcross, & DiClemente, 2013).
- Establishing and maintaining strong therapeutic alliance:
  The successful treatment of patients with BPD requires a strong therapeutic bond and alliance, and agreement about the goals of treatment and manner of achieving the goals (Bordin, 1979).
- Facilitating awareness and understanding of the factors and elements of the patient's undesirable experience:
  Patients with BPD have become stuck in maladaptive ways of relating in part because they have insufficient awareness of what causes their struggle. Sullivan described this as "selective inattention" at a conscious or unconscious level (Sullivan, 1973). A help task in the treatment process is developing a relationship to the patient's "observing ego" to support better awareness of the patient engaged in fault relationship patterns (Freud, 1916/1963). The patient may then witness and develop better awareness and understanding of their thoughts, emotions, behavior patterns, and the interplay of complex interrelations of self and other/object.
- Encouraging and facilitating the patient's engagement in trying out corrective experiences:
  Engagement in new forms of relationship and trying out new experiences increase the likelihood the patient with BPD encounters "emotionally corrective experiences" with the therapist or others (Alexander & French, 1946). The emotionally corrective experience

involves some new understanding and/or interaction that occurs at the corrective cognitive and behavioral level as well, and is considered to be at the core level of change (Brady et al., 1980). For example, object relations-informed treatment will emphasize the awareness of maladaptive patterns of splitting, and encourage the patient to form whole other/object relations out of partially developed and inaccurate ones.

- Encouraging ongoing reality testing in the patient's life (Goldfried, 2019):
  To build upon change from emotionally corrective experiences, the patient is encouraged to maintain this process over time and continually engage in reality testing. Reality testing involves increased awareness of the internal self and perceptions of the external world, and working with supportive others to receive accurate mirroring and feedback.

To summarize the principles of change: patients with BPD will be supported to change when they (1) have hope and expectation to change and maintain optimum levels of motivation, (2) have formed a strong therapeutic alliance with the clinician, (3) increase self awareness of the causes and nature of maladaptive patterns of thinking, feeling and behaving in their lives, (4) take action and create opportunity to test out change in their patterns of thinking, feeling, and behaving, (5) continually engage in reality testing and accurate feedback loops.

Object Relations Theory Treatment Method

In addition to the focus on primary principles that support therapeutic chance, object relations treatment develops specific focus on technique interaction. A primary tenet of object relations-based treatment relates to the general strengthening of the ego and the ability to develop whole self relations and other/object relations. The patient needs to move from lack of identity integration, inconsistent personality/emotional organization, and imbalanced sense of self and other, towards greater states and mechanisms of organization (Kernberg, et al., 1989). While this process unfolds uniquely to the individual, there are corrective-type experiences that assist the patient to trend towards greater states of organization and coherence. Just as we are able to crawl, toddle, walk, and run, the mind's ability to organize itself requires specific support and expectations, and must be tailored to the stage a person inhabits most frequently.

The raising awareness of defense mechanisms can assist the person in digesting more complex experience over time, and strengthens the ego (Hamilton, 1990). Optimal amount of interpretation and the person's tolerance for this activity will vacillate. The task of the clinician is to use accurate empathy and assessment to gauge ability to tolerate. There is a working range: too little is not enough, and too much is too much. Developing the ability to "talk about talking about" difficult experiences can be helpful in clarifying this range with the patient.

Object relations treatment has been described as a series of steps or stages to move through (Kernberg et al., 1989):

Early Phases of Treatment

- Step 1 – Experience and Tolerate the Confusion
- Step 2 – Identify the Actors
- Step 3 – Naming
- Step 4 – Attending to the Patient's Reaction
- Step 5 – Interpreting Primitive Defenses

Step 1 – Experience and Tolerate the Confusion

An initial setting of the framework of therapy may often be confusing, chaotic, and intense when working with patients with BPD. An initial task of the clinician is to sort through and organize their own emotional and cognitive reaction. Demonstrating the ego strength to withstand strong affective states without foreclosing on one or another as "reality" allows the patient to find a center and safe haven within the relationship. Further, the person is encouraged to tolerate intense and opposing feeling states and increases the felt sense of therapeutic alliance.

Step 2 – Identify the Roles

Once the safe, therapeutic atmosphere has been created the task shifts towards understanding the internal objects that inhabit the patient's inner world. Patterns within the patient's interactions with others, including and especially the clinician, provide insight into the nature of the object relations. Just as actors will take on different roles from one script to another, the therapist may notice the subtle and overt shifts in thinking, feeling and behaving within the patient.

For each role taken on by the patient with BPD, there will be a pull for the other person to take on a complementary role, called a role pair. Roles may be played out in alternative ways, wherein the patient takes one side of a complementary pattern and pulls for the other to act accordingly. Switching of roles - at times rapidly - may occur, wherein the clinician now is given the role previously taken by the patient with BPD. For example, common role pairs may be "the controlled child and the controlling parent," "the deprived child and the selfish parent," or "the dependent child and doting parent." These old interactions find new life as rigid patterns and roles projected and identified in current relationships.

The clinician's intuitive feeling-state provides valuable information about the role he or she is in or that the patient wishes them to be in. The therapist may monitor for strong emotion, odd or alien feeling states, intrusive fantasies, desire to withdraw, and uncharacteristic departures from therapeutic role. Noting these shifts and identifying them within the relationship becomes a pivotal step in the therapeutic process.

Step 3 – Naming

After identifying the roles projected and identified with, the clinician may seek to raise the patient's awareness of the pattern in pieces over time. Because the object relation begins as largely unconscious, it takes significant effort over time to increase the awareness. Too much too soon will likely create overwhelm and flight or rejection of emotional insight. To increase the likelihood of the insight and corrective experience to occur, many clinicians use metaphor created from the person's experience as a vehicle to provide an emotionally rich and salient interpretation. The clinician may use the role they find themselves playing, or that they observe the person playing, and then collaborate in creative understanding about the origins and meaning of the pattern.

Step 4 – Attending to the Patient's Reaction

Upon raising awareness and labeling the self and other/object dyad or role pair, the clinician embraces non-hostile curiosity of the patient's response. Agreement or disagreement with the interpretation of the relationship pattern is less important than empathizing with the reaction and response of the patient. Compassionate clinicians seek to increase accurate empathy of the patient's experience, and provide space for the person to respond in any manner of ways. Often, the patient may become more intense and pronounced within the pattern, the roles may interchange, an insight of some degree may occur, the pattern may shift to another role pattern, or the patient may meet the interpretation with blanket denial.

As therapeutic change occurs over time, the process of response and reaction from the person during an interpersonal pattern will shift. Tracking the typical reaction to interpretation allows the therapist and person to identify change in ego strength, observing ego, and emotional tolerance.

Step 5 – Interpreting Primitive Defenses

With a strong therapeutic alliance and increasing understanding of the pattern and process of the object relations, the clinician can interpret the defenses used to manage and sustain the maladaptive psychic conflict of the patient. All defense mechanisms are aimed at relief and management of intrapsychic and interpersonal conflict. The central mechanism of more primitive defenses associated with borderline personality disorder is *splitting.* Splitting involves the isolation of aspects of self and other/object from overall integrated awareness. Further defenses are omnipotent control, projective identification, primitive idealization, devaluation, and denial that allow splitting to occur.

Splitting

The defense mechanism of splitting is central to borderline personality disorder and is characterized as distorted perception. The person with borderline personality disorder will split the perception of themselves or others as "all good" or "all bad," with the potential for rapid shift and reversal of the perception back and forth.

Omnipotent Control and Primitive Devaluation

Both omnipotent control and devaluation involve the distorted perception of the self and other/object representation. The self is seen as grandiose and powerful, while the other/object is seen as depreciated and weak/bad.

Projection and Projective Identification

Projected is the mechanism by which a person attributes a repressed internal experiences as being not of the self, but of the other. In addition to projection, projective identification involves 4 steps. 1) the experience of a repressed impulse projected onto the other person, 2) fear of the other person who is now seen as under the influence of the projected impulse, 3) the need to now control the other person to manage the fear, 4) and the unconscious propensity to create the feared projected impulse in the unsuspecting other person.

Primitive Idealization

Involves the perception of unrealistic, "all good and powerful" image of the self and other/object.

Denial

The denial defense mechanism supports splitting in the person with borderline personality disorder by suppressing the appropriate response or having complete lack of reaction to emotionally important events. The emotional experience can be partially or totally removed from awareness of the person as a defense against anxiety-producing experience.

Advanced Stages of Object Relations Treatment

The key indicator of treatment success and progress is understood as the shift from primary and maladaptive use of primitive defense mechanisms (such as splitting, omnipotent control, projective identification, and primitive idealization and devaluation) towards more mature and adaptive ones. Additionally, the patient will demonstrate more integrated self and other/object representations, and the ability to appreciate complexity in relationship rather than black and white/all-good all-bad thinking.

A patient who is in more advanced stages of treatment will often indicate the shift by relying less on action to cope with anxious internal states, increasingly verbalizing their experience. There is an increased ability to anticipate behavior patterns, due to the awareness of the pattern in previous interactions. The patient often internalizes the clinician and uses the introjected other to support better awareness and decision-making.

The clinician observes better mental representations of self and other/object, and the patient will become more nuanced and detailed in their descriptions. The patient will practice seeing the clinician as a more whole person, and develop realistic observations and understanding of the therapeutic relationship. The therapeutic relationship becomes a point of mutual connection from which the patient recalls interactions from the past and a sense of shared history. With the development of the observing ego and increased ego strength there is a decrease in chaotic and violent shifts from one emotional state to another, and a new sense of emotional expression and depth emerge. The patient will often become more autonomous in their use of the therapeutic space, become more self-directive, and reveal new information that was previously withheld at the beginning stages of the work.

Much of the work may have been focused on here-and-now interactions between the clinician and patient. Over time, the patient may be more able to understand links between past interactions, and even dreams, and the relation to current relationship patterns. This indicates a shift from more ego supportive type interventions towards ego expressive.

SUMMARY AND CONCLUSION

Object relations theory created a lexicon and operational treatment objectives that provided the first effective treatment for BPD. Object relations theory has also given the field of psychotherapy useful metrics to indicate shifts in the belief systems and behaviors of patients with BPD, and a representational map of the internal and external dynamics that are often found in treatment. An integrationist approach with appreciation and implementation of the empirically supported principles of change makes object relations theory a useful addition to the clinician's repertoire. The time required to work through the stages of object relations theory-based psychotherapy to achieve enduring positive outcome might not fit with time-limited models of treatment preferred by third-party payers. Outcome research continues to demonstrate the utility of object relations theory in the treatment of BPD.

REFERENCES

Alexander, F. & French, T. (1946). *Psychiatric therapy: Principles and applications.* New York, NY: Ronald. https://doi.org/10.1002/1097-4679(194610)2:4<401::AID-JCLP2270020418>3.0.CO;2-L.

American Psychiatric Association. (1980). *Diagnostic and statistical manual of mental disorders* (3rd ed.). Washington, DC: Author.

Bordin, E. (1979). The generalizability of psychoanalytic concept of the working alliance. *Psychotherapy: Theory, Research and Practice*, *16*, 252-260. http://dx.doi.org/10.1037/h0085885.

Brady, J. P., Davison, G. C., Dewald, P. A., Egan, G., Fadiman, J., Frank, J. D. & Strupp, H. H. (1980). Some views on effective principles of psychotherapy. *Cognitive Therapy and Research*, *4*, 271-306.

Bromberg, P. M. (1991). On knowing one's patient from the inside out: The aesthetics of unconscious communication. *Psychoanalytic Dialogues*, *1*, 399-422. https://doi.org/10.1080/10481889109538911.

Bromberg, P. M. (1998). *Standing in spaces: Essays on clinical process, trauma, and dissociation.* Hillsdale, NJ: Analytic Press.

Erikson, E. H. (1968). *Identity: Youth and crisis.* New York: Norton.

Fairbairn, W. R. D. (1952). *An object relations theory of personality.* New York: Basic Books.

Freud, S. (1964). New introductory lectures on psycho-analysis. In J. Starchy (Ed. And Trans.), *The Standard edition of the complete psychological works of Sigmund Freud* (Vol. 22). London: Hogarth Press. (Original work published 1933).

Freud, S. (1961). Ego and the Id. In J. Starchy (Ed. And Trans.), *The Standard edition of the complete psychological works of Sigmund Freud* (Vol. 19). London: Hogarth Press. (Original work published 1923).

Fromm-Reichmann, F. (1950). *Principles of intensive psychotherapy.* Chicago: University of Chicago Press.

Goldfried, M. R. (1980). Toward the delineation of therapeutic change principles. *American Psychologist, 35*, 991-999. http://dx.doi.org/10.1037/0003-066X.35.11.991.

Goldfried, M. R. (Ed.). (1982). *Converging themes in psychotherapy: Trends in psychodynamic, humanistic, and behavioral practice.* New York, NY: Springer.

Goldfried, M. R. (2019). Obtaining consensus in psychotherapy: What holds us back? *American Psychologist, 74*, 484-496. http://doi.org/10.1037/amp0000365

Gay, P. (1985). *Freud for historians.* New York, NY: Oxford University Press.

Grinder, R. R., Werble, B. & Drye, R. C. (1968). *The borderline syndrome: A behavioral study of ego functions.* New York: Basic Books.

Hamilton, N. G. (1988). *Self and others: Object relations theory in practice.* Lanham, MD, US: Jason Aronson.

Hartmann, H. (1958). *Ego psychology and the problem of adaptation.* New York, NY: International Universities Press.

Hoch, P. H. & Polatin, P. (1949). Pseudoneurotic forms of schizophrenia. *Psychoanalytic Quarterly, 23*, 248-276.

Jablensky, A. (2007). Living in a Kraepelinian world: Kraepelin's impact on modern psychiatry. *History of psychiatry. 18*, 318-8. http://doi.org/10.1177/0957154X07079690.

Kernberg, O. F. (1975). *Borderline conditions and pathological narcissism.* New York: Jason Aronson Inc.

Kernberg, O. F. (1976). *Object relations theory and clinical psychoanalysis.* New York: Jason Aronson Inc.

Kernberg, O. F., Selzer, M. A., Koenigsberg, H. W., Carr, A. C. & Appelbaum, A. H. (1989). *Psychodynamic psychotherapy of borderline patients*. New York, NY: Basic Book, Inc.

Klein, M. (1964). *Contributions to psychoanalysis, 1921-1945*. New York: McGraw Hill.

Kohut, H. (1977). *The restoration of the self.* New Yor: International Universities Press.

Kohut, H. (1984a). *The analysis of the self.* New York: International Universtites Press.

Kohut, H. (1984b). *How does analysis cure?* Chicago: University of Chicago Press.

Kraepelin, E. (1913). *Lectures on clinical psychiatry.* London: Bailliere, Tyndall, & Cox.

Masterson, J. F. (1976). *Psychotherapy of the borderline adult.* New York: Brunner/Mazel Inc.

McWilliams, N. (2011). Psychoanalytic diagnosis: *Understanding personality structure in the clinical process* (2nd ed.). Guilford Press.

Mitchell, S. A. (1988). *Relational concepts in psychoanalysis: An integration.* Cambridge, MA: Harvard University Press.

Ormont, L.R., Hunt, M. & Corman, R. (1964). *The Talking Cure.* New York: Harper and Row.

Prochaska, J. O., Norcross, J. C. & DiClemente, C. C. (2013). Applying the stages of change. In G. P. Koocher, J. C. Norcross, & B. A. Greene (Eds.), *Psychologist's desk reference* (pp. 176-181). http://dx.doi.org/10.1093/med:psych/9780199845491.003.0034.

Racker, H. (1968). *Transference and countertransference.* New York: International Universities Press.

Rosse, I. C. (1890). Clinical Evidences of borderland insanity. *Journal of Nervous and Mental Diseases, 17*, 669-683.

Sterba, R. F. (1934). The fate of the ego in analytic therapy. *International Journal of Psycho-Analysis, 15*, 117-126.

Sullivan, H. S. (1973). *Clinical studies in psychiatry.* New York, NY: Norton.

Winnicott, D. W. (1949). Hate in the countertransference. In *Collected papers* (pp. 194-203). New York: Basic Books, 1958.

Stern, A. (1938). Psychoanalytic investigation of and therapy in the borderline group of neuroses. *The Psychoanalytic Quarterly*, *7*, 467-489.

Stone, M. H. (1976). The borderline syndrome: evolution of the term, genetic aspects, and prognosis. *American Journal of Psychotherapy, 31*(3), 345-365.

Swenson, C. R. & Choi-Kain, L. W. (2015). Mentalization and dialectical behavior therapy. *American Journal of Psychotherapy, 69*(2), 199-217. http://doi.org/10.1176/appi.psychotherapy.2015.69.2.199.

Thorne, F. C. (1955). Diagnostic classifications. In Principles of Psychological Examining: A Systematic Textbook of Applied Integrative Psychology. Brandon, VT, US: *Journal of Clinical Psychology*, pp. 83-109.

In: Borderline Personality Disorder
Editor: Charles M. Lepkowsky
ISBN: 978-1-53618-021-3

Chapter 6

TREATMENT OF BORDERLINE PERSONALITY DISORDER USING DIALECTICAL BEHAVIOR THERAPY

Joanna L. Fava*[*]*, PhD
***and Madelaine Ellberger*[†]**
Center for Cognitive and Dialectical Behavior Therapy,
Lake Success, New York, US

ABSTRACT

Individuals with Borderline Personality Disorder (BPD) have been called "untreatable patients." High risk and impulsive behaviors, interpersonal difficulties, and frequent intense emotion dysregulation can make it difficult for clinicians to maintain an effective therapeutic relationship with BPD patients. Marsha Linehan's Dialectical Behavior Therapy (DBT) has provided structure and mechanisms that allow for effective and compassionate care for BPD patients. The main components of DBT are presented, providing an overview of the standard treatment

[*] Corresponding Author's E-mail: jfava@ccdbt.com.
[†] Corresponding Author's E-mail: mellberger@ccdbt.com.

model for adults, as well as adaptations for other populations. Research supporting the model is summarized. Consideration is given to clinician stance, risk assessment, crisis management, and clinician burnout and self-care. Case examples and sample intervention tools are presented as practical examples of the treatment model and its use.

Keywords: Linehan, stigma, dialectical behavior therapy, skills training, crisis management, risk assessment, clinician burnout

INTRODUCTION

Individuals with Borderline Personality Disorder (BPD) exhibit the following traits: emotion dysregulation, difficulty managing anger, difficulties maintaining healthy and stable relationships, fear of abandonment, impulsive behaviors, suicidal and/or non-suicidal self-injurious (NSSI) behaviors or threats, fluctuating sense of self, feelings of emptiness, and difficulty thinking clearly when stressed. In addition, individuals with BPD often have comorbid disorders including depression, anxiety, posttraumatic stress, substance abuse/dependence, eating disorders, and physical health issues (American Psychiatric Association [APA], 2013). The combination of interpersonal difficulties often exhibited by individuals with BPD, and the complexity of presentation with other comorbid issues, has led many clinicians to label an individual with BPD the "untreatable client." Clinician bias toward this population has increased the stigma around treating personality disorders, and has led to inadequate and unjust treatment for those with BPD (Ferguson, 2016; Sheehan, Nieweglowski, & Corrigan, 2016).

Ironically, this stigma and unfair treatment by providers limits patients' access to effective and useful treatment options. This is particularly problematic as impulsive behavior, a cornerstone symptom of BPD, places individuals without effective treatment at a higher risk for harm. The scientific literature provides abundant evidence that one of the biggest predictors of therapeutic success, regardless of disorder, therapeutic orientation or research method, is the trusting and caring relationship between the patient and clinician (Choi-Kain, Finch, Masland, Jenkins, & Unruh, 2017; Flückiger, Del Re, Wampold, Symonds, & Horvath, 2012; Woolcott, 1985). The value of the therapeutic relationship is particularly salient for those with BPD, who often have a history of complex trauma, interpersonal problems, and chronic invalidation from others. Clinicians who are rejecting, judgmental, and cold towards patients with BPD could further harm these patients (Ferguson, 2016).

More than 30 years ago, Woolcott (1985) looked at the indicators suggestive of good versus poor prognosis in the treatment of BPD. His conclusion was that a therapist who likes their patient is more likely to help them, and the quality of the therapeutic relationship is indicative of better outcomes. A more recent study at a one-day General Psychiatric Management workshop showed that attendance improved clinicians' attitudes regarding patients with BPD, and clinicians' reportedly felt more hopeful, willing, and competent to treat BPD (Keuroghlian et al., 2015). These studies suggest that clinicians without adequate training, understanding, and competence in treating individuals with BPD should either refer these patients to clinicians who are competent in this area, or seek out the necessary trainings, workshops, and/or supervision to ensure they can effectively treat these individuals with patience, compassion, and dignity. There are several evidence-based treatments available now for BPD, making treatment more accessible to patients and allowing clinicians to find an option that works for them, thus increasing the likelihood of more successful outcomes.

This chapter focuses on one evidence-based treatment for BPD, Dialectical Behavior Therapy (DBT). The goal of the chapter is to provide an overview of DBT including the components of the treatment, summary of the research supporting its use and effectiveness, guidelines for managing high-risk behaviors that are often present with DBT patients, and ways for clinicians to attend to their own needs while providing care for high-risk individuals. Throughout the chapter, case studies will be in italics and serve to bring the discussion to life using clinical examples. Names and identifying information have been altered to maintain confidentiality.

DBT: Biosocial Theory and Basic Concepts

Over the last 25 years, stigma towards individuals with BPD has reduced, largely due to the development of Dialectical Behavior Therapy (DBT) by Dr. Marsha Linehan in 1993. In its advent, DBT offered a new empirically-validated, comprehensive, and straightforward approach for treating chronically suicidal adult patients suffering from BPD. DBT blends cognitive-behavioral strategies, which focus on identifying and changing ineffective thoughts and behaviors, with validation strategies, which involve communicating to individuals that their thoughts, feelings, and behaviors make sense in particular contexts. DBT also emphasizes "dialectics;" the concept that two seemingly opposite things can both exist and be true at the same time. Dialectical strategies can help depolarize conflicts, reduce black-and-white thinking patterns, and identify solutions that honor both sides of an interpersonal or intrapersonal conflict. One of the core dialectics in DBT is the balance of acceptance (a construct found in Zen Buddhism) and change, highlighting the notion that a person is doing the best they can and, at the same time, can be doing better, trying harder, and be more motivated to change (Linehan, 1993).

Within the context of DBT, BPD is conceptualized as the result of a transaction between biological vulnerabilities and environmental factors. There are three components to the biological contribution: 1) high sensitivity - reactions to the environment are quick and require little provocation; 2) high reactivity - individuals' emotions spike more intensely than others' to the same stimuli; and 3) slow return to baseline - emotions last for a long period of time and decline slowly, making a person more vulnerable to the next emotional event. From an environmental standpoint, invalidating environments contribute to more intense emotional reactions and difficulty trusting one's own internal cues and reactions. An invalidating environment is any environment that communicates to a person that his or her emotions are not valid and do not make sense. Examples of invalidating statements include "Stop making such a big deal about this" or "Just get over it." Individuals who experience strong emotions live in a culture that often does not know how to respond appropriately to the level of their emotions and that is unable to respond to those emotions effectively. Over time, the experience of consistent invalidation leads to a sequelae in which a person experiences their own emotions as wrong, believes others do not or cannot understand, and experiences the world as a dangerous and isolating place (Linehan, 1993).

It is difficult to be a person with strong emotions living in a world that does not always tolerate those emotions. Yet, despite the invalidation a person may experience from their environment, it is still important for them to function effectively in the world. DBT therefore seeks to turn people into experts on their internal experience so that they can cope with and manage their emotions in more functional and effective ways. By recalibrating an individuals' internal compass through self-validation and skill use, the treatment helps people learn to experience their emotions to their benefit. As a result, ineffective and dangerous behaviors (e.g., self-harm) used to erase emotions are replaced with skillful and goal-directed behaviors to effectively manage and regulate emotions (Linehan, 1993).

The structure of DBT makes the treatment predictable for patients, which helps to maintain engagement and collaboration in the treatment. The construct of validation as well as the underlying assumptions of DBT serve to build rapport and communicate a compassionate understanding of the patient's behavior and the emotional function it serves. They also assist the clinician in maintaining a non-judgmental stance, crucial in effectively implementing cognitive-behavioral strategies for change, such as functional behavior analyses. A fundamental change strategy is the behavior chain analysis. The behavior chain analysis breaks down an incident where the target behavior was exhibited in order to pinpoint problem areas and highlight opportunities for new skillful behavior. Thus, the comprehensiveness of DBT balances acceptance of the patient while also pushing for change. These elements will be discussed in greater depth later in this chapter.

EVIDENCE REGARDING DBT

A large body of evidence suggests that DBT is a successful treatment for individuals who meet criteria for BPD. Specifically, research has found DBT to be successful in reducing suicidality, non-suicidal self-injury (NSSI), impulsivity, psychiatric hospitalizations, emergency room visits, as well as symptoms of comorbid depression and anxiety (Bedics, Atkins, Comtois, & Linehan, 2012; Cristea et al., 2017; Williams, Hartstone, & Denson, 2010). Its efficacy has been studied in a variety of settings with adult, adolescent, and child populations.

Adults

Randomized controlled trials with adults diagnosed with BPD indicate that compared to psychotherapy by clinicians not trained in DBT (referred to as "treatment as usual"), standard DBT significantly reduces suicidality, self-harm, hospital admissions, emergency room visits, anger outbursts, and hopelessness (Feigenbaum et al., 2012; Linehan, Armstrong, Suarez, Allmon, & Heard, 1991; Linehan, Heard, & Armstrong, 1993; Verheul et al., 2003). This finding has been validated with adult populations being treated in outpatient clinics, on inpatient units, and in forensic institutions. According to the Cochrane Collaborative Review, DBT is the only treatment adequately supported by data to be deemed an effective, empirically supported treatment modality for BPD (Stoffers et al., 2012). DeCou, Comtois, and Landes (2019) recently conducted a meta-analysis indicating that DBT was more effective than "treatment as usual" (including individual and/or group psychodynamic psychotherapy, psychoeducation, relational therapy, supportive therapy, substance abuse treatments, or wait-list conditions) for reducing self-directed violence and the use of psychiatric crisis services. DBT has also been identified as a primary or supplementary treatment modality for individuals with substance disorders (Pennay et al., 2011; Lee, Cameron & Jenner, 2015), eating disorders (Harned et al., 2008), and posttraumatic stress disorder (Harned, Korslund, & Linehan, 2014). In addition, DBT's effectiveness with individuals who exhibit impulsive behaviors, including perpetrators of domestic violence (Fruzetti & Levensky, 2000) and those arrested for harassment or stalking (Rosenfeld et al., 2012) has also been indicated in the literature.

Linehan et al., (2015) evaluated the components of DBT to determine whether a less intensive form of treatment for BPD might also be effective. Standard DBT (including weekly individual therapy and group skills training, consultation team for the clinicians, and phone coaching), as well as DBT-S (group skills training without coaching) yielded similarly significant reductions in self-harm, anxiety, and depression. DBT individual therapy, without group skills training, was not as effective. Although current data offer limited support for less intensive DBT program structures, continued efforts to research such models might help determine whether adaptations can be made to potentially allow treatment to be more practical and attainable for patients in need.

Adolescents

Rathus and Miller (2002, 2015) adapted DBT for use with adolescent patients (DBT-A). Similar to the adult model, adolescent patients attend skills group in addition to individual therapy. The main difference in DBT-A is that the patient must attend group with one or more caregivers. Caregivers complete homework assignments along with the adolescent to maximize skills use in the home and ensure that caregivers and teens are speaking the same "language." In addition, when caregivers use skills in their own lives, they serve as a model throughout the week for the adolescent, and can help generalize the material to real-world situations (Rathus & Miller, 2015).

A substantial body of research supports the efficacy of DBT-A for reducing self-harm, suicidal ideation, depression, and other BPD symptoms in adolescent populations (McCauley et al., 2018; Mehlum et al., 2016; Rathus & Miller, 2002). An inpatient study comparing standard DBT-A (individual and group DBT plus coaching for the patient) to intensive treatment as usual (TAU; individual, family and group therapy utilizing other treatment modalities besides DBT) demonstrated that patients who received DBT had significantly fewer constant observation hours for self-injury; fewer incidents of suicide attempts and/or self-injury; less need of restraints during the inpatient stay; and fewer days hospitalized than those in the TAU group. A cost analysis indicated that the difference in constant observation hours saved over $250,000 on staff time for those in the DBT group compared to the TAU group (Tebbett-Mock, Saito, McGee, Woloszyn, & Venuti, 2019). Utilizing DBT with high-risk adolescents in Germany, Fleischhaker et al., (2011) reported reduction in BPD symptoms including self-harm, with no additional suicide attempts, during the 1-year treatment phase and 1-year follow up phase of their study. A review of the literature on the use of DBT with adolescents suggests that DBT-A is a promising treatment for adolescents with symptoms of BPD, aggressive or impulsive behaviors, and comorbid disorders including depression and eating disorders (Groves, Backer, van den Bosch & Miller, 2011). Adolescents receiving DBT-A were also hospitalized less frequently than adolescents in other treatments. A study looking at three-year follow up data comparing outcomes of adolescents treated with either DBT-A or enhanced usual care (EUC) indicated that adolescents who received DBT-A demonstrated significantly lower rates of NSSI and were able to maintain remission of self-harm behaviors longer than those adolescents receiving EUC (Mehlum et al., 2019). EUC was defined in this study as non-manualized psychodynamic or cognitive-behavioral therapy occurring weekly with a therapist trained in suicide risk assessment and management, but not trained in DBT. Research has also shown that adolescents with significantly more frequent and severe BPD symptomatology at the start of treatment remain in DBT longer than adolescents with fewer or less life-threatening behaviors, suggesting that DBT retains impulsive and struggling adolescents in treatment, which in turn increases the likelihood of symptom reduction (Byrnes, Fava, Feinman, & Harari, 2013).

STANDARD DBT

An adherent DBT program involves four components: individual therapy, skills group, phone coaching, and consultation team. All components work together to help the clinician provide the best care and to help the patient learn and generalize more skillful approaches to situations that elicit intense emotions or ineffective urges or behaviors. The ultimate goal of DBT is to help the patient create a "life worth living" - one that is both tolerable and satisfying.

Individual Therapy

The purpose of individual therapy in DBT is to help patients identify patterns of ineffective responses and connect to goals that motivate them to make necessary changes to achieve a more rewarding, comfortable, healthy and/or productive life. The various DBT skills, primarily taught in skills group, are tools to help patients build a more personally satisfying life. One of the primary goals of individual therapy is to assist clients in applying the skills to specific situations in the patient's daily life. More specifically, individual therapy helps replace unhealthy coping or communication strategies with healthy and effective ones.

Individual therapy sessions are structured based on a three-tier target hierarchy. Any threats to safety are the first targets addressed in individual therapy sessions. These include any life-threatening behaviors and urges such as suicide, self-harm behaviors, or urges to harm others. Every individual therapy session assesses for and addresses first-tier targets to help establish and build a commitment to safety. This practice also encourages discussion about, and disclosure of, any life-threatening information, thereby normalizing open conversation about these topics, which often have been discouraged by others in their lives.

Second-tier targets are any behaviors by the patient or the clinician that interfere with or destroy treatment. This target sets the precedent that effective treatment is collaborative, and that the patient and clinician must work together to problem solve any barriers to treatment that arise. At the outset of treatment, the patient and clinician identify and discuss potential therapy-interfering behaviors so they can be mindful of these behaviors throughout the course of treatment. These could include lateness to sessions, not doing assignments, arguing with or invalidating each other, or ineffective communication such as using threats. Good therapy cannot occur if there is not willingness by both the clinician and patient to change and repair ineffective behaviors that destroy the treatment or the therapeutic relationship. In addition, openly discussing and collaboratively problem-solving therapy interfering behavior allows patients to rehearse skillful behavior in the therapy room. Thus, these targets are important to be aware of and to address as soon as possible when they arise.

The third-tier targets include any behaviors that interfere with a patient's quality of life, contribute to keeping a patient stuck, and prevent movement toward life-worth-living goals. Examples include substance abuse, binge eating, isolating, avoidance due to anxiety, and other impulsive behaviors that a patient would like to decrease. It can also include effective behaviors that a patient would like to increase, such as searching for a job, saying "no" to others when necessary, or socializing in a healthy way.

Diary Cards

In individual therapy, clinicians work collaboratively with patients to develop a "diary card." A diary card is a weekly log in which patients track and rate their emotions, urges, and behaviors throughout the week. The specific emotions, urges, and behaviors are custom tailored for each patient based on the individual's own personal struggles and goals for treatment. The diary card helps ensure that the clinician is not missing important information and can target any behavior or urge that would be important to discuss during the session. Diary cards can be customized on the computer and printed each week for the patient to take home, complete between sessions, and bring back to the next individual session. Alternatively, the DBT app allows clinicians and patients to customize the dairy card on the patient's smartphone and then the patient can complete it in the app and email it to the clinician prior to session each week.

DBT DIARY CARD		**Name: Mia**						
Month: July Year: 2019		23	24	25	26	27	28	29
Day:		Tues	Wed	Thur	Fri	Sat	Sun	Mon
EMOTIONS								
Sadness	(0-5)	1	0	0	0	1	1	4
Anger	(0-5)	1	0	0	0	1	1	5
Shame	(0-5)	2	3	0	0	2	2	5
Happiness	(0-5)	2	3	3	4	3	3	0
URGES								
Self-Harm	(0-5)	1	0	0	0	1	2	5
Binge Eat	(0-5)	1	3	0	0	2	2	4
Suicide	(0-5)	0	0	0	0	0	0	4
BEHAVIORS								
Self-Harm	(#, Y/N)	N	N	N	N	N	N	1, Y
Binge Eat	(#, Y/N)	N	Y	N	N	N	N	N
Apply for Jobs	(#, Y/N)	3, Y	2, Y	N	Int!	N	N	N

= Number of times, Y = Yes, N = No, Int! = designated a job interview.

Figure 1. Portion of a sample DBT diary card.

Sessions are structured to address the three target areas in a way that prioritizes safety and the therapeutic relationship. If the diary card indicates that a problem behavior existed in between sessions, the clinician may conduct a behavior chain analysis to better understand the function and nature of the target behavior in the patient's life.

Behavior Chain Analyses (BCA)

Once a target is identified, the clinician utilizes behavior chain analyses in sessions to identify relationships between prompting events and subsequent ineffective behaviors or urges. The chain analysis involves the patient identifying and recording each discrete thought, feeling, body sensation, behavior, and event that occurred between the prompting event and the ineffective response. The BCA helps the patient become an objective observer of the situation and see how the situation progressed the way it did. The thorough nature of the chain analysis enables the clinician to pinpoint exactly where and how an individual could use DBT skills along the chain of events in order to elicit different future outcomes. The chain functions to build awareness of the various contributors in the emotional system, to validate an individual's reaction based on the context of the behavior, and to consider the vulnerability factors and consequences that possibly contributed to engaging in the target behavior. Over time, the patient and clinician are able to observe patterns of particular triggers for ineffective responses, such as events, vulnerabilities, thoughts, or emotions that increase the likelihood of acting impulsively or ineffectively. A patient might not get to discuss a tier-three life-worth-living goal in session if they engaged in a tier-one life-threatening behavior the previous week, as the session will involve breaking down that event to understand what happened and what the patient could have done differently in the moment. From a behavioral perspective, the experience of a behavior chain is considered a "natural consequence" to engaging in a problem behavior, and may serve to encourage patients to abstain from self-harm in order to avoid a chain analysis. Sticking to the structure, while potentially annoying to a patient at times, makes the session predicable and reinforces the idea that nothing supersedes a patient's safety. The case example below highlights this point:

> Mia arrived to session on Tuesday excited to talk about a job interview she had on Friday. Her diary card indicated that she had cut herself on Monday. While I really wanted to hear about the interview, she had a tier-one target that needed to be addressed first. When I said to Mia that we had to do the behavior chain of the self-harm and then, if time permitted, we could talk about her interview, she got very annoyed. "Why do we have to do these behavior chains so much? They're stupid. If you cared about me, you'd want to hear about my interview that I'm really excited about and couldn't wait to tell you about!" she exclaimed. I validated how frustrating it was and how excited I was to hear all about it. However, because she engaged in self-harm, we needed to address that first. "Safety above everything else. If we can stop the self-harm behaviors, we can get to your

life-worth-living stuff. So let's really try to figure this out and see what you can do differently when urges arise this week because I'd rather be talking about your job interview too."

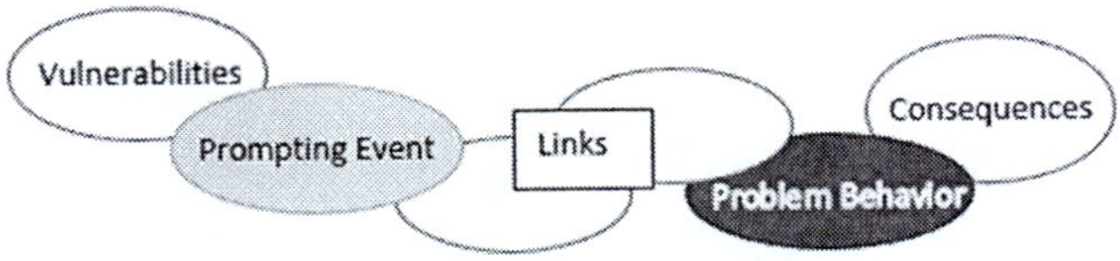

Vulnerability factors: sitting around waiting, feelings of boredom and loneliness, husband's deadline
Prompting event: text from husband
Problem Behaviors: impulsive texting, making threats, cutting

Label* (T, F, B, E)	Description (Chain of Events)	Alternative (Solution Analysis)
E	Sitting at home alone on Monday night at 6pm waiting for my husband	**
F	Bored (3) and Lonely (5)	**
E	Got a text from my husband that he needed to work late and wouldn't be home until 9 or 10pm	**
F	Angry (5)	
T	He doesn't care about me	**
F	Sad (4)	
T	He is probably cheating on me. I'm not good enough.	**
F	Scared (5) and Shame (5)	
T	He's just like everyone else. No one cares. Men are jerks.	**
F	Angry (5)	**
S	Blood rushing to my face, feeling hot, muscles tense	**
B	Texted him multiple times, calling him names, threatening to hurt myself	**
TARGET BEHAVIOR	Got the scissors, cut, and texted him a picture	**
E	He came home	Positive Consequence
F	Calmer because he was home; not lonely, bored, or scared	Positive Consequence
E	He was really angry at me, calling me crazy, slept on the couch and didn't want to speak with me	Negative Consequence
F	Shame (5) and Fear (4)	Negative Consequence
T	I'm so stupid. He's going to leave me if I keep acting like this. (ruminated all night)	Negative Consequence

*T = Thought, F=Feeling, B=Behavior, E=Event, S=Body Sensation;

** Critical links where alternatives strategies can be suggested

Figure 2. Sample DBT behavior chain analysis.

The behavior chain analysis for the above case example breaks down the vulnerability factors, thoughts, emotions, and events that led up to the cutting behavior on Monday. In this example, vulnerability factors that made the chain of events more likely to happen that particular day included sitting at home alone, feeling bored and lonely, and her husband's impending deadline at work. Then, the patient identifies the prompting event and all links between that prompt and the target/problem behaviors. Finally, the chain helps recognize the positive and negative consequences and potential reinforcers of the self-harm after it occurred.

Once the situation is broken down into discrete events, the therapist and patient complete a solution analysis. In the solution analysis phase, the patient and therapist identify "critical links" in which using DBT skills could have disrupted the chain of behavior and potentially prevented the problem behavior from occurring. Possible solutions at those critical links might include making plans with friends, reading a good book, or watching a movie or series that she enjoys. An additional critical link is the thought, "He is probably cheating on me. I'm not good enough." In a solution analysis, the therapist would recommend she use the skill "check the facts," which might remind her that he has a deadline for a project at work that he has been working on and very nervous about all week. When she notices the blood rushing to her head from anger, the therapist might suggest using the distress tolerance skills that she learned in skills group. These alternatives would be written onto the chain for future reference. This is particularly useful if this trigger or series of thoughts, emotions, or urges happen regularly. In this manner, the behavior chain analysis becomes an easily accessible cope ahead plan to increase the likelihood of more skillful behavior in the future.

It is important to note that the solutions identified are options the patient is willing to try. It is not helpful to come up with solutions that the patient would not do or does not have access to in these moments. To increase the chances for success, the solution analysis must be very individualized and requires collaboration with the patient to identify strategies that he or she will and can do. In addition, if the patient reaches out for phone coaching in a similar situation, the therapist can reinforce the strategies the patient came up with and agreed to when completing the solution analysis in session.

DBT Skills Group

The DBT skills group is a way of teaching patients new strategies in order to help them identify and understand emotions and urges, cope with emotions in a healthier manner, communicate with others more effectively, and reduce the likelihood of engaging in dangerous or detrimental behaviors in response to strong emotional stimuli. The standard DBT model for outpatient treatment requires that individuals attend weekly skills group, in addition to weekly individual therapy. Research has found that participation in DBT skills group increases the effectiveness of DBT overall (Linehan et al., 2015). It takes approximately six months to complete the entire cycle of DBT skills learned in group. It is recommended that patients complete two full cycles of DBT to maximize the learning and generalization of skills into one's personal life and triggering situations. Therefore, the typical length of phase one DBT is one-year of individual therapy and skills group.

Skills group follows the same structure and pattern at each session. It begins with a brief mindfulness exercise aimed at increasing group members' focused awareness of the present moment. Group leaders, who are trained DBT clinicians and, when possible, different from the individual DBT clinician, then review the previous week's skill by eliciting examples from group members' homework assignment. The weekly homework assignment asks participants to practice the skill taught, and note their experience. After homework review there is a short break followed by skills training, during which the group leaders teach a new skill to group members.

The skills are divided into sections, or modules, that focus on different deficits experienced by those with BPD. The main modules in DBT skills group are: Mindfulness, Distress Tolerance, Emotion Regulation, and Interpersonal Effectiveness. Walking the Middle Path is a fifth module utilized in DBT-A.

Mindfulness

Mindfulness skills are the first skills taught to help individuals observe and describe their internal experiences in order to participate in the moment in a thoughtful and intentional way. They are the core or central skills of DBT and involve maintaining a focused awareness of the present moment. Given that those who meet criteria for BPD suffer from "instability in affect regulation, impulse control, interpersonal relationship, and self-image" (Linehan, 2015, p. 5), mindfulness is a crucial piece of the treatment process (Linehan & Wilks, 2015) and helps an individual identify the internal and external factors contributing to an emotionally-charged situation. Principles of Zen, specifically mindfulness, are included in DBT to promote awareness and being present in the moment (Lynch, Chapman, Rosenthal, Kuo, & Linehan, 2006; Neacsiu, Ward-Ciesielski, & Linehan, 2012). People diagnosed with BPD often view events as dichotomous and label the events as positive or negative. DBT therapists use mindfulness to promote awareness and acceptance of events as they are, without categorizing events or situations as bad or good (Linehan, 2015; Lynch et al., 2006) and highlight how those labels impact one's emotions.

Mindfulness also teaches a person to sit with thoughts and emotions without judgment and without reaction (Brown, Marquis, & Guiffrida, 2013), which allows more time to intentionally choose an effective response. Hanh (2010) believes that a person who practices being mindful will make better decisions because the decisions will be made in a more deliberate manner. Hanh (1991) also remarked mindfulness can simply begin with mindful breathing, which slows down racing thoughts and reduces mentally living in the past or worrying about future events. People who are absorbed in thoughts are not truly present in the current moment. This lack of awareness greatly contributes to the instability in relationships and impulsivity in behavior found in those diagnosed with BPD.

A person who meets the diagnostic criteria for BPD is prone to risk-taking behavior such as promiscuity and irresponsible spending (APA, 2013). Being mindful of risky behaviors can reduce occurrences of those behaviors (Hanh, 2010). Brown, Marquis and Guiffrida (2013) reported that not only is mindfulness critical to the success of DBT, but that DBT's effectiveness in using mindfulness with challenging clients is one of the major reasons that mindfulness has achieved popularity in the fields of counseling and psychology. BPD is diagnosed using criteria that can be ameliorated by applying mindfulness. For example, being mindful of one's anger allows a person to release it effectively and/or use that anger for a more productive response (Hanh, 2010).

Distress Tolerance

Distress tolerance is one's ability to cope with psychological stress (Kiselica, Webber, & Bornovalova, 2014). This set of skills involves accepting that painful events occur in life. This module helps people develop strategies to tolerate and survive crisis moments without engaging in behaviors that make the situation worse. It is an acceptance of reality as it is, including inevitable painful situations, and "learning to bear pain skillfully" (Linehan, 1993, p. 147). It is not about change but rather acceptance of one's situation, emotions, and experiences as they are. The acknowledgement of the pain along with a willingness to tolerate the moment without acting impulsively are the primary functions of distress tolerance skills.

An inability to tolerate difficult events or feelings can lead to increased avoidance of situations that cause distress (such as social situations or work) or impulsive behaviors (such as substance use or self-harm) to reduce or numb out painful emotions. However, distress is a necessary component of change and therefore, individuals with BPD (who need to make significant changes) need tools to tolerate the inevitable distress that will ensue. Radical acceptance of life as it is does not mean approval of the circumstances of the moment. It simply takes away the need to react to, or change, the moment and thus, distress tolerance skills are a natural complement to the mindfulness skills that also focus on acceptance (Linehan, 2015). Being able to correctly understand and identify emotional states, and accept the moment as it is rather than how we want it to be, is important to increase the tolerance of distress. Engaging in the adaptive behaviors taught in DBT, such as self-soothe or distraction, increases distress tolerance (Gaher, Hofmann, Simons, & Hunsaker, 2013), thereby reducing impulsive and maladaptive coping behaviors used to avoid or change distress (Linehan & Wilks, 2015).

Emotion Regulation

Emotion dysregulation is the central feature of BPD. Individuals with BPD frequently experience emotional intensity and lability, and often do not understand the complex system of their emotional experience. This emotional system includes a prompting event, cognitive interpretations of that event, physiological reactions, and behavioral impulses. Any one of these areas can serve to exacerbate the emotional response as one continues to re-trigger the system with ineffective cognitive and behavioral responses. Emotion Regulation skills are two-fold, and involve both understanding and identifying emotions in order to change or modulate them in a given moment, as well as a variety of skills to reduce vulnerability to emotional lability. Emotion regulation skills include problem-solving for potential situations that could trigger high emotions, exposure to emotional stimuli to encourage re-learning (opposite action), as well as a number of behavioral strategies (e.g., accumulating positive experiences) and physical self-care skills (e.g., balanced eating and getting adequate sleep).

Hypersensitivity in reading emotional cues is one of the primary reasons that people with BPD have difficulty establishing and maintaining relationships (Quattrini et al., 2019). Some research indicates that BPD is marked by increased baseline emotional activity (Kuo, Fitzpatrick, Metcalfe, & McMain, 2016; Quattrini et al., 2019). Kuo and colleagues (2016) suggest that people diagnosed with BPD have higher emotional intensity and vulnerability at rest than those without BPD, which makes controlling their emotions more challenging compared to those in control groups. Nevertheless, they found that those with BPD can learn to effectively reduce their emotional reactivity, improve emotional control, reduce the experience of negative emotions and increase the experience of positive emotions. Considering that increasing the ratio of positive emotions to negative emotions is essential for promoting self-perceived happiness (Seligman, 2006), it is possible that those with BPD can improve their sense of happiness through the use of emotion regulation skills.

Dixon-Gordon, Turner, Rosenthal and Chapman (2017) studied the impact of suppressing emotions versus accepting emotions. They asked people diagnosed with BPD to watch a scene involving social rejection. The participants in the study demonstrated more physiological calmness (lower heart rate variability) when suppressing and not dealing with their emotions then they did when accepting and sitting with their emotions. The findings indicate that the maladaptive behaviors of suppressing and avoiding emotions may produce more immediate benefits for BPD patients, while accepting distressful emotions might take more time to learn and appreciate (Chapman, Rosenthal, Dixon-Gordon, Turner, & Kuppens, 2017). The researchers warn therapists to not indulge in teaching avoidance or suppression, as it could validate these maladaptive behaviors in clients and only allow for short term relief. Instead, teaching patients to accept and regulate emotions helps create long term benefits that positively impact functioning (Chapman et al., 2017; Gaher et al., 2013; Neacsiu, Lungu, Harned, Rizvi, & Linehan, 2014).

Interpersonal Effectiveness

This set of skills involves developing strategies for communicating with others in a way that allows individuals to maintain healthy relationships and have their needs met, without damaging relationships or one's self-respect in the process. Interpersonal Effectiveness relates to creating and strengthening healthy relationships, setting boundaries with others, and communicating in a way that upholds one's values. Often, misperceptions and uncontrollable emotions restrict effective communication and therefore, these skills are often used in conjunction with other DBT strategies that help manage emotions in the moment.

Individuals with BPD have learned, through years of invalidation, that others do not react the same way to situations and do not understand their reactions to situations. This has contributed to individuals with BPD feeling misunderstood and therefore using drastic alternative means, such as threats or splitting, to communicate with others (Linehan, 1993). In addition, BPD criterion, such as an intense fear of abandonment, often encourages maladaptive interpersonal behaviors to prevent others from leaving the relationship. Threatening to commit suicide if a partner ends the relationship, for example, may lead to immediate relief of abandonment fears as the partner is scared into staying. Thus, the threatening behavior is rewarded and reinforced and the individual with BPD learns to use this strategy to keep interpersonal relationships. Nevertheless, it is not a healthy relationship pattern, even though it seemingly "works" and, therefore, the interpersonal effectiveness skills of being gentle and honest, and asking for something in a manner that is assertive, fair, and maintains self-respect serve to replace these maladaptive strategies (Linehan, 2015).

Walking the Middle Path

Walking the Middle Path skills were initially developed for use in DBT-A as a fifth and separate module of skills group specifically for teens and family members. This set of skills focused on changing behaviors within the family. The main skills of this module include dialectical thinking, validation, and finding a middle path solution in conflictual situations. Dialectical thinking allows parents and teens to see that each side has truth and validity. Using validation helps to stop the tug-of-war where each is vehemently trying to prove one's own point, and can de-escalate arguments by helping others to acknowledge each other's perspective. Finding a middle path helps to honor the truth in each person's side of a conflict and seeks to come to a resolution that directly addresses these dialectical truths. For example, if a teenage wants to come home at 2am and a parent wants the teen's curfew to be 10pm, Walking the Middle Path skills help the parent and teen discuss the situation from each one's perspective and to come to an arrangement that is mutually acceptable. Therefore, if a parent is concerned about the teen's safety and the teen is concerned with not missing out on the festivities, a compromise of coming home at midnight does nothing to honor the truths in each of their perspectives and both will likely feel dissatisfied with this solution. A Walking the Middle Path solution might include the teen checking in regularly throughout the night in order to stay later, or the parent wanting to pick the teen up personally to ensure they get home safely. Alternatively, the solution might be that the teen has to come home earlier however, some friends can sleep over so they can continue the festivities where the parents can personally supervise activities. These possible solutions honor the parent's truth of wanting the teen to be safe while also honoring the teen's truth of not wanting to miss out on all the fun.

Despite being developed as a set of skills for families as part of DBT-A, the strategies of dialectical thinking, validation, and finding a middle path solution to conflicts are important in most relationships and therefore, these skills were added to Linehan's 2015 revision of DBT and included as part of the Interpersonal Effectiveness module. Walking the Middle Path skills help improve relationships with healthier communication, increased collaborative problem-solving, and reduced conflict overall (Linehan, 2015; Rathus & Miller, 2002, 2015).

Phone Coaching

Another component of standard DBT is telephone skills coaching. DBT clinicians understand that in moments of high emotion dysregulation, it is difficult for patients to immediately apply the new strategies learned in skills group and individual therapy. As a result, clinicians provide patients with telephone coaching so that a client can contact a therapist and receive help practicing and applying the skills during real-life situations as they are happening. Some examples of when it might be appropriate to use phone coaching include:

1. When a patient is in crisis and having high urges to engage in ineffective behaviors, such as self-injury or suicide,
2. When a patient is in a situation where one could use skills but is not sure which skills to use, or
3. When a patient has done something skillfully and wants to share good news (Linehan, 1993).

Phone coaching intends to help patients solve their problems in effective ways. A phone coaching call should be brief, no more than 10 minutes, and focused on skill generalization. If a patient is having urges for suicide and self-harm, it is critical to encourage patients to call for coaching *before* acting on urges. If a patient does self-harm, a "24 hour rule" goes into effect to avoid reinforcement of the behavior via additional care and attention from the clinician (Linehan, 1993). The "24 hour rule" means that the patient cannot have any unscheduled contact with the clinician for 24 hours following any suicidal or self-harm behavior. If a patient does call the clinician following a suicide attempt or self-injury, the clinician will conduct a brief assessment for safety and help the patient get to the hospital if necessary before ending the call. The clinician will then conduct a more thorough assessment using the behavior chain analysis during the following scheduled session. Upon the initial individual DBT session, the patient and therapist will create and commit to a crisis plan that includes strategies to utilize to delay and prevent acting on urges. This plan is vital as clinicians might not always be available at the particular moment a patient calls for skills coaching. This plan can be implemented and skills can be practiced until the clinician is available to return the call.

Consultation Team

The final component of standard DBT is a weekly consultation team meeting. The purpose of the consultation team is to ensure that each clinician is doing the best work possible with each patient. Every DBT patient is a patient of the whole team, not just of the individual clinician. The team provides the clinician with valuable feedback on how to best help the patient. In addition, the consultation team serves as "therapy for the therapist" to help the clinician deal with their own therapy-interfering behaviors, emotions, thoughts, or burnout. This process ensures that each clinician does the very best work and that the patient receives high quality care.

DBT Assumptions

In developing DBT, Marsha Linehan spelled out assumptions of treatment that are meant to guide clinicians in providing effective, compassionate care. These assumptions help a clinician maintain a mindful and non-judgmental stance of their patients' ineffective behaviors, and builds a humanistic understanding of the borderline patient. For example, in Linehan's second edition of the skills training manual (2015) she adds the following assumption, "Figuring out and changing the causes of behavior is a more effective way to change than judging and blaming – while this is hard, it is more likely to provide long-term benefit" (p. 53). Operating under this assumption helps the clinician maintain a non-judgmental stance and uphold the behavioral tenants of the treatment. The symptoms of borderline personality can be challenging to treat and can often create emotions within the clinician throughout treatment. Clinicians are able to lean on the assumptions to help them tolerate, process, and repair difficult moments such as a suicide attempt or a rift in the patient-therapist relationship. For example, it is helpful particularly in the beginning of treatment, when most skills have not been generalized, to abide by the assumption that, "patients are doing the best they can" in any given moment (Linehan, 2015, p. 53). Therapists can also use the assumptions to guide interventions, or as interventions in and of themselves. The assumption, "Patients may not have caused all of their own problems, but they have to solve them anyway" can be particularly useful in helping a patient both accept the reality of their pain and at the same time work to change what they can in order to feel better and do better in the moment.

Managing Crises in DBT

Often what brings individuals to DBT are severe problems in their lives that are either dangerous or significantly interfering with their quality of life. Family members, loved ones, or patients themselves recognize their self-injurious behavior and/or suicide attempts and ideation as problematic, dangerous, and out-of-control. These patients are suffering and these behaviors help them regulate, either personally or by rallying others to help or reassure them in moments of intense distress. To help curtail these behaviors, therapists need to identify and validate the function of the behavior, in order to work collaboratively to develop alternative healthy strategies to meet those needs instead.

Non-Suicidal Self-Injury (NSSI)

NSSI is non-fatal, intentional injury to oneself often used to regulate emotions or to communicate distress. NSSI includes scratching, cutting, or burning oneself, hitting oneself with one's fists or other objects, smashing one's head or body into walls, or taking pills that are not prescribed or in a way other than how they are prescribed. Proper assessment of previous NSSI behavior is essential and includes asking about the triggers for NSSI, how the behavior occurred, with what means, immediate positive and negative consequences of the behavior, prior need for medical attention, who else was present or involved, presence of suicidal ideation at the time, and any conscious intentions of the behavior. For example, if a new patient has a history of cutting, questions upon initial assessment might include: when cutting started, when the last episode of cutting occurred, how often the patient cuts, what tools have been used to cut, how many cuts are made in an episode, how deep has the person cut in the past, were stitches or other medical interventions ever needed, has the patient ever cut as a suicide attempt or contemplated doing so, do they still have access to means for cutting, and so on.

Reasons for self-harm frequently identified by patients include: to feel physical pain that they know how to handle versus emotional pain that feels unmanageable, to communicate to someone how much distress they are in, to get the "release" that comes following NSSI, or because they feel "numb" afterwards. Patients report that NSSI occurs in moments of intense emotional distress, and the self-harm is used to manage or regulate emotions. NSSI is almost always done alone, in a private place (e.g., one's bedroom, a car, or a bathroom) and using an easily accessible item (e.g., a razor, pencil sharpener blade, scissor, or kitchen knife for cutting; one's own body for scratching or punching oneself). Self-harm usually starts out of desperation to regulate painful emotions. When relief occurs or results in a person feeling more in control, the behavior is reinforced and therefore, maintained. As such, it might be difficult for the patient to consider or try alternatives that might not relieve their distress as quickly as NSSI. This is the reason for phone coaching, to help patients in these moments to consider alternative strategies and motivate them to try something different.

Confidentiality

One of the initial questions asked by patients who come to DBT, especially adolescents, involves what the confidentiality policy is regarding NSSI. Therapists must have these conversations very early in treatment, so that if confidentiality is breached, the patient does not consider it a violation of trust, or a surprise. Whatever the therapist's limits are regarding confidentiality need to be clearly outlined for the patient at the outset of treatment. This might include every instance of NSSI being disclosed to a parent for an adolescent patient, disclosing if there are more than a certain number of episodes per week, disclosing when there are deep and potentially dangerous cuts that increase the likelihood of infection or that warrant medical attention, or when it is done with suicidal intent. Good therapy does not involve surprises, but rather patients know what to expect and can predict the consequences of their actions. Thus, the patient knows from the start of treatment what the conditions are that would warrant a breach in confidentiality. Of note, when a situation warrants disclosing the information (for example, to a parent, spouse, or psychiatrist), it is most helpful to do so with the patient and to coach the patient on how to say it themselves. This models healthy and assertive communication and creates an opportunity to practice skillful behavior, including acting opposite to the urge to avoid, using gentle and honest communication, and effectively managing emotions that arise before, during, or after the disclosure using various distress tolerance strategies.

Suicidality

Suicidal threats or ideation similarly serve an emotion regulation function. Prior to treatment, threats or suicidal thoughts may serve an escape function, allowing individuals to feel that there was a way out of emotional hell. It may give the patient hope that the suffering might end. Threats may have prevented loved ones from leaving or ending a relationship altogether, thus reducing the fear of abandonment and the experience of unbearable loneliness. Assessing the function of suicidal behaviors is necessary to understand the patient's motivation in those moments in order to identify the best potential alternative strategies to get these needs met more effectively.

Although suicidal threats may "work" to accomplish short-term goals, such as avoiding loneliness as mentioned above, suicidal ideation or behaviors distract patients and clinicians from problem solving that could actually help solve the underlying causes of suffering. In addition, it likely causes relationship problems, diminishes self-esteem and self-agency, and burns out the support system, including the therapist. Radically genuine, and nonjudgmental, communication of the impact of these behaviors on the therapist and others can be helpful and can guide patients toward more effective strategies for changing distressing situations in their lives.

As with NSSI, suicidal ideation, threats or attempts require in-depth assessment. Upon intake, the clinician must get a history of suicidality including a detailed account of what happened in each attempt, such as: the trigger, what the patient tried to do, what the outcome was, whether it was planned or impulsive, and how they feel about it now. In addition, it is crucial to assess a patient's intent including asking about a suicide plan and the means to carry it out, if the patient has written suicide letters, and the function of suicidal ideation. A risk assessment is completed at the start of treatment and is continued as necessary throughout treatment to determine changes in risk and protective factors for suicide (see the Linehan Risk Assessment and Management Protocol, LRAMP, for one example of a comprehensive suicide risk assessment measure, available online).

If a patient reports that he or she is considering suicide, the therapist needs to assess the immediate risk and determine "method and means." What method is the patient intending to use and do they have the means to carry out that plan? If the patient states that he wants to shoot himself and has access to a firearm, risk is significantly higher and warrants much more immediate intervention than if he does not have access to any weapons. In addition, will the patient be alone at all that day or over the next few days? Are there individuals that can be available to stay with the patient? What skills or strategies are they willing and able to use at that moment to avoid acting on the urge? The goal is to gather information necessary to properly assess risk and ensure safety. If means are available to carry out a suicide plan, the first priority is to remove access to those means. When the patient is in session and has brought the suicide means to the office, the clinician can ask for it and remove the immediate risk. Our clinic has a locked drawer for sharps, ropes, pills, and other items that patients turn over in session. Clinical staff can then properly dispose of the items. If the patient is not in the office, and risk is determined during a coaching call, the clinician can insist that the patient removes access to means while on the phone. Guns and ammunition can be locked up in a weapon case or trunk of a car and the key given to someone safe; drugs or pills can be flushed down the toilet; razors or sharps can be disposed of in a dumpster or bin outside of the patient's home so they cannot easily access them; ropes can be cut up and disposed of in the trash; and/or the patient can leave the place where the means are available and go someplace else. When possible, it can be helpful to verify that means have been removed by either speaking with someone else who is with the patient or watching (via FaceTime, WhatsApp, Skype, Zoom or any other software that allows for video calls) while the patient follows through on the plan to remove access.

> Marty called in tremendous distress after breaking up with his girlfriend. He felt abandoned, unlovable, and lonely. He was catastrophizing and telling himself that he would never find someone because no one "would ever love a loser like [him]." He had scoured his cabinets and found cleaning supplies, such as bleach and ammonia. He was sitting in his kitchen crying, supplies on the table nearby, wanting to end his life because he could not handle the pain anymore. Marty called to say goodbye and thank you. He initially did not want coaching. He was home alone. After some initial attempts at coaching were not immediately successful, I asked if Marty, who I knew loved soccer, was willing to turn the television on and tell me who was winning the World Cup game. After some hesitation, he agreed to do so. When he saw that his team was playing, he got a little less entrenched in his misery. He was willing to describe the game and do a play-by-play for a few minutes. Although still distraught, he was calmer. He was not willing to go to a friend's house to watch the game. He wanted to sit home and be alone for a little bit. He indicated that his risk was lower and he felt slightly better. However, he would be alone for a while before his roommate returned from work. Uncomfortable with Marty being alone, thinking, and still having access to his means, I insisted that Marty dump the cleaning supplies he had found. I watched via Zoom as Marty poured out the chemicals he wanted to ingest. Reducing the access to dangerous means made both of us feel safer. Marty agreed to check in with updates about the soccer game over the next hour. Within that hour, Marty's friend texted him to hang out and he did not feel as lonely or unlovable. We completed a full behavior chain in the next session about the event and a new risk assessment to determine whether he could be safe between sessions.

If the patient is not willing to use skills or is not collaborative in providing answers to the therapist's assessment questions, the risk increases and therefore, the therapist should follow an emergency protocol. In such a case, the clinician should call an ambulance and/or 911 and report the patient's location, identifying information, and indicate that the individual is feeling suicidal and requires emergency intervention to get them to a hospital to ensure safety and receive further assessment. Knowing the patient's location is imperative and, therefore, it is a good habit to begin a coaching call by getting the patient's location in case the situation escalates. If the patient is in a city or crowded location, it might also be useful to know what they are wearing or how someone might be able to identify them if necessary.

> During consultation team, a clinician received an urgent text from a patient's mother indicating that the patient had stormed out of the apartment after an argument and stated that she would never see her again. The clinician called the patient and learned that she was walking to a bridge and intended to jump to her death. She would not indicate which bridge and was very distressed. The clinician encouraged the patient to stay in the present moment and to describe what she saw around her as she walked. This served as both a distraction from the emotions and provided us with information about the patient's potential whereabouts. Meanwhile, another clinician on the team reached out to the patient's mother and asked her to locate her daughter through the tracker app on her phone. In addition, information was gathered regarding what the patient was wearing when she left the apartment. While the clinician remained on the phone with the patient, the other team member notified the area police with the information, including what the patient was wearing and the potential bridges she might be headed towards based on the information we had at the time. The clinician remained on the phone with the patient the entire time and was able to convince her to willingly go with the police once they were on the scene. The officers were able to bring the patient to the hospital for further assessment and care. In the following session after discharge from the hospital, the clinician completed a full behavior chain with solution analysis as well as addressed the therapy-interfering behavior of not being forthcoming regarding her location at the time of the incident.

Higher Level of Care

In DBT, hospitalizations are avoided when possible, and it is one of the goals of treatment to reduce emergency room visits or hospitalizations. The treatment provides alternative strategies for dealing with stressors in the patient's environment, which means the patient will learn the most if they are able to remain in their environment. When symptoms or urges arise, DBT views this as an opportunity to learn and apply new behavior. To learn skills or discuss alternatives in the hospital setting where patients are not experiencing real-world stressors is not viewed as an effective course of action, but rather a break in the treatment (Linehan, 1993). That said, short-term hospitalization or longer-term residential placement are not always avoidable and there are times when the patient warrants a higher level of care than outpatient treatment. Some situations that may lead to the recommendation for a higher level of care include, when:

1. a patient is not responding to treatment and has significant risk factors for suicide,
2. a patient continues to be unsafe with escalating threats or high-risk behaviors,
3. a patient is in a psychotic state and threatening suicide,
4. the risk of suicide outweighs the risk of inappropriate hospitalization, or
5. the therapeutic relationship is significantly strained creating additional risk of suicide (or a reduction in protective factors against suicide).

Hospitalization ensures momentary safety and allows additional consultation from inpatient providers regarding the treatment course and direction. It can also allow for a medication adjustment in a quicker and more effective manner with careful observation. Residential placement may allow the patient to receive the necessary DBT skills training more quickly, or provide treatment for the underlying issue that triggers suicidal urges (e.g., trauma or eating disorders) in a safer environment. The following case example highlights this benefit:

> Terry was struggling with debilitating anxiety. As a business owner, spouse, and parent, they were often overwhelmed and would have regular panic attacks. The fear that something was terribly wrong and that they would die of a heart attack was very high and Terry often thought of suicide as a way out of the daily anxiety and stress. Terry also met criteria for borderline personality disorder and needed DBT. Terry had been to many treatment providers and all had hospitalized at some point because of the frequent suicidal threats and gestures. Terry would tie ropes around their neck and go to rooftops where they would consider jumping. While Terry needed DBT for relationship problems and emotional dysregulation, the frequent and debilitating panic attacks made it impossible to target anything else in the treatment. Without reducing the panic symptoms, the suicidal urges would not dissipate; however, it was incredibly difficult to do panic treatment or exposures with the suicidal gestures present. While learning DBT skills was a priority, Terry needed panic-specific treatment to alleviate the underlying cause of the suicide urges and doing so in an outpatient clinic was proving ineffective. Recommendation was made for a residential facility where Terry could receive intensive, evidence-based panic treatment in a quick and safe way, where they were under constant observation and did not have means to harm oneself. Terry then returned to an outpatient level of care for DBT and the remaining treatment goals were able to be discussed with the panic symptoms disrupting progress.

Self-Care for DBT Clinicians

Burnout

Patients who come to DBT often exhibit a complex clinical picture and high-risk behaviors that warrant considerable time and energy to manage. In addition, they often lack effective communication skills and have limited tools to manage their intense emotional experiences. This combination of clinical complexity, high risk, and poor coping and communication strategies increase the chances for burnout and compassion fatigue in the treating clinicians (Dimeff & Linehan, 2001; Ditty, Landes, Doyle & Beidas, 2015; Linehan, 1993). Understanding the weight of the clinical burden on DBT clinicians, Linehan designed DBT with a component meant to help support the therapist during the course of treatment, the consultation team. DBT clinicians are expected to work with a clinical consultation team who can help validate their stress, identify therapy-interfering behaviors including inadvertently reinforcing problematic patient behaviors, and support the therapist during difficult treatment moments. Consultation is considered "therapy for the therapist" in DBT.

In addition to consultation team, skill use amongst DBT providers was found as a significant predictor of lower burnout (Jergensen, 2017). In teaching emotional awareness, mindfulness, and coping strategies to manage distress and reduce emotional vulnerability, DBT practitioners have access to and knowledge of a large repertoire of adaptive and skillful behaviors. When clinicians utilize consultation and practice what they preach with regard to skills, they are less likely to experience burnout or compassion fatigue.

> In our center, consultation team is weekly for 2 to 3 hours, clinician burnout is targeted in team, and no clinician works more than a 4-day work week or on the weekends. This helps us focus on our own life worth living goals outside of work and provides adequate time for rest and relaxation. In addition, a regular mindfulness practice is encouraged, healthy foods are stocked in our office pantry, and therapists and staff check in on each other often throughout the workday to offer support, validation, or distraction from clinical stressors. Copies of risk assessments and behavior chains are readily available, and phone numbers for local hospitals, patient information and emergency contacts are all kept in folders on an accessible secure server so that clinicians do not have the added stress of making copies or finding phone numbers during crises. Front desk staff are all psychology graduate students or working in the mental health field (e.g., part-time school psychologist, crisis center volunteer) and receive basic training including knowledge and understanding of BPD and some assumptions and strategies from DBT to help manage patients over the

phone or if a crisis erupts in the office. These things make a tremendous difference.

When the work is already stressful, it is important to not have added obstacles that could be avoided. Having additional support and good self-care are extremely helpful to ensure longevity as a DBT clinician and limit burnout. Focusing on the progress of various patients or successful moments in treatment also help reduce burnout by keeping in mind the benefits and purpose of the difficult work.

Limit-Setting

One of the fundamental relationship problems with individuals with BPD is poor boundaries. Patients either put up a guard to protect themselves from potential abandonment or rejection, or so desperately want to be understood, validated, and liked that they flood the therapist with information and seek attention or assistance regularly. Often, the patient vacillates between these extremes making the therapeutic relationship a wonderful example of interpersonal problems or deficits, and providing the therapist with opportunities for radical genuineness, effective communication, and limit setting. Modeling how to set boundaries with others is an important tool for both the therapist, to avoid burnout, and for the patient, to learn more appropriate interpersonal strategies.

There are no rigid rules about specific limits in DBT; however, it is important to the sustainability of the treatment with each patient as well as the long-term sustainability of the clinician doing DBT to be mindful of limits. The therapist must decide if they want to be available 24/7 for phone coaching or between certain hours, such as 7am and 11pm. In addition, the therapist determines boundaries regarding coaching as far as their preference for patients to call, email, or send a text message. It is up to the clinician to determine what works for them, for the relationship, and for the intended goal. Some clinicians prefer text or email for scheduling issues or good news but want a live telephone call for coaching - to be able to hear the person's voice, collaborate more quickly, and avoid misinterpretations that can occur through written text. As far as frequency of communication or words that a patient might use, a clinician must be mindful of what crosses their limits. In session, what behaviors are intolerable or reduce the clinician's connection with the patient? The more mindful that a clinician can be about how the patient pushes limits or what specific behaviors help or hurt the connection, the better the treatment will be because specific interpersonal targets can be explored and discussed. In addition, by ignoring a patient's behaviors that cross one's limits or boundaries, the clinician is more likely to burn out and be less effective in the treatment. Therefore, mindfulness of one's limits is necessary and adjustment of limits as needed is also important to the clinician's self-care and the longevity of the treatment.

Mindful Preparation

Patients who come to DBT often report NSSI and/or suicidal ideation, therefore, it is imperative to have an emergency contact on file of those who either live with the patient or nearby, the current address of the patient, nearest emergency room information, psychiatrist contact information, and the patient's cell phone number, and to keep this information readily available to ensure the patient's safety in case of emergency. Having copies of suicide risk assessments, behavior chains, authorization forms for release of information, and diary cards readily available helps clinicians have whatever they might need in a given session accessible and easily located. DBT is difficult enough. Make sure the easy stuff, like copies and access to necessary information in a crisis, does not add any additional burden.

Clinicians who are thoughtful about what they might need during the week can plan accordingly and avoid some unnecessary stress. For example, if a clinician's highest risk patients come on Tuesday evenings and the clinician knows they are emotionally dysregulated afterwards, the clinician might plan to go to the gym or to call a funny friend on the way home Tuesday nights. If a clinician engages in crisis management with a newer patient every week, that clinician might want to plan a break after that session to take a walk, go to the bathroom, or consult with a colleague instead of scheduling another patient immediately afterwards. While it is often necessary to schedule back-to-back appointments, a clinician must be mindful and honest about how that is affecting them and adjust accordingly to be able to deliver quality care and prevent burnout.

SUMMARY AND CONCLUSION

Dialectical Behavior Therapy offers a straightforward and comprehensive approach to treating individuals with BPD who were once considered "untreatable." Acceptance combined with the mindful and intentional use of skills makes DBT effective. Structured individual psychotherapy and group skills training, phone coaching for support in the moment of crisis, and consultation team for the treating therapist are all necessary components of an adherent DBT program. Since the time of Linehan's initial publication in 1993, numerous randomized control trials have demonstrated DBT's efficacy. Linehan (2015) and others have found that DBT treatment of at least twelve months produces the greatest and most enduring symptom reduction.

Research has begun to explore the effectiveness of less intensive versions of DBT (without all four components) to determine whether similar reductions in self-harm, impulsivity, hospitalizations, emergency room visits, depression, and emotion dysregulation can still be achieved. If so, more patients might benefit from DBT with greater cost containment. At present, however, data indicate that time-limited versions of DBT appear to be less effective for enduring symptom reduction. This is an important consideration in the context of increasing pressure from third-party payers to contain costs by employing brief treatment models. Fiscally-driven models of care have yet to demonstrate robust clinical outcomes for BPD. In the future, longitudinal research is suggested to clarify the relative cost effectiveness of standard DBT treatment versus time-limited DBT treatment for patients with BPD.

Given that the therapeutic relationship has been a well-known supported component of effective treatment, it is important for the relationship between the patient and clinician to be a focus of the treatment. Therapy interfering behaviors on the part of either the patient or the clinician must be explored and discussed in session and/or in consultation team to prevent disruption in the treatment process. Clinicians must also practice what they preach and establish self-care routines and mindful preparation strategies to reduce burnout and to ensure high quality care.

References

American Psychiatric Association. (2013). *Diagnostic and statistical manual of mental disorders* (5th ed.). Arlington, VA: American Psychiatric Association. https://doi.org/10.1176/appi.books.9780890425596.

Bedics, J. D., Atkins, D. C., Harned, M. S., & Linehan, M. M. (2015). The therapeutic alliance as a predictor of outcome in dialectical behavior therapy versus nonbehavioral psychotherapy by experts for borderline personality disorder, *Psychotherapy, 52*(1),67-77. https://doi.org/10.1037/a0038457.

Brown, A. P., Marquis, A., & Guiffrida, D. A. (2013). Mindfulness-based interventions in counseling. *Journal of Counseling and Development, 91*(1), 96. https://doi.org/10.1002/j.1556-6676.2013.00077.x.

Byrnes, J., Fava, J., Feinman, L., & Harari, E. (2013, November). The relationship between emotion regulation and treatment completion in an adolescent DBT sample. Poster session presented at the *Annual Conference of the International Society for the Improvement and Teaching of Dialectical Behavior Therapy*, Nashville, TN.

Chapman, A. L., Rosenthal, M. Z., Dixon-Gordon, K., Turner, B. J., & Kuppens, P. (2017). Borderline personality disorder and the effects of instructed emotional avoidance or acceptance in daily life. *Journal of Personality Disorders, 31*(4), 483-502. https://doi.org/10.1521/pedi_2016_30_264.

Choi-Kain, L. W., Finch, E. F., Masland, S. R., Jenkins, J. A., & Unruh, B. T. (2017). What works in the treatment of borderline personality disorder, Current Behavioral Neuroscience Reports, *4*(21). https://doi.org/10.1007/s40473-017-0103-z.

Cristea, I. A., Gentili, C., Cotet, C. D., Palomba, D., Barbui, C., & Cuijpers, P. (2017). Efficacy of psychotherapies for borderline personality disorder: A systematic review and meta-analysis, *JAMA Psychiatry*. *74*(4), 319–328. https://doi.org/10.1001/jamapsychiatry.2016.4287.

DeCou, R. C., Comtois, A. K., & Landes, S. (2018). Dialectical behavior therapy is effective for the treatment of suicidal Behavior: A meta-analysis. *Behavior Therapy*, *50*(1), 60-72. https://doi.org/10.1016/j.beth.2018.03.009.

Dimeff, L. & Linehan, M. (2001). Dialectical behavior therapy in a nutshell. *The California Psychologist, 34*(3), 10-13. https://doi.org/10.1177/0011000011421023.

Ditty, M. S., Landes, S. J., Doyle, A., & Beidas, R. S. (2015). It takes a village: A mixed method analysis of inner setting variables and dialectical behavior therapy implementation. *Administration and Policy in Mental Health and Mental Health Services Research, 42*(6), 672-681. https://doi.org/10.1007/s10488-014-0602-0.

Dixon-Gordon, K. L., Turner, B. J., Rosenthal, M. Z., & Chapman, A. L. (2017). Emotion regulation in borderline personality disorder: An experimental investigation of the effects of instructed acceptance and suppression. *Behavior Therapy, 48*(6), 750-764. https://doi.org/10.1016/j.beth.2017.03.001.

Feigenbaum, J. D., Fonagy, P., Pilling, S., Jones, A. H., Wildgoose, A., & Bebbington, P. (2012). A real-world study of the effectiveness of DBT in the UK National Health Service. *The British Journal of Clinical Psychology, (51)*2, 121-41. https://doi.org/10.1111/j.2044-8260.2011.02017.x.

Ferguson, A. (2016) Borderline personality disorder and access to services: A crucial social justice issue, *Australian Social Wor*k, *69*(2), 206-214. https://doi.org/10.1080/0312407X.2015.1054296.

Fleischhaker, C., Böhme, R., Sixt, B., Brück, C., Schneider, C., & Schulz, E. (2011). Dialectical behavioral therapy for adolescents (DBT-A): A clinical trial for patients with suicidal and self-injurious behavior and borderline symptoms with a one-year follow-up. *Child and Adolescent Psychiatry and Mental Health*, *5*(1), 3. https://doi.org/10.1186/1753-2000-5-3.

Flückiger, C., Del Re, A. C., Wampold, B. E., Symonds, D., & Horvath, A. O. (2012). How central is the alliance in psychotherapy? A multilevel longitudinal meta-analysis, *Journal of Counseling Psychology, 59*(1), 10-17. https://doi.org/10.1037/a0025749.

Fruzzetti, A. E., & Levensky, E. R. (2000). Dialectical behavior therapy for domestic violence: Rationale and Procedures. *Cognitive and Behavioral Practice, 7*(4), 435-447. https://doi.org/10.1016/S1077-7229(00)80055-3.

Gaher, R., Hofman, M., Simons, N., & Hunsaker, L. (2013). Emotion regulation deficits as mediators between trauma exposure and borderline symptoms. *Cognitive Therapy and Research, 37*(3), 466-475. https://doi.org/10.1007/s10608-012-9515-y.

Groves, S., Backer, H. S., Van den Bosch, L., & Miller, A. (2011). Dialectical behaviour therapy with adolescents. *Child and Adolescent Mental Health*, *17*(2), 65-75. https://doi.org/10.1111/j.1475-3588.2011.00611.x.

Hanh, T. N. (1991). *Peace is every step: The path of mindfulness in everyday life.* New York, NY: Bantam Books.

Hanh, T. N. (2010). *You are here: Discovering the magic of the present moment.* Boston, MA: Shambala.

Harned, M. S., Chapman, A. L., Dexter-Mazza, E. T., Murray, A., Comtois, K. A., & Linehan, M. (2008). Treating co-occurring Axis I disorders in recurrently suicidal women with borderline personality disorder: A 2-year randomized trial of dialectical behavior therapy versus community treatment by experts. *Journal of Consulting and Clinical Psychology, 76*(6), 1068-1075. https://doi.org/10.1037/a0014044.

Harned, M. S., Korslund, K. E., & Linehan, M. (2014). A pilot randomized controlled trial of dialectical behavior therapy with and without the

Dialectical behavior therapy prolonged exposure protocol for suicidal and self-injuring women with borderline personality disorder and PTSD. *Behaviour Research and Therapy*, *55*, 7–17. https://doi.org/10.1016/j.brat.2014.01.008.

Jergensen, Kate. (2017). Practice what you preach: An exploration of DBT Therapists' personal skill utilization in burnout prevention. *Clinical Social Work Journal. 46*(5). https://doi.org/10.1007/s10615-017-0633-6.

Keuroghlian, A. S., Palmer, B. A., Choi-Kain, L. W., Borba, C. P., Links, P. S., & Gunderson, J. G. (2016). The effect of attending good psychiatric management (GPM) workshops on attitudes toward patients with borderline personality disorder. *Journal of personality disorders*, *30*(4), 567–576. https://doi.org/10.1521/pedi_2015_29_206.

Kiselica, A. M., Webber, T., & Bornovalova, M. A. (2014). Stability and change in distress tolerance and its prospective relationship with borderline personality features: A short-term longitudinal study. *Personality Disorders: Theory, Research, and Treatment*, *5*(3), 247–256. https://doi.org/10.1037/per0000076.

Kuo, J. R., Fitzpatrick, S., Metcalfe, R. K., & McMain, S. (2016). A multi-method laboratory investigation of emotional reactivity and emotion regulation abilities in borderline personality disorder. *Journal of Behavior Therapy and Experimental Psychiatry*, *50*, 52-60. https://doi.org/10.1016/j.jbtep.2015.05.002.

Lee, N. K., Cameron, J., & Jenner, L. (2015). Review of treatment for substance use and borderline personality disorder. *Drug and Alcohol Review*, *34*, 663-672. https://doi.org/10.1111/dar.12267.

Linehan, M. M., Armstrong, H. E., Suarez, A., Allmon, D., & Heard, H. L. (1991). Cognitive behavioral treatment of chronically parasuicidal borderline patients. *Archives of General Psychiatry, 48*(12), 1060-1064. https://doi.org/10.1001/archpsyc.1991.01810360024003.

Linehan, M. (1993). *Cognitive behavioral treatment of borderline personality disorder*. New York, NY: Guilford Press.

Linehan, M. M., Heard, H. L., & Armstrong, H. E. (1993). Naturalistic follow-up of a behavioral treatment for chronically parasuicidal borderline patients. *Archives of General Psychiatry, 50*(12), 971-974. https://doi.org/10.1001/archpsyc.1993.01820240055007.

Linehan, M. M. (2015). *DBT Skills Training Manual* (2nd ed.). New York, NY: Guilford Press.

Linehan, M., Korslund, K. E., Harned, M., Gallop, R. J., Lungu, A., & Neacsiu, A., McDavid, J., Comtois, K., & Murray-Gregory, A. (2015). Dialectical behavior therapy for high suicide risk in individuals with borderline personality disorder: A randomized clinical trial and component analysis. *JAMA psychiatry*, *72*(5), 475-482. https://doi.org/10.1001/jamapsychiatry.2014.3039.

Linehan, M. M. & Wilks, C. (2015). The course and evolution of dialectical behavior therapy. *American Journal of Psychotherapy, 69*(2), 97-110. https://doi.org/10.1176/appi.psychotherapy.2015.69.2.97.

Lynch, T. R., Chapman, A. L., Rosenthal, M. Z., Kuo, J. R. and Linehan, M. M. (2006). Mechanisms of change in dialectical behavior therapy: Theoretical and empirical observations. *Journal of Clinical Psychology, 62*(4), 459-480. https://doi.org/10.1002/jclp.20243.

Mccauley, E., Berk, M., Asarnow, J. Adrian, M., Cohen, J., Korslund, K., Avina, C., Hughes, J., Harned, M., Gallop, R., & Linehan, M. (2018). Efficacy of dialectical behavior therapy for adolescents at high risk for suicide: A randomized clinical trial. *JAMA Psychiatry*, 75*(8), 777-785.* https://doi.org/10.1001/jamapsychiatry.2018.1109.

Mehlum, L., Ramberg, M., Tørmoen, A., Haga, E., Diep, L., Laberg, S., Larsson, B. S., Stanley, B. H., Miller, A. L., Sund, A., & Groholt, B. (2016). Dialectical behavior therapy compared with enhanced usual care for adolescents with repeated suicidal and self-harming behavior: Outcomes over a one-year follow-up. *Journal of the American Academy of Child and Adolescent Psychiatry*, *55*(4), 295-300. https://doi.org/10.1016/j.jaac.2016.01.005.

Mehlum, L., Ramleth, R., Tørmoen, A. J., Haga, E., Diep, L. M., Stanley, B. H., Miller, A. L., Larsson, B., Sund, A. M. and Grøholt, B. (2019). Long term effectiveness of dialectical behavior therapy versus enhanced usual care for adolescents with self-harming and suicidal behavior.

Journal of Child Psychology and Psychiatry, (in press). https://doi.org/10.1111/jcpp.13077.

Neacsiu, A. D., Lungu, A., Harned, M. S., Rizvi, S. L., & Linehan, M. M. (2014). Impact of dialectical behavior therapy versus community treatment by experts on emotional experience, expression, and acceptance in borderline personality disorder. *Behaviour Research and Therapy, 53*(1), 47-54. https://doi.org/10.1016/j.brat.2013.12.004.

Neacsiu, A. D., Ward-Ciesielski, E. F., & Linehan, M. M. (2012). Emerging approaches to counseling intervention: Dialectical behavior therapy. *Counseling Psychologist, 40*(7), 1003-1032. https://doi.org/10.1177/0011000011421023.

Pennay, A., Cameron, J., Reichert, T., Strickland, H., Lee, N. K., Hall, K., & Lubman, D. I. (2011). A systematic review of interventions for co-occurring substance use disorder and borderline personality disorder. *Journal of Substance Abuse Treatment*, *41*(4), 363-373. https://doi.org/10.1016/j.jsat.2011.05.004.

Quattrini, G., Pini, L., Pievani, M., Magni, L. R., Lanfredi, M., Ferrari, C., Rossi, R. (2019). Abnormalities in functional connectivity in borderline personality disorder: Correlations with metacognition and emotion dysregulation. *Psychiatry Research: Neuroimaging, 283*, 118-124. https://doi.org/10.1016/j.pscychresns.2018.12.010.

Rathus, J. H., & Miller, A. L. (2002). Dialectical behavior therapy adapted for Suicidal adolescents. *Suicide and Life-Threatening Behavior, 32*(2), 146-157. https://doi.org/10.1521/suli.32.2.146.24399.

Rathus, J. H., & Miller, A. L. (2015). *DBT skills manual for adolescents*. New York, NY, US: Guilford Press.

Rosenfeld, B. Galietta, M., Ivanoff, A., Garcia-Mansilla, A., Martinez, R., Fava, J., Fineran, V., & Green, D. (2007). Dialectical behavior therapy for the treatment of stalking offenders. *International Journal of Forensic Mental Health. 6*. 95-103. https://doi.org/10.1080/14999013.2007.10471254.

Seligman, M. P. (2006). *Learned optimism: How to change your mind and your life.* New York, NY: Vintage Books.

Sheehan, L., Nieweglowski, K. & Corrigan, P. (2016). The Stigma of Personality Disorders, *Current Psychiatry Reports*, *18*(11). https://doi.org/10.1007/s11920-015-0654-1.

Stoffers-Winterling, J. M., Völlm, B. A., Rücker, G., Timmer, A., Huband, N., & Lieb, K. (2012). Psychological therapies for people with borderline personality disorder. *Cochrane Database of Systemic Reviews, 8*(CD005652). https://doi.org/10.1002/14651858.CD005652.pub2.

Tebbett-Mock A. A., Saito E., McGee M., Woloszyn P., & Venuti M. (2019). Efficacy of dialectical behavior therapy versus treatment as usual for acute-care inpatient adolescents, *Journal of the American Academy of Child & Adolescent Psychiatry,* in press. https://doi.org/10.1016/j.jaac.2019.01.020.

Verheul, R., van den Bosch, L. M. C., Koeter, M. W. J., De Ridder, M. A. J., Stijnen, T., & Van Den Brink, W. (2003). Dialectical behaviour therapy for women with borderline personality disorder: 12-month, randomised clinical trial in The Netherlands. *The British Journal of Psychiatry, 182*(2), 135-140. https://doi.org/10.1192/bjp.182.2.135.

Williams, S. Hartstone, M., & Denson, L. (2010). Dialectical behavioural therapy and borderline personality disorder: Effects on service utilization and self-reported symptoms. *Behaviour Change, 27*(4), 251-264. https://doi.org/10.1375/bech.27.4.251.

Woolcott, P. Jr (1985) Prognostic indicators in the psychotherapy of borderline patients. *American Journal of Psychotherapy*, 39, 17-29. https://doi.org/10.1176/appi.psychotherapy.1985.39.1.17.

In: Borderline Personality Disorder
Editor: Charles M. Lepkowsky
ISBN: 978-1-53618-021-3

Chapter 7

CONSTRUCTIONIST APPROACHES TO TREATING BORDERLINE PERSONALITY DISORDER

***Stephen Bacon**, PhD**
Independent Practice, Santa Barbara, California, US

ABSTRACT

The results of significant new research meta-analyses using the contextual model have challenged basic assumptions about how psychotherapy works. These changes have led to new perspectives on how to treat different diagnoses and specifically, suggest innovative approaches to treating Borderline Personality Disorder (BPD). The basics of the contextual model are presented, with an explanation of findings from a social constructionist perspective. Both the BPD diagnostic category and the concept that extant treatment approaches have inherent power are examined and decontructed. Specific constructionist interventions for BPD are discussed and recommended.

---

* Corresponding Author's E-mail: stephen@drstephenbacon.com.

Keywords: psychotherapy, theories of psychotherapy, borderline personality disorder, contextual model, constructionism

INTRODUCTION

There is a rich history of how the psychotherapy field has responded to the Borderline Personality Disorder (BPD) diagnosis, including increasingly specific diagnostic criteria, detailed individual therapy protocols, and manualized group therapy models. The BPD diagnosis and its treatment can be viewed from an alternative perspective, that of social constructionism and the contextual model. The contextual model group coalesced around efforts to create a psychotherapeutic paradigm that was more congruent with the outcome research than the ruling paradigm of the medical model. The medical model begins with an assessment leading to a diagnosis, for which the therapist uses an evidence-based technique to resolve the issue. The medical model is both diagnostic-centric and technique-centric. Conversely, the contextual model (Duncan, Miller, Wampold, & Hubble, 2010) begins with a review and a fresh analysis of the outcome literature. Based on the results of those analyses, some surprising and provocative conclusions can be made. Contextual authors argue that psychotherapeutic techniques lack inherent power and are actually rituals (Anderson, Lunnen, & Ogles, 2010), that therapists fail to get better as a result of experience (Miller & Hubble, 2011), that our training models, including graduate education, workshops, continuing education, and supervision, fail to enhance outcomes (Thomas, 2014), and that the field as a whole is generating the same results as it did forty years ago with no indications that there has been any progress or evolution (Miller, Hubble, & Duncan, 2007). If these arguments are valid, they will have an enormous impact on the treatment of BPD, and on the entire field of psychotherapy, making it necessary to understand the essence of the contextual model arguments.

The contextual model arguments are essentially contained in two seminal works, *The Heart and Soul of Change: Delivering What Works in Therapy* (Duncan, Miller, Wampold, & Hubble, 2010) and *The Great*

Psychotherapy Debate (Wampold & Imel, 2015). Supplemental arguments and the constructionist perspective come from additional recent work (Bacon, 2018). The lack of training effects is one of the major findings supporting the contextual model. Training effects are common and robust in most professions. However, this is not true of the field of psychotherapy. The initial article raising doubts about training effects was the famous Strupp and Hadley (1976) study, which showed that untrained college professors were capable of achieving equivalent positive outcomes in comparison to experienced, licensed therapists. That study was recently replicated when Anderson, Crowley, Himawan, Holmberg, and Uhlin (2016) compared the outcomes of advanced clinical psychology graduate students with graduate students in non-helping fields (e.g., history or biology). The authors found that both groups achieved equivalent positive results with normal neurotics. While these were relatively small studies, they have huge implications. Are therapeutic outcomes really so easy to achieve that the untrained can match the trained and experienced?

Unfortunately for the credibility of the psychotherapy field, review articles on training have supported these conclusions. Malouff (2012), in his review of training in psychology graduate programs, noted that, "There appears to be no evidence to suggest that coursework and research completion, which make up a great deal of required psychology training, have any value to future psychotherapy clients of the students (p. 31)." His evaluation of training programs as a whole concluded, "Overall, research findings provide little support for the idea that typical professional training of psychologists leads to better outcomes for their psychotherapy clients (p. 29)."

Hill and Knox (2013), in their review article on training, find a variety of outcomes. Some showed small effects for the benefits of training, a couple showed a negative effect from training, and most showed no significant effects. This pattern of results is found when researching a factor that has small, negligible, or no effects. This is widely at variance with the training effects seen in most professions. Hill and Knox also found evidence that students can be trained in specific skills, such as applying a manualized treatment program, but there was no evidence that these skills translated into better client outcomes and there was additional evidence that this kind of skill acquisition faded over time. Here is their summary statement about the effects of training:

> The results of these studies certainly do not provide direct evidence for the effectiveness of training; in fact, they call into question the very necessity of this training. … No differences were found, however, between trained experienced therapists and friendly college professors or lay helpers, nor between clinical psychology graduate students and graduate students in nonhelping professions who were equally matched in terms of facilitative levels. (p. 799)

The lack of training effects is one of the provocative and peculiar findings in the outcome literature analysis. It is certainly does not arise from a dearth of effort. There are literally thousands of books and articles designed to contribute to professional psychotherapeutic knowledge and a myriad of trained, motivated, and competent professionals and academics who work unceasingly in the area. The sum of their efforts is what might be termed psychotherapy's privileged knowledge: the knowledge that characterizes the profession, the knowledge that must be mastered to succeed at the profession. If all this effort has failed to establish potent privileged knowledge, there must be something different about the field of psychotherapy, something that precludes establishing the robust knowledge base belonging to fields such as chemistry or engineering.

The second major area with provocative negative findings is the question of whether experience enhances effectiveness in psychotherapy. This is also an area where one would expect to find robust effect sizes. Experienced surgeons get better outcomes than beginners, tennis players with years of experience beat players with weeks of experience. In most fields the experienced best the inexperienced. However, in psychotherapy, this experience factor is notably absent.

The relationship between experience and outcome can be tested. Psychology has performed hundreds of treatment outcome studies which have also included measurements of therapist experience. The data, whether bundled together in large meta-analyses or taken individually, have consistently failed to find a relationship between experience and outcome. For example, Lambert & Ogles state (2004):

> ...overall, the meta-analytic reviews of psychotherapy that have provided correlational data find little evidence for a relationship between experience and outcome. (p. 169)

In a 2013 review article Hill and Knox summarize the same material by citing two seminal studies:

> Two recent analyses of very large numbers of therapists perhaps provide the most definitive evidence about therapist experience. Wampold and Brown (2005) found no effects for therapist experience level (years of practice) when they analyzed the outcomes of 6,146 clients seen by 581 therapists in a managed care setting (all therapists were postdegree). Similarly, Okiishi et al. (2006) found no effects of therapist experience level (pre-internship, internship, post internship) on the speed of client improvement in their study of more than 5,000 clients seen by 71 therapists at a university counseling center. (p. 797)

"Practice makes perfect" is a cliché, but a cliché that is based in reality. This finding suggests that psychotherapy differs markedly from other professions that have a typical relationship to experience. It also suggests that psychotherapists must be doing something during practice that blocks their ability to learn from experience.

The third and final research finding is the so-called "Dodo bird" effect, the finding that different schools of therapy achieve equivalent positive results.

> The conclusion of most, but not all, of these reviews is similar to that drawn by Luborsky, Singer, and Luborsky (1975) who suggested a verdict similar to that of the Dodo bird in Alice in Wonderland: "Everyone has won and all must have prizes."... However, meta-analytic methods have now been extensively applied to large groups of comparative studies, and these reviews generally offer similar conclusions, that is, little or no difference between therapies. (Lambert & Ogles, 2004, p. 161)

This finding is robust and frequently replicated. It has stood up against a variety of critiques. However, of the three arguments marshalled by the contextual model group, the Dodo bird effect is the most debatable. This is due, of course, to the fact that there are literally hundreds of studies that have found one technique superior to another, at least in certain circumstances. In response, the Dodo bird defenders cite metanalyses and research design flaws to account for the seeming superiority.

The Dodo bird debate is essentially a discussion about whether there are any specific factors in psychotherapy. The effects of psychotherapy are divided between common factors, most often portrayed as a relationship with a wise and caring therapist, and specific factors, the innately powerful techniques and ideas developed by each different psychotherapy system. When the Dodo bird conclusion is accepted so that each school is seen as achieving equivalent, positive results, it implicitly destroys the argument for specific factors. This is due to the obviously irrational idea that every school has "coincidentally" developed specific factors that account for an equivalent amount of the variance in outcome. In other words, given that each school has very different theories and very different interventions, is it feasible that they would generate the exact same size positive effects? That is highly unlikely, leading to the conclusion that therapy consists of nothing but common factors. The differing interventions, it can be concluded, are simply therapeutic rituals. The rituals must be convincing and believable but, in truth, their form and structure are unimportant, mere empty vehicles powered by expectations.

Accepting the stance that psychotherapeutic interventions are placebos/rituals makes psychotherapy "unscientific", feels counter-intuitive, and reduces the status of the profession. It is easy to see how the debate over the validity of the Dodo bird finding rages on: the entire reputation of our profession is at stake. It seems unlikely that the debate will be settled by simply looking at the outcome research. As long as one side can say "meta-analyses and poor research design" and the other can say "but many studies show superiority" a consensual decision cannot be reached.

Fortunately, there are three other arguments that support the Dodo bird theory that collectively have the capacity to resolve this debate. The first argument is the "absence of failure" finding. It appears that virtually every system of therapy (and there are over 400 of them) (Arkowitz & Lilienfeld, 2012) generates positive, measurable results. This bias to the positive is well illustrated by the problems discovered when researchers attempted to create a placebo psychotherapy, an approach that appears to be therapeutic but which fails to generate client improvements (Wampold, 2010). Actual ineffective approaches were quickly recognized by the research subjects as placebo/false therapy. When these placebos were made more credible, they generated the same positive results as the "active" intervention. The following quote from Wampold (2010) summarizes this sense that everything credible works.

> Clinical trials comparing two treatments should be discontinued. Much money has been spent on clinical trials, with the same result: "Both treatments were more effective than no treatment, but there were no differences in outcomes between the two treatments." (Kindle Locations 2089-2092)

The second argument supporting the Dodo bird finding is the no training effect finding. If Dodo bird is false, and specific factors do contribute to psychotherapy outcomes, then techniques and knowledge of systems have inherent power. Put another way, knowing techniques, because they are inherently powerful, gives the knower an edge over the ignorant. However, because there are no training effects, neither knowledge of systems nor knowledge of specific techniques creates superiority. Hence, the Dodo bird finding is confirmed and the specific factors theory is unsupported. The third argument is the no experience finding. Experienced therapists know more systems and techniques than the inexperienced and have practiced them more assiduously. However, because there are no experience effects, it can be concluded that techniques and systems have no inherent power.

In sum, the Dodo bird finding was already credible simply by analyzing the outcome research. Combining the three arguments of everything works and that there are no training and experience effects, the Dodo bird finding appears a better explanation than the specific factors theory. Something unusual is going on in psychotherapy. One explanation is that our vaunted therapeutic procedures are actually rituals powered by client and therapist beliefs and expectancies. This is an old discussion in psychotherapy. One form it has taken is the conceptualization of psychotherapists as "placebologists" (Lambert & Ogles, 2004). Therapy works but not because of the inherent power of techniques. Instead, it appears that it works because of common factors: the therapeutic relationship/alliance and the associated power of rituals, beliefs and expectancies.

This argument can be made less abstract by considering concrete examples. Imagine that two different cultures believe that spirit possession is the primary explanation for mental health problems. In the first culture, there are real spirits and the possession really does cause the mental health symptoms. Exorcists, after much experimentation, have developed a number of effective techniques that tend to drive the spirits out. Many other techniques have failed to remove the spirits. Study of the spirits has led to theories that predict additional techniques that might work. While most of these also fail, the ones that work tend to improve outcomes and there is a sense that the field is evolving. Trained exorcists best the untrained because they are using proven and inherently powerful techniques. In addition, more experienced exorcists best less experienced as they become more proficient with the techniques and master more of them.

While the second culture also believes in spirit possession, in this instance the spirits are not real; rather, they are shamanic constructs. In this world, the exorcists also use techniques to banish the "spirits;" significantly, all the different techniques work as long as the client believes in them. The exorcists become attached to the interventions they have developed and argue about whether their interventions, foe example, painting someone blue versus sprinkling them with holy water, are superior to the competing exorcists' interventions. In most cases the exorcism succeeds in that the client reports feeling the spirit leave her body and, as a result, the mental health symptoms remit. Both exorcist and client believe that the spirits are real and the interventions have inherent power. Partly because everything works and partly because the interventions seem logical by that culture's standards, the question of whether the spirits are constructs or real and whether their interventions are rituals or techniques never seems to arise.

One can use these imaginary cultures to understand the outcome research results. The first culture has big training effects because they have something to teach new exorcists. The first culture exorcists tend to get better with experience because they are paying attention to factors which directly affect outcomes and because they can contrast failure with success and learn from the difference. While having a good relationship with their clients helps facilitate the outcomes, the power of the techniques makes the real difference; hence, relationship is secondary.

Conversely, the second world exorcists would not show a training effect. When everything works, beginners match the well-trained. It is difficult to learn from experience in the second world because the exorcists are focusing on the wrong factors. They should focus on how persuasive they are and how well the rituals fit the clients. Instead they are focusing on the "techniques", the constructed rituals. The exorcist/client relationship is much more important. When techniques lack inherent power, the relationship becomes definitive.

Returning to abstract thinking, research results imply that psychotherapeutic reality is much more similar to the second world than the first. The main difference between the two is the actual reality of the spirits. The secondary difference is the reality of the symptoms. While it is true that the symptoms in both worlds are equally painful, and in that sense they are equally real, in the second world they arise secondary to a misconstrual. Symptoms arising from misconstruals are more malleable and fluid than symptoms arising from "real" malevolent spirits.

The two worlds example illustrates the way in which rituals powered by expectancies and beliefs are primarily effective on misconstruals and constructed symptoms. Even though the power of lacebo is well understood, how many people would believe that a broken leg will heal well if intervention is limited to a ritual, when the leg also needs the techniques of being reset and casted? Problems in the material world are solved with techniques with inherent power. Problems in a constructed world (problems that live in the dimension of beliefs, assumptions and expectancies) are amenable to ritual solutions.

Constructionism

The contextual model analysis has essentially turned the basic assumptions of psychotherapy upside down. Almost all psychotherapy research is focused on amassing more privileged knowledge. The finding that this knowledge fails to improve outcomes is disheartening. Psychotherapeutic training and continuing education are based on the assumptions that psychotherapy's theoretical systems are getting better and better at explaining the factors that underly mental health, and that the techniques derived from these systems are seen as having inherent power and essentially determine what happens in the therapy room. The contextual model results indicate that all of these assumptions are misconstruals. The field of psychotherapy is as confused as the exorcists in culture 2.

While the contextual model arguments are rationally convincing, they simply don't "feel" true. Therapists might believe that their training prepared them to be therapists. Most therapists believe that they are better therapists because of their years of experience. Psychotherapists might also absolutely respect the value of the systems and techniques they have studied. Although psychotherapists understand that research shows that these feelings are unfounded, that simply seems wrong to them. What can explain why the results are so profoundly incongruent with their feelings?

Enter constructionism, a philosophic system which concerns itself with the meaning or connotation added to experience by a person or social group. The connotations are so powerful that constructionism suggests that different cultures actually create different realities.

> It is an ethnological commonplace that the ways of becoming and being human are as numerous as man's cultures. Humanness is socio-culturally variable. ... While it is possible to say that man has a nature, it

> is more significant to say that man constructs his own nature, or more simply, that man produces himself. (Berger and Luckmann, 1966, p. 49)

When Berger and Luckmann (1966) wrote their seminal work, *The Social Construction of Reality,* constructionism was a relatively new idea. Since then, constructionism and its close cousin, postmodernism, have become pervasive in western culture. It is not an exaggeration to state that many psychotherapeutic systems have incorporated constructionist elements and ideas and that some systems are highly constructionistic in orientation. Even with that sense that constructionism has become somewhat familiar, it is still worth reviewing Berger & Luckmann's main ideas about psychotherapy and psychopathology. Essentially, they believe that every culture is committed to inducting all cultural members into a shared vision of reality. Despite that intention, every culture has its share of "deviants", individuals who fail to internalize the desired worldview. Treating these deviants requires that every culture have a group of professionals, shamans, doctors, priests, whose job is to develop explanations for the deviancy and treatment methods capable of resolving the deviancy. The symptoms of deviancy are culture specific: spirit possession for some cultures, the evil eye in others, and neuroses in others. Berger and Luckmann argue that all of these mental health models were constructed. Each was valid inside its own culture but would look like superstition and misconstruals from the outside. Note the following quote illustrating the difficulties associated with applying a foreign mental health construction to an indigenous culture.

> Psychology... has created the mass abnormalization of Maori people by virtue of the fact that Maori people have been... recipients of English defined labels and treatments... Clinical psychology is a form of social control... and offers no more "truth" about the realities of Maori people's lives than a regular reading of the horoscope page in the local newspaper. (Lawson-Te, 1993)

The medical model had no problem with the initial part of the Berger and Luckmann argument. It also believed that previous culture's mental health models were built on superstition and irrationality. In contrast, for the first time in the history of humanity, a mental health model was going to be built on science, finally escaping the relativity and misconstruals of all the previous, "primitive" cultures. The contextual model research just reviewed has blown a hole in that argument. Western psychotherapy is as constructed as all the other culture's mental health models. As an illustration, examine the following quote from famous psychotherapist, Irving Yalom, arguing that all of our vaunted psychotherapeutic systems are invented.

> The superego, the id, the ego; the archetypes, the idealized and the actual selves, the pride system; the self system and the dissociated system, the masculine protest; parent, child, and adult ego states-none of these really exists. They are all fictions, all psychological constructs created for semantic convenience, and they justify their existence only by virtue of their explanatory power... . (Yalom & Leszcz, 2008, Kindle Locations 4852-4867)

Yalom is not a formal constructionist, although he is aware of the postmodern trends in western culture. When he wrote the passage, he did not have the benefit of the contextual model analysis. Instead he relied on his many years of doing therapy, his innumerable explanations to clients, listening to their varied beliefs about what made them sick and better, and intimate knowledge of the psychotherapeutic literature and he simply said: "none of these really exist". It is only useful because it helps people improve and this improvement is based on beliefs and expectations.

Returning to the culture 1 & 2 metaphor, labels can be used to describe each culture's reality. Culture 2 clearly represents Berger and Luckmann's version of a mental health model. It has a theory explaining deviant symptoms (spirit possession) and a culturally-approved method of resolving those symptoms (exorcism). The procedure helps most but not all cultural members. From the outside, it is apparent that their entire model is constructed. From the inside they would argue that it is real and true. If it didn't seem real and true, it would lose the power to help those possessed by "malevolent spirits".

Knowing that these spirits and the symptoms are constructed gives the awakened exorcist vast powers compared to the standard exorcist. First, the awakened exorcist sees this sort of constructed reality as much more fluid and malleable than the standard exorcist; if it's "all made up" then there is reason to be optimistic about prognosis and outcomes. It's much easier to improve symptoms based on false beliefs than to treat symptoms arising from actual spirit possession.

Second, the awakened therapist is clear that the best way forward is to concentrate on two factors: how well the ritual offered fits the client and her own ability to be persuasive and charismatic. Since no ritual has inherent power, the concentration is on what makes the ritual believable and what raises expectations. Conversely, the focus of the standard exorcist is entirely on the next technique: yes, sprinkling with holy water didn't remove the spirit but perhaps painting sacred designs on their chest will. All the creativity and focus of the standard therapist is on the imagined inherent power of the techniques; the client fit factor and the therapist charisma factors are neglected or ignored. Ignoring the active factors and favoring the misconstruals is unlikely to lead to better outcomes.

It should be noted that the kind of simple or pragmatic constructionism discussed in Berger and Luckmann and embodied in the culture 1 & 2 metaphor is not the only form of constructionism. Since Berger and Luckmann's day there has been ongoing development of postmodern thought; current conceptualizations of constructionism especially focus on issues such as linguistics, discourse, philosophy, and power relationships (Gergen, 2009a; Burr, 2003). Many current constructionists argue that the material world can never be experienced objectively and that the very use of language impels us into constructed reality. Put another way, these sorts of constructionists might argue that the world of culture 1 had as many constructed elements as the world of culture 2, at least from a discursive point of view.

While these more complex constructionist arguments are both useful and interesting, how a constructionist might treat BPD will be based on the more limited version of constructionism contained in the Berger and Luckmann arguments and the culture 1 & 2 metaphor. This level of pragmatic constructionism and the provocative implications of the contextual model will carry the discussion forward all on their own.

Deconstructing Borderline Personality Disorder

In order to take full advantage of the insights and possibilities revealed by the contextual model and constructionism, it is necessary to address the compelling nature of specific factors. It takes hard work to conceive of psychotherapy without imbuing techniques with inherent power. For example, even after reviewing the contextual model research, it is challenging to imagine addressing BPD without thinking of techniques that are specially designed to treat BPD. In this sense many therapists might mention DBT, others would emphasize the trauma aspect and talk about EMDR, and others with a more psychodynamic bent might discuss Trauma Focused Psychotherapy (TFP). Before we can examine a constructionist approach to BPD, we have to root out and deconstruct our residual assumptions about BPD.

The contextual model has already accepted that all of these approaches work, that they all get equivalent results, and that none of them are the "superior" treatment for BPD. Scott Miller (Walt, 2007) comments.

> Also, and more importantly, when the appropriate analyses of the research are done between so-called "evidence-based practices" and any other approach that's intended to be therapeutic—now listen to that—any approach that's intended to be therapeutic, you don't find any difference in outcome between those approaches. I know this can be hard to believe given the current zeitgeist. Unfortunately, at the state and federal oversight level, and for an increasing number of clinicians, it has somehow become "known" that certain treatments work best for clients with certain diagnoses. For people diagnosed with so-called "Borderline Personality Disorder," Dialectical Behavior Therapy is the "best practice" when, in fact, available evidence indicates that it works as well as everything else. …
>
> Now, I'm not saying that DBT is not effective or that therapists shouldn't learn about it, or other approaches. Rather, the point here is something that most therapists know intuitively: all approaches work with some people some of the time. The challenge for the practicing clinician

> is, therefore, not figuring out what approach works for which diagnosis, but what will work for this person sitting with me on this day at this stage in their life (p. 85).

This is one of the essential arguments of the contextual model: everything works but no treatment is superior to another. It has been demonstated that this is true with general psychotherapy, and here Miller applies it to BPD. Miller's argument can be extended by taking a closer look at the EMDR literature. EMDR was chosen because it is another treatment that is "known" for being a superior method for treating PTSD and because trauma is closely associated with BPD. Examine the following summary statement from Wampold & Imel (2015) regarding the effectiveness of EMDR versus cognitive therapies for trauma.

> There is more disturbing evidence imbedded in treatments for PTSD. All of the meta-analyses discussed above that have examined the efficacy of EMDR have found it to be comparable to the best treatments for PTSD (see Seidler & Wagner, 2006). However, EMDR is based on questionable ingredients from a scientific perspective. It has been labeled as pseudoscience (e.g., Herbert et al., 2000) and compared to Mesmerism (McNally, 1999) by Medical Model adherents. Clinical scientists have been annoyed by unjustified claims of efficacy and efficiency and the way it is publicized and disseminated (see also Davidson & Parker, 2001; Rosen, 1999). Herbert et al. (2000) asserted that "the promotion of EMDR provides a good illustration of pseudoscience in general and of how pseudoscience is marketed to mental health clinicians, some of whom may be relatively unfamiliar with the published research on EMDR" (p. 955). Yet this purportedly pseudoscientific treatment is as effective as the "scientific" evidence-based treatments for PTSD.
>
> The evidence from PTSD clinical trials creates multiple issues from a Medical Model perspective, but is entirely consistent with the Contextual Model. It appears that treatments with a variety of ingredients are equally effective, including CBT without exposure, PCT, and EMDR. (Kindle Locations 3354-3364)

In this quote, Wampold & Imel not only highlight the equivalence between EMDR and cognitive therapies but include an interesting discussion noting how shocking that equivalence has been to CBT advocates. The CBT group has had trouble believing that the "pseudoscience" of EMDR could stand up to rigorous testing. The scientific psychologists clearly believe that eye movements are pure placebo; it is upsetting that something so arbitrary and so "obviously invented" will work as well as their own treatments, treatments that are literally supported by hundreds if not thousands of books and research studies. This equivalence essentially shakes the stability of their scientific reality. In this sense, EMDR makes a meaningful contribution beyond the many clients it has helped: its clearly constructed nature reveals the absurdity in believing in the inherent power of techniques.

Consistent with the EMDR research results, the contextual model argues that all psychotherapeutic interventions are placebo delivery devices whether they seem to be rational, like CBT, or seem like constructed pseudoscience.

> … (T)herapeutic change occurs because there is a single theory or rationale that is acceptable or believable to both the healer and client. The specifics of the theory and techniques are for all points and purposes irrelevant…… At the same time, it may be said, paraphrasing Winston Churchill, that never has a subject that contributes so little to outcome received so much professional attention and approbation. ...
>
> As long as a treatment makes sense to, is accepted by, and fosters the active engagement of the client, the particular treatment approach used is unimportant. In other words, therapeutic techniques are placebo delivery devices. …(Moreover), suffice it to say that techniques work, in large part, if not completely, through the activation and operation of placebo, hope, and expectancy. … Fortunately, the evidence indicates that therapists need not spend any time searching for the right treatment for a particular disorder. Instead, the "best" methods are those (a) intended or believed to be therapeutic; (b) delivered with a cogent rationale; and, above all, (c) acceptable to the client. (Anderson, Lunnen and Ogles, 2010, Kindle Locations 3864-3990)

In this quote, Anderson, Lunnen and Ogles, who are part of the contextual model group, argue that every technique is a ritual, no technique has inherent power, and that the effectiveness of any intervention is dependent on the belief of the client. As hope fades that change is secondary to effective techniques, one becomes free to pay attention to the actual factors that enhance outcomes.

Miller sees DBT just as he sees EMDR: an effective treatment but not something that is superior to any other approach. As one would expect, there is lots of evidence that DBT is effective and little or no evidence that it is a superior treatment. Here's a quote about the equivalence of DBT and other therapies from a review article on treating BPD in *Bergin & Garfield's Handbook of Psychotherapy and Behavior Change.*

> Suicidality and anger reduced in patients treated with TFP and DBT, but not in those treated with supportive treatment; all three treatments were effective in reducing depression and in improving global functioning and social adjustment. Thus, although DBT is generally found to be more effective than treatment as usual, superiority over other manualized treatments specifically developed for BPD has not been demonstrated. (Emmelkamp, 2013, p. 372)

Other metanalyses and review articles generally agree although there are some variations in their conclusions. Cristea et al. (2017) found that DBT and psychodynamic treatment models both worked better than standard treatment although these improvements faded over time and were limited by experimental design factors. Stoffers, Rucker, Timmer, Huband, and Lieb (2012) also found that DBT was effective as were a variety of other interventions that addressed BPD but failed to find sufficient well-designed studies to conclude that DBT was superior to other methods. In sum, the literature confirms Miller's and Wampold's contextual model analysis: everything works and nothing works better.

This moves us to the next major point: the necessity of deconstructing the seriousness of the psychopathology. From the medical model perspective, psychopathology is considered to be both real and internalized: it is part of the person. The contextual model and constructionism demonstrate that this assumption of the stability, reality, and seriousness of psychopathology is a cultural construct that is no more real than the imagined spirits of culture 2. Deconstructing psychopathology—especially when working with BPD where the psychopathology seems so ingrained and pervasive—is an essential prerequisite to working gracefully and effectively with any personality disorder.

To that end, examine the quotes below from constructionist, Vivian Burr.

> Since the social world, including ourselves as people, is the product of social processes, it follows that there cannot be any given, determined nature to the world or people. There are no essences inside things or people that make them what they are. … It is important to stress the radical nature of the proposal that is being put forward here. (Burr, 2003, p. 5-6)

Later in her book, she expands this point further.

> Social Constructionism, then, replaces the self-contained, pre-social and unitary individual with a fragmented and changing, socially produced phenomenon who comes into existence and is maintained not inside the skull but in social life. (Burr, 2003, p. 104)

In these quotes Burr lays out the essential constructionist position. There is no determined nature nor are there essences inside people, hence, no internalized stable psychopathology. Certainly there are fluid and mobile constructions, some of which are more stable than others and some which cause pain and suffering, but none of these are more real than the constructed spirits of culture 2. They are as real as one believes and as real as others believe but they have no independent existence. This understanding is central for empowering a therapist to deal with BPD.

Moreover, Burr suggests that the individual is fragmented and changing and maintained in social life. This opens the door for framing BPD the same way, as something that is fragmented, changing and maintained in social life. More specifically a therapist can conceive of BPD as only a part or ego state of a client and not the entire client. BPD can be understood as operating in only certain social situations, for example, in intimate relationships and not at work; or as a chosen behavior designed to maximize secondary gains. This is a process of "unreification", the effort to make something fluid that has been solidified and concretized. Given that psychotherapists are in the change and transformation business, anything that makes psychopathology less solid, dense and immobile is welcome.

In sum, deconstructing BPD begins with understanding that psychotherapy has no particular expertise when it comes to treating BPD. The interventions used with BPD work but there are no interventions that work any better than any other. The BPD diagnosis is heavily reified in western culture; in terms of treatment, it is considered one of the most difficult and demanding syndromes. Unreifying/deconstructing these implicit assumptions—and replacing them with ideas connected to fragmented, changeable, and socially sustained identities—creates a much more favorable milieu for transformation.

Treating Borderline Personality Disorder

Treating BPD begins with understanding a famous Scott Miller quote: "…far more important than what the therapist is doing is who the therapist is" (Duncan, Miller, Wampold, & Hubble, 2010, Kindle Locations 385-386). Psychotherapy for BPD is effective. It is not as effective as the standard psychotherapeutic outcome because clients are only defined as BPD when they have symptoms and behaviors that are more severe than average. Even with this caveat, from a constructionist perspective every approach that is used with BPD is effective and all approaches will have equivalent outcomes. It follows that attempts to achieve superior outcomes must focus not only on developing new techniques. To the degree that the therapist feels stronger, clearer, more centered, and more connected than the average therapist, superior outcomes will be achieved.

BPD clients are famous for having a negative effect on the therapist. They tend to attack the therapist, exhaust the therapist with needy demands, disappoint the therapist as apparent gains are discarded and old behaviors emerge, switch from idealizing the therapist to disparaging the therapist, and terrify the therapist with self-harm and suicidal behaviors. If a therapist can block the impact of these dispiriting behaviors, and continue to use whatever approach they prefer, such "immunized" therapists should be able to achieve superior results. Put another way, many therapists become exhausted, hopeless, judgmental or disdainful when working with BPD clients; if they can remain resilient, connected, optimistic, creative and centered, outcomes should be affected positively.

Looking at these BPD behaviors from the client perspective, they can be conceptualized as attempts to maintain identity stability by using strategies that create an expected reality. Constructionism postulates that identity is sustained and reinforced by every interaction with another person. For example, a shy person presents as shy and thereby creates a limited set of responses in the other; the other can be judgmental, dismissive, hierarchical, warm, reassuring or kind. They aren't likely to respond with submission, respect, or obsequiousness. At the end of the encounter, the identity of the shy person is reinforced and stabilized. In addition, the shy person's view of the world is also reinforced; allowing for some oversimplification to make the point, for a shy person the world consists of people that are dismissive or dominant alternating with people that are kind and empathetic.

What kind of people make up the BPD client's world? Again, from an oversimplified perspective, it is populated by people that are unsafe, aggressive and unjust. This alternates with people that look sympathetic in the beginning but who fail to come through in the long run as the borderline demands go on and on. As a BPD individual, one can attract people but, in the end, they will be exposed as individuals that are never really there for the BPD person. They will construed as people who make promises they have no intention of keeping, and people that overtly or covertly will take advantage of or abuse the BPD person. The secret to one's stability is to have strategies that turn everyone into the people that one expects them to be.

In this sense, one way to describe the goal of BPD therapy is that the therapist creates an identity and a relationship that refuses to fulfill these parameters and expectations. Put poetically, the therapist understands that the BPD client is attempting to bewitch the therapist into acting in the predicted manner; the therapist resists the "trance state", understands the underlying strategies, and, instead of cooperating, creates a new reality.

Therapists design, propose, and co-create client interventions with the goal of serving client needs. It is possible to expand the scope of the interventions so they also serve therapist needs. Following is a list of reasonably common interventions that are used both with typical clients and BPD clients. However, they will be presented in an unusual manner; the interventions will be described from the therapist perspective and analyzed as rituals that will help therapists resist the "borderline ensorcelment". More specifically, what follows are a series of interventions and frames that are designed to help the therapist stay centered in their own sense of being an ethical, compassionate and effective helper. As will be made clear, every suggested intervention has a double purpose: the potential positive impact on the therapist, and the potential positive impact on the client. The client-centered aspects will be discussed at the end of this section.

Diagnosis

Many clients have already received a borderline diagnosis before meeting the current therapist and many of those clients are aware of the negative connotations of the diagnosis. It tends to be useful to dispute or moderate the diagnosis early in therapy. For example, the therapist can make statements such as, "Yes, I agree that you have BPD but it seems to be limited to only one part of your psyche and is interspersed with healthy and high functioning parts." Or one might say, "Yes, you have BPD but it's a rather rare type. It's clear to me that you only adopted BPD strategies to help your sister and this rare, 'altruistic' type of BPD has a much better prognosis than standard BPD."

Therapists, of course, are concerned about authenticity and many would feel wrong about simply making up diagnostic permutations that are not generally endorsed by the field. These therapists might feel more comfortable with a more standard definition of BPD, something like, "you have BPD because you had a traumatic childhood leading to impaired brain development (Schore, 2012) and you will tend to default to dysfunctional strategies in all your relationships."

Constructionism, of course, sees all three definitions as equally valid and equally wrong. The "truest" definition of BPD might be one thing if one is taking a test in graduate school; conversely, an alternative definition might be more accurate if the goal is client empowerment. Recall that the contextual model research demonstrates that knowledge of diagnostic categories fails to enhance outcomes. More specifically, it can be argued that many of the mental health diagnoses are arbitrary. Can it be verified that there are exactly 10 personality disorders? Why not eight or thirteen? Moreover, the precise way of seeing BPD varies from one therapist to another depending on their personality, training and experience. Accepting that the current diagnostic system is no more valid than ones generated by other cultures allows the therapist significant freedom when it comes to interpreting diagnoses in a way that benefits the client.

The question of authenticity and being honest with clients simply scratches the surface of the "how real is BPD" question. In the material reality symbolized by culture 1 with real spirits and interventions with inherent power, reality is relatively easy to define. In culture 2, where the spirits and the interventions are made up, only the level of suffering is real; everything else is constructed. Understanding that most of psychotherapy operates in constructed reality—culture 2—allows the therapist creative freedom when shaping rituals, defining terms and prognoses, and predicting outcomes. Learning to exercise that kind of freedom in service to the client's needs often starts with the ability to work with the therapeutic beginning point: the diagnosis. Feeling empowered to adjust the meaning of the diagnosis, the prognosis, the symptoms, and the signs of improvement is one of the early indications that a therapist is beginning to understand the malleability and fluidity of reality inherent in constructionism.

Recall that each of these interventions is designed to help the therapist resist the BPD "bewitchment". When the therapist can see diagnoses—particularly BPD—as fluid and malleable, this vision goes a long way towards the underlying goal of helping the therapist stay centered, relaxed, and confident. The BPD diagnosis itself can unnerve a therapist; to achieve superior outcomes, those negative connotations must be resisted at a minimum or, even better, be transformed into opportunities.

Self as a Social Construction

Burr made the point above that identity is maintained in social relationships. Put another way, constructionism believes that the Self exists in the space between me and the other (Burr, 2003; Gergen, 2009a). The apollonian view of the self is that it exists within me and is essentially the same across encounters. The constructionist perspective, however, implies much more variability; in fact, it sees "me" as potentially having a different identity with every different person. A BPD client could have been a difficult mother but be a beloved grandmother. A BPD teacher can be effective with their students and still be a difficult spouse.

When the therapist includes others in therapy, either literally by bringing significant others into the room, or figuratively by hearing stories and creating "what if" scenarios, there is an opportunity to witness these identity shifts. Witnessing this ability to shift supports the therapist's feelings that the BPD client is mobile and this perception of mobility expands the range of possibilities in therapy. These encounters with others also tend to support the idea that the BPD client has a wider range of social skills than previously acknowledged. The goal of therapy moves from "acquiring skills" to deciding when skills should be employed. As the therapist sees the BPD client as more skillful and as more mobile and flexible, these experiences can be used to dispute the common feeling that BPD clients are hopeless, unchangeable, and use primitive and regressive skill sets. In sum, looking for variability in behaviors and pathology across different social encounters is a primary way to avoid BPD bewitchment.

BPD and Ego States

Ego state therapy (Watkins, 1993) and internal family systems (Engler & Fulton, 2012) are two similar models that function as personality theories and as schools of psychotherapy. These approaches conceptualize the Self as a conglomeration of multiple parts or ego states. The number of states, their age and gender, their objective and goals, and their styles and personalities vary across clients; in fact, one of the benefits of an ego state approach is that it is so malleable, parts can be invented/constructed spontaneously. After the parts are identified, therapy consists of dialog—similar to an internalized family discussion—between the parts with the aim of reducing conflict, integrating repressed and rejected parts, and helping the disparate parts work together as a cohesive team.

With BPD clients, the therapist can identify a BPD part and a series of healthy parts; another possibility might be to identify a desperate/needy part, an angry part, and a series of healthy parts. Various themes can be explored including: 1) what cues elicit the BPD part? 2) What are the secondary gains? 3) What strategies might work better than BPD strategies? As part of this exploration, the client will spend significant time identifying with healthy parts and seeing the BPD part or parts as "other". This dissociative strategy often empowers the client in terms of symptom management and affective regulation; it also supports the therapist in that the therapist has repeated experiences where the client functions as a "co-therapist". Witnessing the client acting as a helpful and insightful co-therapist supports the therapist's respect for the client and inoculates the therapist against seeing the entire client as BPD.

Behavioral Interventions

One of the most prominent features of BPD is the continued use of self-destructive and ineffective strategies in life in spite of ongoing negative feedback. When a therapist finds, or can structure, exceptions to this feature, it helps them see the BPD client as more functional. Perhaps, the most common exception is found in the work environment. The same BPD client who is a nightmare at home can be a functional co-worker on the job. Also, many BPD clients are very attractive, even charismatic, when first encountered. They can begin relationships well, but often have trouble sustaining those same relationships. One might say that BPD clients have above average social skills in terms of relationship initiation, and simply need to expand those skills into the relationship sustaining area. Similarly, in doing couples therapy with BPD women in particular, their partners sometimes report that, when things are going well, the BPD clients are the most giving and present romantic partners they have ever known. These men sometimes say something like, "when it's good, it's the best relationship I've ever had; when it turns bad, it's a nightmare."

Understanding this range of functioning is helpful, but it can be even more helpful when the therapist is able to see the BPD client as altering their behavior in response to rewards and punishments. Changing personal strategies to fit the environment is an adaptive response that is characteristic of high functioning individuals; in addition, it suggests a level of control in the BPD client that is either conscious or close to conscious.

One of the most important rituals/interventions that arises out of this sense of choice and control is to directly impose consequences on the BPD client, similar to ones imposed by an employer. Since the therapist has no direct control over the client, imposing consequences for BPD behaviors must come from significant others. For example, the therapist, with the client's permission, could encourage a spouse could require the BPD client to rent a hotel room for the night whenever certain target BPD strategies are employed. If the "price" for using the BPD strategies exceeds the "cost" (temporary expulsion from the relationship plus the financial penalty of renting the hotel room), there can be a diminishment of BPD strategies. Such simple approaches often fail at the beginning of treatment but can be quite helpful to the therapist and the client as treatment progresses. The opportunity to see BPD clients responding appropriately to behavioral consequences inoculates against BPD bewitchment.

Summary

These four interventions are not intended to be exhaustive; rather, they offer concrete examples of the types of interventions that can help therapist resist BPD ensorcellment. Once the characteristics of such interventions are internalized, other examples arise, particularly examples that are custom designed to fit the specific therapeutic needs of each unique BPD client. In choosing these interventions, perhaps the most important therapeutic tool is the therapist's ability to monitor her own internal state. When therapists finds themselves frightened of, angry at, or frustrated with a BPD client, they need some kind of intervention to recover their centeredness. Another sign is the urge to retreat behind the diagnosis. When one begins to think of the BPD client as a diagnosis instead of as a unique person, it is another indication of losing one's center and succumbing to the bewitchment.

Recall that the basic argument underlying this section is that superior results are achieved merely by executing any kind of reasonable therapeutic approach while resisting enchantment. This is, indeed, a simple argument in itself. What makes it profound is the understanding that therapy occurs in constructed reality and that all interventions truly are equal to each other. Fully integrating these ideas provides a meaningful foundation for this approach. Accepting that BPD clients will improve if the therapist does anything helpful and simultaneously stays centered creates a sense of lightness and optimism. It is aligned with the Miller dictum to focus on the therapist and not the technique. For all of these reasons, this strategy enhances the probability of improved client outcomes.

Rituals versus Techniques

While each of these interventions is designed to center the therapist, they all have the dual function of simultaneously impacting the client in a positive manner. In this sense, they can be seen as a list of "techniques" that are specially designed to help BPD clients. This feeling of "techniques" is, of course, in conflict with the contextual model research showing that techniques lack inherent power. In this sense, the four approaches create the opportunity to understand the difference between techniques and rituals. Moreover, the deconstruction of the concept of techniques opens new doors for developing enhanced outcomes.

The four interventions above—disputing the diagnosis, self exists between people, dissociation and ego state therapy, and BPD is behaviorally functional—all have the capacity to elicit positive outcomes in BPD clients. So do many other interventions not listed above: EMDR for trauma, existential interventions focused on empowering the authentic self, DBT's tool bag of techniques for affective regulation; and the psychodynamic exploration of historical precursors to maladaptive behaviors. It is easily possible to add twenty-five or thirty additional interventions that would have a positive impact on the BPD client.

The literal goal with a BPD client arises from the diagnostic criteria. Ideally they will stop their self-destructive behaviors, regulate their affect, control their interpersonal attacks, and feel that they are a normal person. Since simply saying that is unlikely to achieve those goals, rituals are created or co-created that allow the BPD client to address the direct goals gradually and metaphorically. In other words, the rituals provide a justification for change.

The constructionist therapist who understands that he is using rituals instead of techniques has a number of advantages over the standard therapist. The first advantage is that the lack of belief in techniques allows the constructionist to assess the client relatively free of "technique bias". Technique bias is the tendency to prefer certain interventions above others and to apply them to most or all clients. Colloquially this is described as, "If I only have a hammer, everything is seen as a nail".

Limiting one's interventions to a relatively small range of techniques that "I believe in" forces one to "sell" those techniques to the client whether they fit well or not. Conversely when therapists are unlimited by any allegiance to a set of techniques, they start building their interventions/rituals by paying attention to the client first. It makes a big difference whether our first thought is "which technique should I choose from my armamentarium" versus "what does this client actually need?" In this sense, the lack of any attachment to any techniques—an evenhandedness that rests on the knowledge that all techniques are actually rituals—allows the therapist to "hear" the needs of the client more clearly and respond accordingly.

The second advantage of a constructionist therapist over a standard therapist is the ability to understand and to feel that the pathology is as constructed as the techniques. Put another way, the ability to see the client as a person rather than perceiving them through a diagnostic/ psychopathology lens positions the constructionist to feel the situation is relatively malleable and fluid. Returning to our culture 2 metaphor: is it easier to exorcize an imaginary malevolent spirit or a real one?

Pathology and the concept of inherent power of techniques are inextricably linked. In the culture 1 metaphor, "real" spirits can only be changed by "real" techniques. Conversely, if a ritual is sufficient to create change, by definition the associated psychopathology must be constructed. A real broken leg requires the real techniques of resetting and casting; simply preforming a ritual on the broken leg might enhance the patient's mood but will create inferior outcomes. Rituals imply constructed problems; problems in material reality require techniques with inherent power.

Understanding and integrating these two principles, the client-centered position and the ephemerality of psychopathology, allows the constructionist therapist to have a relatively light, confident, and creative style when conducting therapy. Returning again to the culture 2 metaphor, how would an exorcist in the know differ from one who believed in spirits and exorcisms? The aware exorcist would take client suffering seriously, but all of the interventions, the expectations, and the relationship would be infused with the knowledge that, in the end, everything will turn out given that all of the suffering is founded on misconstruals. This kind of confidence is numinous and pervasive, and is communicated to the client on a nonverbal level. In sum, the constructionist therapist, via the freedom to fit the ritual to the client and via the nonverbal communication of optimistic prognoses, has significant opportunities to enhance outcomes with BPD clients.

Another important edge the constructionist has over the standard therapist arises from the definition of "common factors". The contextual model group has sometimes been described as the common factors group because they were arguing against the "specific factors" group's beliefs in techniques with inherent power. While there can be many definitions of common factors in psychotherapy, the most well-known summary of common factors is "a relationship with a wise and caring therapist". Virtually every school, recognizing the power of common factors, recommends that therapists cultivate wisdom and caring. Because everyone recommends this approach, it is difficult to become a superior therapist simply by cultivating wisdom and caring. Because everyone is already trying to be wiser and more caring, one's attempts in this area fail to give one a meaningful edge. Put another way, one can't achieve superior client outcomes by intentionally practicing wisdom and caring. (Miller, 2004)

Constructionism introduces a new perspective on these two therapist qualities, a perspective that can open doors in terms of enhancing wisdom and caring. Wisdom can be viewed as having two qualities, wisdom embedded in the culture and constructionist wisdom. Cultural wisdom consists of items such as knowledge of developmental processes, definitions of success, honor and integrity, and sexual identity issues. Constructionist wisdom is the understanding that most of those factors are constructed and vary from culture to culture. Knowing that one is in culture 2 and not culture 1 is part of constructionist wisdom. Constructionists have full access to standard wisdom but, in addition, they have an opportunity to supplement that wisdom with constructionist insights. Exploration of the implications of constructionism is a new and relatively undeveloped way to cultivate wisdom beyond that available to the standard therapist.

Similarly, constructionism provides an ability to enhance the "caring" aspect as well. The most significant critique of constructionism goes something like, "if everything is constructed, how can we know what's true and good? Is there any solid place to stand?" In this sense, it is appropriate to argue that any serious constructionist must inevitably encounter the existential abyss and respond to its implicit challenges of chaos, meaninglessness, and emptiness. The constructionist *therapist*, however, can essentially escape this challenge by finding a place to stand in the authentic needs and goals of the client. Serving the needs of the client provides a sense of meaning and purpose similar to raising a child or caring for the ill. Such activities are numinous in their own right; they cut through the chaos and emptiness inherent in deconstructionism run amuck. In this sense, the constructionist "cares" more about the client and her needs and goals than the standard therapist. The standard therapist is less invested in the client given that existential dilemmas can be avoided by aligning with diagnoses, therapeutic systems, and a variety of cultural assumptions about the "right way to live life".

In addition, the social constructionist definition of the self as fragmented, variable, and existing in the relationship between people opens additional possibilities in the "caring" area. Examine the following quote from Kenneth Gergen (2009b, p. xv)).

> My attempt is to generate an account of human action that can replace the presumption of bounded selves with a vision of relationship. I do not mean relationships between otherwise separate selves, but rather, a process of coordination that precedes the very concept of the self. My hope is to demonstrate that virtually all intelligible action is born, sustained, and/or extinguished within the ongoing process of relationship. From this standpoint there is no isolated self or fully private experience. Rather, we exist in a world of co-constitution. We are always already emerging from relationship; we cannot step out of relationship; even in our most private moments we are never alone.

With this quote Gergen introduces a second category of "caring", a kind of epistemology of the heart. People are not separate selves; instead, the self exists in the dialectical space between. Alienation and separation are revealed as confused misconstruals. People are always connected and interdependent whether they are conscious of it or not. Constructionist wisdom rests on the discernment between the constructed and the material. Constructionist compassion and caring rest on the discernment between the bounded self and the relational self.

The concept of the relational self is just as radical as the constructionist version of wisdom and discernment. It is not limited to caring about clients and it is not the same as imbuing the relationship with a sense of unconditional positive regard. Laudable as both those goals might be, they are still restricted by the bounded self. One's confusion about being a bounded self parallels one's confusion about the nature of reality; awakening to the relational self opens the door to developing another level of caring. Martin Buber (1970) differentiates between these two types of caring via his famous categories of the "I-It" relationship versus the "I-Thou" relationship. In "I–It", we attempt to reach across loneliness with caring and love to equally isolated selves. In "I–Thou" there is the recognition of an always, already present connectedness; in fact, I only exists in connection to Thou.

The constructionist ability to extend "wisdom and caring" is not limited to BPD; it applies to all clients regardless of diagnoses. The important thing to emphasize is that a constructionist perspective opens the door for a differential development of wisdom and caring. It is now possible to develop those common factors concepts effectively and bypass the standard objection that, "everyone is already trying their best to be wiser and more connected." Not limited to working with BPD clients, the development of wisdom and caring is especially central with BPD given the ongoing attempts of those clients to remove wisdom and caring from their world.

Summary and Conclusion

No one can convincingly argue that the contextual model and constructionism have dethroned the medical model. Regardless of how compelling the literature results and the deductions may be, it takes time and effort to accomplish a paradigm shift. Nonetheless, the arguments against techniques and specific factors are powerful, and the benefits of constructionism, with its attendant mobility, its optimistic prognoses and its ability to focus on what makes a difference in outcomes, suggests that the perspectives offered by the contextual model are going to make a significant contribution.

The contextual model/constructionist analyses and their implications give constructionist therapists a genuine edge over standard therapists. They are allowed to assess client fit without being distracted by confusing assumptions about what BPD clients are like. They can develop their own charisma, persuasiveness and connectedness without being seduced by the imagined power of techniques, and they can cultivate a sense of fluidity and malleability because they understand that psychotherapy operates in constructed reality. Most importantly, constructionist therapists have a new set of possibilitiesfor treating BPD bsed on the common factors of wisdom and compassion.

References

Anderson, T., Crowley, M., Himawan, L., Holmberg, J. & Uhlin, B. (2016). Therapist facilitative interpersonal skills and training status: A randomized clinical trial on alliance and outcome, *Psychotherapy Research*, 26 (5), 511-529. Retrieved fromhttp://dx.doi.org/10.1080/10503307.2015.1049671

Anderson, T., Lunnen K. M. & Ogles, B. M. (2010). Putting models and techniques in context. In B. L. Duncan, S. D. Miller, B. E. Wampold & M.A Hubble's *The heart and soul of change* (Kindle Locations 3795-4399). Retrieved from https://www.amazon.com/Heart-Soul-Change-Second-Delivering-ebook/dp/B004T9YTEG

Arkowitz, Hal & Lilienfeld, Scott. (2012, August 1) EMDR: Taking a Closer Look. *Scientific American*. Retrieved from https://www.scientificamerican.com/article/emdr-taking-a-closer-look/

Bacon, S. (2018). *Practicing psychotherapy in constructed reality: Ritual, charisma, and enhanced client outcomes*. New York, NY: Lexington Books.

Berger, P., & Luckmann, T. (1966). The Social Construction of Reality: A Treatise in the Sociology of Knowledge. Garden City, NY: Doubleday.

Buber, M. (1970). *I and thou*. (W. Kaufmann, Trans.) New York, NY: Scribner's.

Burr, V. (2003). *Social constructionism* (2nd edition). New York, NY: Routledge.

Cristea IA, Gentili C, Cotet CD, Palomba D, Barbui C, Cuijpers P. (2017) Efficacy of Psychotherapies for Borderline Personality Disorder: A

Systematic Review and Meta-analysis. *JAMA Psychiatry.* 74(4):319-328. http://dx.doi.org/10.1001/jamapsychiatry.2016.4287

Duncan, B. L., Miller, S. D., Wampold, B. E., & Hubble, M. A. (2010). *The heart and soul of change: delivering what works in therapy* (2nd edition). Retrieved from https://www.amazon.com/Heart-Soul-Change-Second-Delivering-ebook/dp/B004T9YTEG

Emmelkamp, Paul. (2013). Behavior therapy with adults. In *Bergin and Garfield's Handbook of psychotherapy and behavior change* (6th ed.). New York: John Wiley & Sons.

Engler, J. & Fulton, P. (2012). Self and no-self in psychotherapy. In C. K. Germer & R. D. Siegel (Eds.) *Wisdom and compassion in psychotherapy: deepening mindfulness in clinical practice,* (pp. 35-47). Retrieved from https://www.amazon.com/Wisdom-Compassion-Psychoherapy-Deepening-Mindfulness-ebook/dp/B007W4ED6O

Gergen, K. J. (2009a). *An invitation to social construction* (2nd edition). Los Angeles, CA: SAGE Publications Ltd.

Gergen, Kenneth J. (2009b). *Relational Being: Beyond Self and Community.* Oxford University Press. Kindle Edition.

Hill, C. E., & Knox, S. (2013). Training and supervision in psychotherapy. In *Bergin and Garfield's Handbook of psychotherapy and behavior change* (6th ed.). New York: John Wiley & Sons.

Hubble, Mark; Duncan, Barry; Miller, Scott & Wampold Bruce. (2010) Introduction. In Wampold, Bruce E.; Duncan, Barry L.; Miller, Scott D. (Eds). *The Heart and Soul of Change, Second Edition: Delivering What Works in Therapy*. Retrieved from https://www.amazon.com/Heart-Soul-Change-Second-Delivering-ebook/dp/B004T9YTEG

Lambert, M. & Ogles, B. M. (2004). The efficacy and effectiveness of psychotherapy. In *Bergman and Garfield's Handbook of Psychotherapy and Behavior Change* (5th Ed.). New York: John Wiley & Sons.

Malouff, John. (2012). The need for empirically supported psychology training standards, *Psychotherapy in Australia*, 18:3, 28-32. https://search.informit.com.au/documentSummary;dn=316992349249508;res=IELHEA

Miller, SD. (2004) Losing faith: arguing for a new way to think about therapy. *Psychotherapy in Australia*, 10 (2), Feb: 44-51. https://search.informit.com.au/documentSummary;dn=547331565542521;res=IELHEA

Miller, S., & Hubble, M. (2011). The road to mastery. *Psychotherapy networker*, 35 (3). https://www.psychotherapynetworker.org/magazine/article/328/the-road-to-mastery

Miller, S., Hubble, M., & Duncan, B. (2007). Supershrinks: what is the secret to their success? *Psychotherapy networker*, 31 (6). Retrieved from http://dx.doi.org/10.1037/e526322010-003

Miller, Scott, Hubble, Mark & Chow, Daryl. (2017) Professional development: From oxymoron to reality. In Rousmaniere, Tony; Goodyear, Rodney K.; Miller, Scott D. & Wampold, Bruce E. (Eds). *The Cycle of Excellence: Using Deliberate Practice to Improve Supervision and Training*. Retrieved from https://doi.org/10.1002/9781119165590.ch2

Schore, A. N. (2012). *The science of the art of psychotherapy*. Retrieved from https://www.amazon.com/Science-Psychotherapy-Norton-Interpersonal-Neurobiology-ebook/dp/B005LW5K2U

Stoffers, J. M., Vollm, B. A., Rücker, G., Timmer, A., Huband, N. and Lieb, K. (2012) Psychological Therapies for People with Borderline Personality Disorder. *Cochrane Database of Systematic Reviews,* 8, CD005652. http://dx.doi.org/10.1002/14651858.CD005652.pub2

Strupp, H. H., & Hadley, S. W. (1979). Specific vs nonspecific factors in psychotherapy. A controlled study of outcome. *Archives of General Psychiatry,* 36 (10), 1125-1136. http://dx.doi.org/10.1001/archpsyc.1979.01780100095009

Thomas, J. (2014) Therapy: No Improvement for 40 Years. *The National. Psychologist*. 23 (1).

Walt, J. (2007, February). The future of mental health: an interview with Scott D. Miller, Ph.D. *The Therapist*, 81-87.

Wampold, Bruce E. (2017). What should we practice? A contextual model for how psychotherapy works. In Rousmaniere, Tony; Goodyear, Rodney K.; Miller, Scott D. & Wampold, Bruce E. (Eds). *The Cycle of*

Excellence: Using Deliberate Practice to Improve Supervision and Training. Retrieved from https://doi.org/10.1002/9781119165590.ch3

Wampold, Bruce. (2010). The research evidence for the contextual model models: A historically situated perspective. In Wampold, Bruce E.; Duncan, Barry L.; Miller, Scott D. (Eds). *The Heart and Soul of Change, Second Edition: Delivering What Works in Therapy*. American Psychological Association. Retrieved from http://dx.doi.org/10.1037/12075-002

Wampold, B. E., & Imel, Z. E. (2015). *The Great Psychotherapy Debate: The Evidence for What Makes Psychotherapy Work (2nd edition).* New York: Routledge.

Watkins, H. (1993). Ego-state therapy: an overview. *American Journal of Clinical Hypnosis*, 35 (4), 232-240. Retrieved from https://doi.org/10.1080/00029157.1993.10403014

In: Borderline Personality Disorder
Editor: Charles M. Lepkowsky
ISBN: 978-1-53618-021-3

Chapter 8

THE STIGMA OF BORDERLINE PERSONALITY DISORDER

Charles M. Lepkowsky*[*], *PhD
Independent Practice, Solvang, California, US

ABSTRACT

Historically, the Borderline Personality Disorder (BPD) diagnosis has carried a stigma that can negatively impact the BPD person's self-image, employment opportunitues, physical health, and the perceptions and effectiveness of the psychotherapist. The stigma of BPD manifests in the community, among health care providers, and within one's self. Identification of biological correlates of BPD and their utility in evaluating the effectivess of evidence-based treatment methodologies for BPD have had some impact on the stigma of BPD. Additional advances in understanding and treating BPD have also impacted the ways in which the stigma associated with BPD is recognized and addressed.

Keywords: borderline personality disorder, BPD stigma, BPD self-stigma, BPD Therapist Stigma

[*] Corresponding Author's E-mail: clepkowsky@gmail.com.

INTRODUCTION

The term "stigma" is defined as "a mark of shame or discredit: a stain" (Merriam-Webster, 2020). Social stigmatization is understood as stereotyping, prejudice and discrimination (Stull, McGrew, Salyers, & Ashburn-Nardo, 2013). Members of stigmatized groups are viewed as tainted or having less value, and as a consequence are discounted by others and experience social and emotional isolation (Goffman, 1963). People respond to stigmatization with cognitive, emotional, psychological and behavioral responses that are often unconscious or involuntary (Miller & Kaiser, 2001).

Emotionally unregulated unconscious or involuntary cognitive, emotional, psychological and behavioral responses manifesting as emotional dysregulation, interpersonal difficulties, and negative self-concept are hallmark symptoms of Borderline Personality Disorder (BPD) (American Psychiatric Association [ApA], 2013). Historically, BPD has been characterized by health care providers as difficult to treat (Ferguson, 2016; Dingfelder, 2004). This is due in part to the complexity of BPD. BPD is defined by the following features: emotion dysregulation, difficulty managing anger, difficulties maintaining healthy and stable relationships, fear of abandonment, impulsive behaviors, suicidal and/or non-suicidal self-injurious (NSSI) behaviors or threats, fluctuating sense of self, feelings of emptiness, and difficulty concentrating under stress (ApA, 2013). Seventy-five percent of people diagnosed with BPD have comorbid conditions, including depression, anxiety, post-traumatic stress disorder (PTSD), complex post-traumatic stress disorder (CPTSD), substance abuse/dependence, eating disorders, and physical health issues (Sauer-Zavala, Bentley, & Wilner, 2016).

The BPD diagnosis is associated with more severe and persistent impairment in social functioning than major depressive disorder (MDD) or other personality disorders, with greater utilization of mental health resources and use of antidepressant, anxiolytic or mood stabilizing medication (Bender et al., 2001). Compared with other personality disorders, a significantly higher percentage of BPD patients have a history of individual and group therapy, day and residential treatment, psychiatric hospitalization, participating in self-help groups, and use of psychoactive medications. BPD patients are significantly younger when initiating these treatments, and spend significantly more time in individual therapy, psychiatric hospitals, and on medications, with a significantly higher number of psychiatric hospitalizations, lifetime number of psychoactive medication prescriptions, and number of psychotropic medications taken at the same time (Zanarini, Frankenburg, Khera, & Bleichmar, 2001).

Estimates of the prevalence of BPD in outpatient clinics varies widely depending on the setting and methodology, ranging from 7% to 27% (Korzekwa, Dell, Links, Thabane, & Webb, 2008). Much of the literature on BPD states that up to seventy percent of BPD patients drop out of treatment (Gunderson, 2009; Dingfelder, 2004), despite a systematic meta-analysis finding that only between sixteen and twenty-five percent of BPD patients drop out of treatment (Barnicot, Katsakou, Marougka, & Priebe, 2011). BPD symptoms are often viewed by clinicians as challenging or difficult, producing a stigma for BPD that is greater than that associated with other mental health diagnoses (Aviram, Brodsky, & Stanley, 2006).

Based on characterizations emphasizing BPD's complex symptom picture, high rate of comorbidity, high frequency of interpersonal difficulties, and low rate of successful treatment outcomes, many health care professionals view BPD negatively and decline to work with BPD patients. A priori clinician decisions to decline to treat people with BPD can be viewed as stereotyping, prejudicial, discriminating, and stigmatizing (Aviram, Brodsky, & Stanley, 2006). Although poor BPD treatment outcomes have been associated with the employment of ineffective methodologies, negative clinician attributions and the accompanying bias and stigma regarding BPD persist (Gunderson et al., 2011). Ironically, clinician stigma toward BPD leading to inadequate and unfair treatment increases the likelihood of poor outcomes and risk for impulsive behavior leading to self-harm, 'validating' negative clinician attributions about BPD in what might be characterized as a self-fulfilling prophecy (Ferguson, 2016; Sheehan, Nieweglowski, & Corrigan, 2016).

During the past twenty years, BPD has surfaced into the awareness of the lay population, with both positive and negative consequences. Potential positive consequences include recognition of characteristic BPD behaviors as possible symptoms of a diagnosable and treatable condition, so that people with BPD may be accurately diagnosed and enter treatment earlier than if their condition had gone unrecognized (Dimeff & Linehan, 2001). Potential negative consequences include labeling and stereotyping by members of the lay community in ways that can be stigmatizing, even affecting employment and opportunities for advancement for the person with BPD (Juurlink et al., 2019). Similarly, people who self-identify with BPD might benefit from early identification and intervention, or might also suffer self-stigma by associating their diagnosis with negative characterizations of BPD (Corrigan, Larson, & Rüsch, 2009).

Increased awareness of BPD over the last few decades is also reflected by increased research and clinical interest in the diagnosis, producing novel conceptualizations and treatment modalities for BPD. These include increasing knowledge of biological correlates of BPD, which have contributed to the understanding of BPD's relationship with trauma and CPTSD. Increased understanding of BPD has promoted specific training in novel and effective methodologies for the treatment of BPD. Each of these advancements has demonstrated effectiveness in improving the attitudes of health care providers toward patients with BPD, which might eventually lead to reductions in the stigma associated with BPD.

BPD Stigma in the Community

Stigma in the community, or public stigma, is expressed in the form of stereotypes, prejudice, and discrimination (Corrigan, Larson, & Rüsch, 2009). Stereotypes can be understood as belief systems held by the majority of members of one group and applied to members of other groups (Major & O'Brien, 2005). Prejudice or "prejudgment" is the consequence of making decisions about others based on stereotypes (Hilton & von Hippel, 1996; Devine, 1995). The behavioral manifestation of prejudice is discrimination

(Crocker, Major, & Steele, 1998), which is expressed toward stigmatized persons through loss of opportunities (including vocation and access to housing), coercion (e.g., decision-making authority is taken from the individual who is considered incapable), and segregation (e.g., in the past, placement in state mental hospitals, and in the present, homelessness) (Corrigan, 2005).

Stereotypes applied to people with mental health diagnoses include assignment of blame, dangerousness and incompetence (Corrigan & Kleinlein, 2005). Historically, American culture has stigmatized people with mental health diagnoses. Systematic reviews of the research literature on the stigma applied to people with mental health diagnoses indicate that public stigma of mental illness in the U.S. remains widespread (Parcesepe & Cabassa, 2013; Corrigan, Morris, Michaels, Rafaczm, & Rüsch, 2012), despite increasing public understanding of the biological correlates of mental illness (Schomerus et al., 2012).

Poor community understanding of mental health issues and the associated stigma affect the person with BPD in numerous ways throughout the lifespan. A growing body of research evidence indicates that BPD features can be identified during childhood and can interfere with early academic and social functioning. In a longitudinal study, 1,116 pairs of same-sex twins were followed from birth through age 12 years. BPD characteristics at 12 years of age were found to be highly heritable, and more common in children who had exhibited poor cognitive function, impulsivity, and more behavioral and emotional problems at age 5 years. BPD characteristics also co-occurred with symptoms of conduct disorder, depression, anxiety, and psychosis (Belsky et al., 2012). A short-term longitudinal study of 400 fourth through sixth grade children supported the validity of the Borderline Personality Features Scale for Children (BPFS-C), with girls scoring higher for BPF than boys (Crick, Murray-Close, & Woods, 2005). In both instances, BPD characteristics were found to interfere with academic performance and social functioning. Without an understanding of BPD, teachers and school administrators interpret characteristic BPD behaviors in negative terms (poor cognitive function, impulsivity, conduct disorder, depression, anxiety, and psychosis) that contribute to stigma, which might also generalize to stigmatization by other children. Retrospective self-reports of past experiences of childhood abuse and neglect indicate that compared with other populations, BPD patients report a higher prevalence of physical abuse by peers (Laporte, Paris, Guttman, Russell, & Correa, 2012).

BPD stigma is likely to increase after high school. Psychological distress in the general college population has been increasing over the past four decades. College students experiencing higher levels of distress than the general population, and increased distress is associated with increased disability (Stallman, 2008). Over half of college students report at least one mental health issue during their first year in college, increasing to sixty percent after two years, with fewer than half receiving treatment (Zivin, Eisenberg, Gollust & Golberstein, 2009). At-risk college student behaviors associated with the experience of stress include alcohol consumption, unhealthy diet, physical inactivity, tobacco smoking and cannabis use (Deasy, Coughlin, Pironom, Jourdan & McNamara, 2015). In a study of 2,261 college students, rumination, alexithymia, and emotional regulation were predictors of dysregulated behaviors associated with BPD including self-harm, substance use and aggression. College students with BPD experience significantly greater than average emotional distress and risk for self-injurious behaviors that interfere with academic and social functioning, also increasing the stigma associated with BPD (Meaney, Hasking & Reupert, 2016).

With or without post-secondary education, BPD is associated with higher than average rates of unemployment and impaired vocational functioning. Vocational barriers for people with BPD have been categorized into three subsets: characteristics of BPD, stigma, and lack of vocational support. Characteristics of BPD including low self-image, difficulty with interpersonal boundaries, difficulty regulating emotions, externalization, overestimation of competencies, and lack of structure have been identified as primary barriers to employment. These BPD characteristics contribute to the stigma and inadequate vocational support that have also been identified as significant barriers to employment or career advancement for people with BPD (Juurlink et al., 2019; Link, 1982).

BPD has been linked to eating disorders, including obesity, a significant health problem that bears a stigma of its own. Among people with obesity, the prevalence of BPD is over 26% (Sansone & Sansone, 2013a). BPD is also found in 22% of people with anorexia nervosa (restricting type), 25% of people with anorexia nervosa (bingeing and purging type), and 28% of people with bulimia nervosa (Sansone & Sansone, 2011). Although the general prevalence of personality disorders among people with eating disorders is not known, BPD is the most common personality disorder in binge-eating/purging type anorexia nervosa and bulimia nervosa, each of which bears a stigma as well (Sansone, Levitt & Sansone, 2005; Sansone & Sansone, 2010a).

BPD is also associated with a higher than average frequency of negative interactions with law enforcement and the legal system. Law enforcement officers typically receive little or no training in personality disorders (PDs). In most communities, there is poor coordination between law enforcement and mental health systems. When attempting to refer people with PDs to mental health services, law enforcement officers express frustration, anger, powerlessness and resignation. Law enforcement officers often view hospital emergency departments as reluctant to assess people with PDs, with emergency staff often stating that the PD person does not meet criteria for admission. If admitted, the PD person is often quickly discharged, consuming considerable law enforcement resources. Largely due to lack of education and training in working with people with personality disorders, law enforcement officers frequently experience people with PDs as frustrating, uncooperative or difficult, negative attributions consistent with the stigma associated with BPD (Martin & Thomas, 2015).

BPD Stigma in Popular Culture

Relatively unknown to mainstream American culture over the last century, during the past decade BPD has become a household expression. The increase in public awareness of BPD is largely attributable to the emergence of media portrayals of BPD in film and television, self-help literature describing BPD, and online access to BPD information and support groups. Most self-help literature concerning BPD is intended not for the person with the diagnosis, but for their friends and family. A well-known best-seller is the book "Stop Walking on Eggshells -- Taking Your Life Back When Someone You Care About Has Borderline Personality Disorder" (Mason & Kreger, 2010). As the title indicates, the book's target audience is the person in a relationship with someone with BPD. The book provides a description of BPD and the experience of the BPD person, but its emphasis is "taking your life back," suggesting that someone with BPD takes over the lives of people around them. However well-intended, the implication is that other people suffer or endure people with BPD, consistent with negative characterizations of BPD that reinforce the stigma associated with the diagnosis.

Other popular literature focused on helping the reader understand the BPD person includes "I Hate You--Don't Leave Me: Understanding the Borderline Personality" (Kreisman & Straus, 2010) and "Loving Someone with Borderline Personality Disorder" (Manning, 2011). Although these books intend a more sympathetic and respectful look at the BPD person and their experience of the world and people around them, their premise is that the potential rewards of maintaining a relationship with someone with BPD might outweigh the emotional discomfort and effort required – an equation which itself bears a negative connotation. The naïve reader is likely to come away viewing people with BPD as moody, manipulative, difficult, challenging, and difficult to love.

Media portrayals of BPD have varied from sympathetic to extremely negative and stigmatizing. The motion picture *Fatal Attraction* (Paramount Pictures, 1987) tells the story of a man who has a casual affair with a woman with BPD who becomes increasingly clingy, desperate, and aggressive, stalking and terrorizing the man and his family (the film is perhaps best remembered for the scene in which the BPD woman boils the family's pet rabbit). *Fatal Attraction*'s characterization of BPD is perhaps the most widely known in motion pictures, and has been criticized as stigmatizing, negative and damaging, even by actress Glenn Close, who played the BPD character in the film (Desta, 2017). In *Play Misty for Me* (The Malpaso

Company, 1971) and *The Crush* (Morgan Creek Entertainment, 1993) women with BPD are also portrayed as seductive and dangerous stalkers of male love objects. Research indicates that a relatively small minority (between 4% and 15%) of stalkers in forensic studies have a diagnosis of BPD (Harmon, Rosner, & Owens, 1995; Kienlen, Birmingham, Solberg, O'Regan & Meloy, 1997; Purcell, Pathé & Mullen, 2001). A retrospective study of psychiatrists indicated a BPD prevalence rate of 15% among stalkers (McIvor, Potter, & Davies, 2008), and only one retrospective study where no criminal charges were filed indicates that a larger percentage (45%) of stalkers have a diagnosis of BPD (Meloy & Boyd, 2003). These data suggest that repeated media portrayals of people with BPD as dangerous stalkers is an inaccurate and stigmatizing exaggeration (Sansone & Sansone, 2010b).

Other motion pictures that portray people with BPD in ways that might be stigmatizing include *Welcome to Me* (Gary Sanchez Productions, 2014), in which the impulsive main character eventually experiences "a mental breakdown," and several films described as portraying people with BPD, although the diagnosis is never explicitly assigned in the film. More negative characterizations include *Single White Female* (Columbia Pictures, 1992), *Fear* (Imagine Entertainment, 1996), *One Hour Photo* (Searchlight Pictures, 2002) and *Ingrid Goes West* (Star Thrower Entertainment 141 & Entertainment Mighty Engine, 2017). Less dramatic but unsympathetic characterizations include *Margot at the Wedding* (Paramount Vantage, 2007), *Rachel Getting Married* (Demme, Armian & Platt, 2008), *Frances* (Universal Pictures, 1982), *Thirteen* (Searchlight Pictures, 2003) (Allen, 2013), *Eternal Sunshine of the Spotless Mind* (Focus Features, 2004), *Silver Linings Playbook* (The Weinstein Company, 2012), *Prozac Nation* (Miramax, 2001), *Star Wars Episodes II and III* (Lucasfilm Ltd., 2002, 2005) (Virzi, 2017), and *The Crush* (Morgan Creek Entertainment, 1993) (Sansone & Sansone, 2010b). Bui and associates (2011) state that the *Star Wars* character Anakin Skywalker meets the criteria for BPD, and suggest that the films might be useful in educating the general public and medical students about BPD symptoms (Bui, Rodgers, Chabrol, Birmes, & Schmitt, 2011). The suggestion is alarming, to the extent that the character of Anakin

Skywalker murders a tribe of men, women and children in *Star Wars Episode II*, and among other victims, a large number of young children in *Star Wars Episode III.* Murdering men, women and children is not a documented symptom of BPD. The association of the *Star Wars Episodes II and III* character Anakin Skywalker with BPD conveys an inaccurate and stigmatizing view of a person with BPD.

There have also been a number of television series that explicitly or implicitly depict BPD, varying from stigmatizing to sympathetic. These include *One Life to Live* (ABC, 1968-2013), *The Sopranos* (HBO, 1999-2007), *Crazy Ex-Girlfriend* (The CW, 2015-2019), and *Love* (Netflix, 2016-2018). In these series, the BPD person is depicted in ways that vary from sympathetic to terrifying. Often the same character is portrayed as sympathetic and terrifying, like Tony Soprano, the mobster who suffers from panic attacks, develops an emotional fixation on his psychotherapist, and all the while engages in murder and mayhem. Again, these media portrayals convey to the public an overall impression of BPD that is negative and stigmatizing.

BPD Stigma among Health Care Providers

Irv Yalom once wrote, "The word 'borderline' strikes terror in the heart of the middle-aged comfort-seeking psychiatrist" (Yalom, 1989). BPD is viewed more negatively by mental health practitioners than almost any other psychiatric diagnosis (Bodner et al., 2015; Black et al., 2011; Ferguson, 2016). In a sample of 706 psychiatrists, psychologists, social workers and psychiatric nurses, nearly half reported that they preferred to avoid BPD patients (Black et al., 2011). Clinicians often perceive patients with a prior diagnosis of personality disorder (PD) as more difficult and less deserving of care than people with other psychiatric diagnoses, and are regarded as manipulative, attention-seeking, annoying, and in control of their suicidal urges and debts (Lewis & Appleby, 1988). Negative clinician assumptions about people with BPD represent stereotyping and prejudice, and reluctance or refusal to treat people with BPD is discrimination. A meta-analysis found that biogenetic explanations might reduce clinician tendencies to blame patients, but have no impact on social distancing, and are associated with clinician pessimism regarding anticipated outcome. The authors concluded that clinician pessimism might lead to a self-fulfilling prophecy of treatment failure (Kvaale, Haslam, & Gottdiener, 2013).

Psychiatrists are often reluctant to assign psychiatric inpatients the diagnosis of BPD, which can lead to staff confusion and negative behavior in response to characteristic BPD behaviors (Paris, 2015, 2007). The attitudes of psychiatric nursing staff toward patients with BPD have been studied more than any other group of clinicians (Sansone & Sansone, 2013b). Psychiatric nurses are less likely to demonstrate affective involvement in response to BPD patients than schizophrenic patients, and are more likely to offer BPD patients belittling or contradicting responses (Gallop, Lancee, & Garfinkel, 1989; Markham, 2003). Among mental care providers including psychiatrists, psychologists and social workers, psychiatric nurses have the lowest self-ratings on overall caring attitudes toward patients diagnosed with BPD (Black et al., 2011).

Negative countertransference reactions from health care providers occur more frequently toward people with BPD than any other mental health diagnoses (Liebman & Burnette, 2013). Psychotherapists often withhold the BPD diagnosis from BPD patients, citing low confidence in assigning the diagnosis or concern that assigning the BPD diagnosis might be harmful to the patient (Sisti et al., 2016). To the interpersonally sensitive BPD patient, withholding the BPD diagnosis suggests that the psychotherapist perceives the patient as fragile, self-destructive, or suicidal, reflective of negative countertransference. This interpretation is supported by the finding that BPD patients who later learn that their diagnosis had been withheld by their therapists frequently terminate treatment (Sulzer et al., 2016). A systematic review of research literature found that health care professionals frequently stigmatize BPD individuals through the use of derogatory language including the terms "treatment resistant," "complicated," "demanding," "dangerous," "manipulative," and "attention seeking," with the consequence that people with BPD are marginalized in the health care system. The authors attribute negative characterizations of people with BPD within the health care community to a lack of training and clinical supervision (Ociskova et al., 2017).

There is evidence that clinicians with inadequate training in BPD emotionally distance themselves from BPD patients, exacerbating the BPD patient's tendency to perceive rejection and abandonment in relationships (Sansone & Sansone, 2013b). The BPD patient may react by engaging in self-harm or withdrawing from treatment. In turn, the practitioner's emotional distancing increases, possibly out of self-protection. This interaction can become a self-fulfilling prophecy to which both patient and therapist contribute, perpetuating a cycle of stigmatization (Aviram, Brodsky, & Stanley, 2006). Adolescents with BPD are likely to experience even greater stigmatization than BPD adults. Research indicates that among adolescents seeking treatment for Axis I psychiatric diagnoses and/or personality disorders, BPD is the strongest predictor for the experience of stigma, with the most symptomatic BPD adolescents reporting the highest levels of stigma (Catthoor, Feenstra, Hutsebaut, Schrijvers, & Sabbe, 2015).

People with BPD have been described as marginalized or denied access to mental health services due to stigmatizing practices and limited services (Kealy & Ogrodniczuk, 2010; Nehls, 1998). Research data indicate that people with a diagnosis of BPD experience significant discrimination within both public and private health services, findings attributed to pervasive negative attitudes towards people with a diagnosis of BPD (Lawn & McMahon, 2015). The negative stigma associated with BPD among mental health practitioners has been variously described as a natural reaction to dealing with difficult people, a self-protective mechanism, and a form of discrimination (Lawn & McMahon, 2015; Veysey, 2014; Zimmerman, 2015). The stereotype that BPD patients are manipulative might lead to therapists not believing or validating the experience of the patient, who in turn might feel unheard, increasing symptom expression and increasing therapist feelings of inadequacy or failure. Therapists who feel ineffective or a lack of control might assign blame to the BPD patient as a self-protective mechanism against feelings of failure or inadequacy, consistent with findings that stereotypes applied to people with mental health diagnoses include assignment of blame (Corrigan & Kleinlein, 2005). Whatever its basis, clinician stigma regarding BPD has become widely recognized (Bodner et al., 2015; Markham, 2003), and is increasingly considered evidence of a lack of training in or understanding of BPD (Ferguson, 2016; Sansone & Sansone, 2013b).

SELF-STIGMA IN BPD

Self-stigma is the application of stigma to one's self. Self-stigma requires that people are aware of the stereotypes applied by the community to a stigmatized group, agree with the stereotypes, and apply the stereotypes to themselves (Watson, Corrigan, Larson, & Sells, 2007). In a culture with prevailing stereotypes about mental health diagnoses, people with mental health diagnoses are likely to anticipate and internalize those stereotypes, including attitudes that reflect devaluation and discrimination. In this context, devaluation is experienced as an awareness that the community does not accept the person with a mental health diagnosis. Being aware that one is considered unacceptable by the community, agreeing with that stereotype, and applying it to one's self results in self-devaluation, or more fully, self-stigma (Corrigan, Larson, & Rüsch, 2009).

Internalizing stereotypes about mental illness reduces self-esteem and self-efficacy (Link, 1987; Link, Cullen, & Frank, 1987; Markowitz, 1998; Otilingam & Graiales, 2003; Ritsher & Phelan, 2004; Ritsher & Rosenfield, 1997). People with mental health diagnoses report moderate to severe levels of self-stigma, associated with low self-esteem, self-efficacy, and recovery orientation, as well as more severe psychiatric symptoms (Drapalski et al., 2013). People diagnosed with BPD experience significantly greater self-stigma than people with other mental health diagnoses (Corrigan & Calabrese, 2005; Grambal et al., 2016). In women diagnosed with BPD, self-stigma is inversely related to self-esteem, self-efficacy, and quality of life, and women with BPD experience more self-stigma than women with social phobia (Rüsch et al., 2006). This finding might be the consequence of the belief that people with BPD should be able to control their behavior, as if it is bad and purposeful (Aviram et al., 2006).

The way that people perceive, evaluate, memorize, and respond to self-related information is directly influenced by self-conscious emotions including guilt, shame, or self-disgust, as well as self-related motives, including self-enhancement or self-verification. Impairments in self-functioning and identity are considered central features of BPD (ApA, 2013). In people with BPD, self-concept is frequently negative, and self-esteem is low, unstable, and reactive to self-relevant cues. These include negative feelings toward one's self, including self-disgust and shame, which can negatively impact self-related motives (Winter, Bohus, & Lis, 2017). Reduced self-esteem and self-efficacy tied to mental health self-stigma may lead to a "why try" perspective that dissuades people with mental health diagnoses from pursuing opportunities to achieve life goals, and avoid accessing and using evidence-based practices that help achieve those goals. The "why try" effect works on three levels: self-stigma that results from self-applied stereotypes; mediators including self-esteem and self-efficacy; and life goal achievement, or lack thereof (Corrigan, Larson, & Rüsch, 2009). Because stigma functions as a cue to elicit prejudice and discrimination (Goffman, 1963), self-stigma interferes with the attainment of self-determined goals including vocation, housing, education, health and wellness, relationships and recreation, and faith-based aspirations, and can undermine the positive effects of evidence-based psychotherapeutic practices (Corrigan, Larson, & Rüsch, 2009).

People with BPD appear more likely than individuals with other mental health diagnoses to evoke negative countertransference reactions from health care providers (Liebman & Burnette, 2013). Health care providers report that they frequently withhold the diagnosis of BPD from patients, partly due to uncertainty about the diagnosis, and partly out of concern that assigning the stigmatizing diagnosis would be harmful to the patient (Sisti, Segal, Siegel, Johnson, & Gunderson, 2016). People with BPD are acutely aware of how they are regarded by others. Withholding the BPD diagnosis might convey or imply that the therapist believes that the patient is too fragile, self-destructive, or suicidal to accept the BPD diagnosis. Negative countertransference is palpable to people with BPD, and contributes significantly to the negative self-concept, low self-esteem, self-disgust, and deep shame that contribute to self-stigma. BPD patients who later learn that their diagnosis had been withheld by their therapists frequently terminate treatment (Sulzer, Muenchow, Potvin, Harris, & Gigot, 2016). Informing BPD patients of their diagnosis is a more person-centered approach that improves therapeutic trust, rapport, and outcome (Lequesne & Hersh, 2004). For patients with BPD, increases in negative self-concept (self-stigma) correlate with the number of times they have had psychiatric hospitalizations with increased exposure to hospital personal with stigmatizing views of BPD (Aviram, 2006). BPD self-stigma contributes to resistance to seeking treatment, resistance to psychotherapists, and continuation of abusive relationships that "validate" the BPD person's being blamed for the abuse they receive (Usher, 2016).

Information from the media and society also contribute to the self-stigma associated with BPD. Internet access to information about BPD has increased exponentially over the last decade. Information available online ranges from symptom check lists and educational websites to online support groups and chats to vlogs, blogs or other platforms in which negative experiences with or views of people with BPD are shared by others. BPD patients in uncertain therapeutic relationships may turn to the internet for support, only to find angry or accusatory posts by people who believe that they have been mistreated by someone with BPD. Online criticisms and negative characterizations of people with BPD can confirm negative self-stigma for the person with BPD, contributing to feelings of hopelessness that are a key component of suicidal ideation and self-destructive behaviors (Usher, 2016).

Addressing the Stigma Associated with BPD

A stigma, as the root term "stain" suggests, is difficult to remove. A more realistic and achievable goal is to reduce stigma. The stigma clinicians attach to BPD can be reduced by understanding the contributions of genetic and biological influences to BPD, the role of trauma in the etiology of BPD, and the efficacy of evidence-based treatments for long-term symptom remission.

Biological Influences

Biological Correlates of BPD

Advancements in neuroimaging, genetic studies and molecular genetics have made it possible to identify biological correlates of BPD. Using neuroimaging techniques that have previously demonstrated neurobiological differences in people with PTSD (O'Neill & Frodl, 2012), neurobiological differences have also been found in people with BPD (Krause-Utz, Winter, Liedfeld, & Schmahl, 2014). Reduced volume in the amygdala and especially, the hippocampus, are associated with BPD and have been nominated as potential biomarkers for BPD (Ruocco, Amirthavasagam, & Zakzanis, 2012).

People with BPD also demonstrate functional neurological differences from other populations, which can be seen in functional brain imaging studies (Sosic-Vasic et al., 2019). When exposed to stress, reduced functioning in the amygdala, uncus and hippocampus is apparent in people with BPD, which might explain poor inhibitory regulation, exaggerated fear responses and impulsive or aggressive behavior (Phillips & LeDoux, 1992).

Genetic Predisposition to BPD

Whether due to genetics or environment, BPD appears to run in families (Gunderson et al., 2011). Parental histories of mental illness and lifetime Axis I disorders appear to be significant and unique predictors of BPD (Trull, 2001). BPD does, however, appear to have a genetic component. Genetic studies demonstrate that the prevalence of BPD among relatives is 14%, more than three times the 4.9% prevalence rate of BPD in family members of controls (Gunderson et al., 2011). Longitudinal twin studies suggest that the heritability of BPD is between 40% and 70%, and that there are both genetic and environmental factors in the development of BPD (Bornovalova et al., 2018; Skoglund et al., 2019).

Molecular Genetic Research in BPD

Molecular genetic research has found differences in neurotransmitter receptor polymorphism and function, as well as enzyme production and activity in people with BPD. In people with BPD, genetic polymorphisms have been found (Amad, Ramos, Thomas, Jardri, & Gorwood, 2014), affecting serotonin metabolism (Pier, Marin, Wilsnack, & Goodman, 2016) in ways associated with higher levels of aggression, emotional lability, and increased suicidal behavior (Perez-Rodriguez, 2010). Similarly, polymorphisms of dopamine receptors exist in people with BPD (O'Neill & Frodl, 2012), interfering with behavioral inhibition (Aron & Poldrack, 2006; Brown, Manuck, Flory, & Hariri, 2006; Congdon & Canli, 2008). Understanding that people with BPD have genetic predispositions toward symptom expression is one way of reducing blame and stigma from clinicians.

Understanding BPD's Relationship with CPTSD

In 2018, the World Health Organization (WHO) presented the 11th edition of the International Statistical Classification of Diseases and Related Health Problems (ICD-11) (WHO, 2018). ICD-11 introduces a new diagnosis, complex post-traumatic stress disorder (CPTSD), distinct from the diagnosis of post-traumatic stress disorder (PTSD) (Brewin, n.d.). PTSD is typically associated with a specific traumatic event or set of events. CPTSD is associated with prolonged, chronic exposure to traumatic experiences, especially in childhood. CPTSD is a diagnosis not included in the fifth edition of the Diagnostic and Statistical Manual of Mental Disorders (DSM-5, ApA, 2013).

BPD is frequently associated with PTSD (Pagura et al., 2010), giving rise to some controversy about whether or how CPTSD is distinct from PTSD comorbid with BPD. Data support the construct of the CPTSD diagnosis as a distinct entity, which has significant symptom overlap with BPD (Jowett, Karatzias, Shevlin, & Albert, 2020; Rosenfield et al., 2018). CPTSD consists of six symptom clusters, three of which are the PTSD criteria of re-experiencing, avoidance, and hypervigilance. The other three symptom clusters are the three disturbances of self-organization (DSO) symptoms defined as emotional dysregulation, interpersonal difficulties, and negative self-concept. BPD shares these three symptom clusters with CPTSD (ApA, 2013). Significant similarities in neuropsychological deficits between BPD and CPTSD have also been found in psychoendocrinological and neuroimaging studies. Some authors believe that BPD might be a form of CPTSD (Driesen et al., 2002), or that many individuals diagnosed with BPD actually have CPTSD (Walker, 2014).

Evidence of Childhood Trauma in BPD

There is substantial evidence supporting a strong association between BPD and a history of childhood abuse and/or neglect, with estimates of a correlation between forty and ninety-three percent (Ball & Links, 2009; Bandelow et al., 2005; Goodman & Yehuda, 2002; Gunderson et el., 2011; Herman, Perry & Van der Kolk, 1989; Laporte et al., 2012; Merza, Papp, & Szabó, 2015; Ogata, Silk, Goodrich, Lohr, & Hill, 1990; Oldham, Skodol, Gallaher, & Kroll, 1996; Zanarini, Frankenburg, Khera, & Bleichmar, 2001). A recent systematic review of the literature and meta-analysis indicates that people diagnosed with BPD are more than three times as likely to report childhood abuse and/or neglect than people with other psychiatric diagnoses (Porter et al., 2020).

There is some indication that the relationship between childhood abuse or neglect and BPD is causal (Ball & Links, 2009). Specifically, a history of childhood abuse appears to correlate with the BPD diagnostic criteria of unstable relationships, feelings of emptiness, and abandonment fears. A childhood history of neglect correlates with suicidal behavior (Oldham et al., 1996). There is a significant association between childhood sexual abuse (CSA) and BPD (Bandelow et al., 2005; Goodman & Yehuda, 2002; Merza, Papp, & Szabó, 2015; Ogata et al., 1990; Salzman et al., 1993), with evidence that BPD women who experienced biparental abuse or neglect have significantly higher rates of CSA by non-caretakers (Zanarini et al., 2000).

Early research suggested that affective instability, intense anger, and identity disturbance appear uncorrelated with abuse or neglect, suggesting that the affective symptoms of BPD might be unrelated to aversive childhood events, consistent with the concept of a subtype of BPD dominated by affective dysregulation (Oldham et al., 1996). However, more recent research indicates that there is an indirect relationship between childhood emotional abuse and BPD, specifically through difficulties with emotional regulation, a key component of BPD (Kuo, Khoury, Metcalfe, Fitzpatrick, & Goodwill, 2015). Because it is more subtle than physical or sexual abuse, emotional abuse may be largely unrecognized by those who have experienced it as abuse per se. To date, research has focused much less on emotional abuse than physical or sexual abuse, and emotional abuse is rarely included in assessments of adverse childhood experiences. Consequently, emotional abuse is likely to go unreported. Although its developmental contributions to BPD are more difficult to calculate, emotional abuse specifically may have a developmental role in BPD pathology (Kuo et al., 2015).

Cumulatively, the research data strongly suggest that adverse childhood experiences play a significant role in the development of BPD, illustrated by the overlap between BPD and CPTSD on self-report measures of disturbed relationships, suicidality, and latent variables showing childhood interpersonal trauma (Hyland, 2019). Understanding that there are multiple factors contributing to BPD (genetics, biology and experience) might reduce clinician stigma toward BPD.

Evidence-Based Treatment: Specific Training in the Treatment of BDP

Longitudinal research indicates that naturalistic integration of evidence-based treatments (EBTs) for BPD reduces BPD and PTSD symptoms with or without a PTSD-specific intervention (Masland, Cummings, Null, Woynowskie, & Choi-Kain, 2019). Specific training in the treatment of BPD is associated with more positive clinician perceptions of BPD patients and better treatment outcomes (Bedics, Atkins, Harned, & Linehan, 2015; Choi-Kain et al., 2017; Cristea et al., 2017). Training in understanding cognitive processing differences in BPD and techniques for improving cognitive processing in BPD leads to better treatment outcomes (Soloff, White, Omari, Ramaseshan, & Diwadkar, 2015; Zanarini, Frankenburg, Reich, & Fitzmaurice, 2012). Teaching staff working in mental health care settings about the neurobiological underpinnings of BPD produces improvements in attitudes toward BPD patients at post-test and eight-week follow-up (Clark, Fox, & Long, 2014).

Healthcare staff who complete a two-day self-management workshop show positive change in attitudes, therapeutic relationship, and social distance towards people with BPD at post-test and six-month follow-up (Clarke, Taylor, Bolderston, Lancaster, & Remington, 2014). Attendance at "good psychiatric management" or GPM workshops on attitudes toward patients with BPD has demonstrated effectiveness for improving treatment outcomes (Gunderson, 2016; Keuroghlian et al., 2016). Specialized BPD training for clinical psychologists has been associated with increased service provision to and more positive attitudes towards people with BPD (Egan, Haley, & Rees, 2014).

Addressing BPD Self-Stigma

Marsha Linehan's Dialectical Behavior Therapy (DBT) emphasizes understanding the world-view of the person with BPD (Dimeff & Linehan, 2001), which reduces self-stigma and has demonstrated long-term effectiveness for BPD symptom remission (Neacsiu, Lungu, Harned, Rizvi, & Linehan, 2014), acute symptom resolution for adolescent inpatients (Tebbett-Mock, Saito, McGee, Woloszyn, & Venuti, 2019), and long-term reduction of self-injurious or suicidal behavior in adolescents with BPD (Mehlum et al., 2019). Corrigan, Larson and Rüsch (2009) suggest that the "why try" model of self-stigma in BPD can be used to identify and evaluate self-stigma modification approaches. Corrigan and associates advocate empowerment through consumer operated services, group identity and coming out as mechanisms for positive change, as opposed to a dysfunction-based model of change. A first step toward empowerment is cognitive reframing from "what should not be done" to "what might be done" (Corrigan, Larson, & Rüsch, 2009).

Self-stigma can also be reduced by understanding that BPD is not necessarily a chronic, life-disrupting condition. Engaging in EBT with appropriately trained clinicians, participating in consumer operated services, establishing a positive group identity, and coming out in a manner of one's choosing are all strategies associated with long-term symptom remission for BPD. Long-term follow-up studies indicate that although symptoms may periodically increase or decrease, acute behavioral symptoms tend to remit early and rarely recur. The majority of people diagnosed with BPD experience long-term symptom remission (Temes & Zanarini, 2018).

Summary and Conclusion

The evolution of the understanding of BPD, its neurobiological correlates, and its overlap with CPTSD has helped reduce the stigma associated with BPD. The development of appropriate clinician training in humanistic EBTs for BPD has led to better treatment outcomes. Better BPD treatment outcomes have increased clinician optimism for treating BPD, with consequent reductions in clinician stigma toward BPD. Optimism plays an important role in reducing BPD self-stigma, with powerful implications for symptom reduction and maintenance of remission over time.

REFERENCES

ABC. (1968-2013) *One Life to Live.* Television series.

Allen, D. M. (2013). Borderline personality disorder in the movies. *Psychology Today*. Available from: https://www.psychologytoday.com/us/blog/matter-personality/201307/borderline-personality-disorder-in-the-movies.

Amad, A., Ramoz, N., Thomas, P., Jardri, R. & Gorwood, P. (2014). Genetics of borderline personality disorder: systematic review and proposal of an integrative model. *Neurosci Biobehav Rev,40*, 6-19. http://dx.doi.org/10.1016/j.neubiorev.2014.01.003.

American Psychiatric Association. (1980). *Diagnostic and statistical manual of mental health disorders (3rd ed.)*. Washington, D.C.: Author.

American Psychiatric Association. (1994). *Diagnostic and statistical manual of mental health disorders (4th edition)*. Washington, D.C.: Author.

American Psychiatric Association. (2000). *Diagnostic and statistical manual of mental health disorders (4th ed., text revision).* Washington, D.C.: Author.

American Psychiatric Association. (2013). *Diagnostic and statistical manual of mental health disorders (5th ed.).* Arlington, VA: American Psychiatric Association.

Aron, A. R. & Poldrack, R. A. (2006). Cortical and subcortical contributions to stop signal response inhibition: role of the subthalamic nucleus. *Journal of Neuroscience*, *26*(9), 2424-2433. http://dx.doi.org/10.1523/JNEUROSCI.4682-05.2006.

Aronson, T.A. (1985). Historical perspectives on the borderline concept: A review and critique. *Psychiatry: Journal for the Study of Interpersonal Processes, 48*(3), 209-222. http://dx.doi.org/10.1080/00332747.1985.11024282.

Ball, J. S. & Links, P. S. (2009). Borderline personality disorder and childhood trauma: Evidence for a causal relationship. *Curr Psychiatry Rep, 11*, 63–68. http://dx.doi.org/10.1007/s11920-009-0010-4.

Bandelow, B., Krause, J., Wedekind, D., Broocks, A., Hajak, G. & Rüther, E. (2005). Early traumatic life events, parental attitudes, family history, and birth risk factors in patients with borderline personality disorder and healthy controls. *Psychiatry Res, 134*(2), 169–179. http://dx.doi.org/10.1016/j.psychres.2003.07.008.https://doi.org/10.1016/j.psychres.2003.07.008.

Bannon, M. J., Michelhaugh, S. K., Wang, J., & Sacchetti, P. (2001). The human dopamine transporter gene: gene organization, transcriptional regulation, and potential involvement in the neuropsychiatric disorders. *European Neuropsychopharmacology, 11*(6), 449-455. http://dx.doi.org/10.1016/s0924-977x(01)00122-5.

Barnicot, K., Katsakou, C., Marougka, S. & Priebe S. (2011). Treatment completion in psychotherapy for borderline personality disorder – a systematic review and meta-analysis. *Acta Psychiatr Scand, 123*, 327–338. DOI: 10.1111/j.1600-0447.2010.01652.x.

Bedics, J. D., Atkins, D. C., Harned, M. S., & Linehan, M. M. (2015). The therapeutic alliance as a predictor of outcome in dialectical behavior therapy versus nonbehavioral psychotherapy by experts for borderline personality disorder, *Psychotherapy, 52*(1), 67-77. http://dx.doi.org/10.1037/a0038457.

Belsky, D. W., Caspi, A., Arseneault, L., Bleidorn, W., Fonagy, P., Goodman, M., Houts, R. & Moffitt, T. E. (2012). Etiological features of borderline personality related characteristics in a birth cohort of 12-year-old children. *Dev Psychopathol, 24*(1), 251-265. http://dx.doi.org/10.1017/S0954579411000812.

Bender, D. S., Dolan, R. T., Skodol, A. E., Sanislow, C. A Dyck, I. R., McGlashan, T. H., Shea, M. T., Zanarini, M. C., Oldham, J. M. & Gunderson, J. G. (2001). Treatment utilization by patients with personality disorders. *Am J Psychiatry 158*(2), 295-302. http://dx.doi.org/10.1176/appi.ajp.158.2.295.

Black, D. W., Pfohl, B., Blum, N., McCormick, B., Allen, J., North, C. S., Zimmerman, M. (2011). Attitudes toward borderline personality disorder: a survey of 706 mental health clinicians. *CNS Spectr, 16*(3), 67-74. http://dx.doi.org/10.1017/S109285291200020X.

Bornovalova, M. A., Verhulst, B., Webber, T., McGue. M., Iacono, W. G., Hicks, B. M. (2018). Genetic and environmental influences on the codevelopment among borderline personality disorder traits, major depression symptoms, and substance use disorder symptoms from adolescence to young adulthood. *Dev Psychopathol,30*(1), 49-65. http://dx.doi.org/10.1017/S0954579417000463.

Brewin, C. (n.d.). Complex post-traumatic stress disorder: A new diagnosis in ICD-11. *B J Psych Advances*, 1-8. http://dx.doi.org/10.1192/bja.2019.48.

Brown, S. M., Manuck, S. B., Flory, J. D., & Hariri, A. R. (2006). Neural basis of individual differences in impulsivity: contributions of corticolimbic circuits for behavioral arousal and control. *Emotion*, *6*(2), 239-245. http://dx.doi.org/10.1037/1528-3542.6.2.239.

Bui, E., Rodgers, R., Chabrol, H., Birmes, P. & Schmitt, L. (2011). Is Anakin Skywalker suffering from borderline personality disorder? *Psychiatry Res, 185*(1-2), 299. http://dx.doi.org/10.1016/j.psychres.2009.03.031.

Catthoor, K., Feenstra, D. J., Hutsebaut, J., Schrijvers, D., & Sabbe, B. (2015). Adolescents with personality disorders suffer from severe psychiatric stigma: evidence from a sample of 131 patients. *Adolescent health, medicine and therapeutics, 6*, 81–89. http://dx.doi.org/10.2147/AHMT.S76916.

Clark, C. J., Fox, E. & Long, C. G. (2015). Can teaching staff about the neurobiological underpinnings of borderline personality disorder instigate attitudinal change? *J Psychiat Int Care, 11*(1), 43–51. http://dx.doi.org/10.1017/S1742646414000132.

Clarke, S., Taylor, G., Bolderston, H., Lancaster, J. & Remington, B. (2014). Ameliorating patient stigma amongst staff working with personality disorder: randomized controlled trial of self-management versus skills training. *Behav Cogn Psychoth, 43*(6), 692–704. http://dx.doi.org/10.1017/S1352465814000320.

Columbia Pictures. (1992). *Single White Female*. Motion picture.

Congdon, E. & Canli, T. (2008). A neurogenetic approach to impulsivity. *Journal of Personality*, *76*(6), 1447-1484. http://dx.doi.org/10.1111/j.1467-6494.2008.00528.x.

Corrigan, P. W. (Ed.) (2005). *On the stigma of mental illness: practical strategies for research and social change*. Washington: American Psychological Association.

Corrigan, P. W. & Calabrese, J. D. (2005). Strategies for assessing and diminishing self-stigma. In P. W. Corrigan (Ed.), *On the stigma of mental illness: practical strategies* (pp. 239–256). Washington, DC: American Psychological Association. ISBN: 978-1-59147-189-9.

Corrigan, P. W. & Kleinlein, P. (2005). The impact of mental illness stigma. In P. W. Corrigan (Ed.), *On the stigma of mental illness: practical strategies for research and social change* (pp. 11–44). Washington: American Psychological Association.

Corrigan, P. W., Larson, J. E. & Rüsch, N. (2009). Self-stigma and the "why try" effect: impact on life goals and evidence-based practices. *World Psychiatry, 8*(2), 75–81. doi: 10.1002/j.2051-5545.2009.tb00218.x.

Corrigan, P. W., Morris, S. B., Michaels, P. J., Rafaczm J. D. & Rüsch, N. (2012). Challenging the public stigma of mental illness: a meta-analysis of outcome studies. *Psychiatr Serv, 63*(10), 963–973. http://dx.doi.org/10.1176/appi.ps.201100529.

Crick, N. R., Murray-Close, D. & Woods, K. (2005). Borderline personality features in childhood: a short-term longitudinal study. *Dev Psychopathol, 17*(4):1051-1070. PMID: 16613430.

Cristea, I. A., Gentili, C., Cotet, C. D., Palomba, D., Barbui, C., & Cuijpers, P. (2017). Efficacy of psychotherapies for borderline personality disorder: A systematic review and meta-analysis, *JAMA Psychiatry. 74*(4), 319–328. http://dx.doi.org/10.1001/jamapsychiatry.2016.4287.

Crocker, J., Major, B. & Steele, C. (1998). Social stigma. In D. T. Gilbert & S. T. Fiske (Eds.), *The handbook of social psychology, Vol. 2* (4th ed., pp. 504–553). New York: McGraw-Hill.

Crowell, S. E., Beauchaine, T. P., & Linehan, M. M. (2009). A biosocial developmental model of borderline personality: elaborating and extending Linehan's theory. *Psychological Bulletin, 135*(3), 495-510. http://dx.doi.org/10.1037/a0015616.

Deasy, C., Coughlan, B., Pironom, J., Jourdan, D. & Mcnamara, P. M. (2015). Psychological distress and lifestyle of students: implications for health promotion. *Health Promot Int, 30*(1), 77-87. http://dx.doi.org/10.1093/heapro/dau086.

Demme, J., Armian, N. & Platt, M. E. (2008). *Rachel Getting Married*. Motion picture.

Desta, Y. (2017). 30 years later: Why Fatal Attraction never sat right with Glenn Close. *Vanity Fair*, September 18, 2017. Available from: https://www.vanityfair.com/hollywood/2017/09/fatal-attraction-30-year-anniversary-glenn-close.

DeShong, H. L., Grant, D. M., & Mullins-Sweatt, S. N. (2019). Precursors of the emotional cascade model of borderline personality disorder: The role of neuroticism, childhood emotional vulnerability, and parental invalidation. *Personality Disorders: Theory, Research, and Treatment, 10*(4), 317–329. http://dx.doi.org/10.1037/per0000330.

Devine, P. G. (1995). Prejudice and out-group perception. In: A. Tesser (Ed.), *Advanced social psychology* (pp. 467–524). New York: McGraw-Hill.

Dimeff, L. & Linehan, M. (2001). Dialectical behavior therapy in a nutshell. *The California Psychologist, 34*(3), 10-13. http://dx.doi.org/10.1177/0011000011421023.

Drapalski, A.L., Lucksted, A., Perrin, P.B., Aakre, J.M., Brown, C.H., DeForge, B.R. & Boyd, J.E. (2013). A model of internalized stigma and its effects on people with mental illness. *Psychiatr Serv, 64*(3), 264–29. http://dx.doi.org/10.1176/appi.ps.001322012.

Driessen, M, Beblo, T., Reddemann, L., Rau, H., Lange, W., Silva, A., Ratzka, S. (2002). Is the borderline personality disorder a complex post-traumatic stress disorder? - The state of research. *Der Nervenarzt*, *73*(9), 820-829. http://dx.doi.org/10.1007/s00115-002-1296-1

Egan, S. J., Haley, S. & Rees, C. S. (2014). Attitudes of clinical psychologists towards clients with personality disorders. *Aust J Psychol, 66*(3), 175–180. http://dx.doi.org/10.1111/ajpy.12068.

Ensink, K., Biberdzic, M., Normandin, L., & Clarkin, J. (2015). A developmental psychopathology and neurobiological model of borderline personality disorder in adolescence. *Journal of Infant, Child, and Adolescent Psychotherapy, 14*, 46-69. http://dx.doi.org/10.1080/15289168.2015.1007715.

Focus Features. (2004). *Eternal Sunshine of the Spotless Mind*. Motion picture.

Fossati, A., Madeddu, F. & Maffei, C. (1999). Borderline personality disorder and childhood sexual abuse: A meta-analytic study. *J Pers Disord, 13*(3), 268–280. http://dx.doi.org/10.1521/pedi.1999.13.3.268.

Gallop, R., Lancee, W. J., & Garfinkel, P. (1989). How nursing staff respond to the label" borderline personality disorder". *Psychiatric Services, 40*(8), 815-819. http://dx.doi.org/10.1176/ps.40.8.815.

Gary Sanchez Productions (2014). *Welcome to Me*. Motion picture.

Ghiasi, H., Mohammadi, A., & Zarrinfar, P. (2016). An investigation into the roles of theory of mind, emotion regulation, and attachment styles in predicting the traits of borderline personality disorder. *Iran Journal of Psychiatry, 11*(4), 206-213. Available from https://www.ncbi.nlm.nih.gov/pmc/articles/PMC5206322/.

Gill, D. & Warburton, W. (2014). An investigation of the biosocial model of borderline personality disorder. *Journal of Clinical Psychology, 70*, 866-873. http://dx.doi.org/10.1002/jclp.22074.

Gill, D., Warburton, W., & Sweller, N. (2018). The development of borderline personality disorder: beyond the biosocial model. *Journal of Evidence-Based Psychotherapies, 18*(2), 55-75. http://dx.doi.org/10.24193/jebp.2018.2.14.

Godbout, N., Daspe, M. E., Runtz M., Cyr, G., & Briere, J. (2019). Childhood maltreatment, attachment, and borderline personality-related symptoms: gender-specific structural equation models. *Psychological Trauma: Theory, Research, Practice, and Policy, 11*(1), 90-98. http://dx.doi.org/10.1037/tra0000403.

Goffman, E. (1963). *Stigma: Notes on the management of a spoiled identity*. Englewood Cliffs, NJ: Prentice Hall.

Goodman, M. & Yehuda, R. (2002). The relationship between psychological trauma and Borderline Personality Disorder. *Psychiatric Annals 32*(6), 337-345. http://dx.doi.org/10.3928/0048-5713-20020601-08.

Grambal, A., Prasko, J., Kamaradova, D., Latalova, K., Holubova, M., Marackova, M., Ociskova, M., & Slepecky, M. (2016). Self-stigma in borderline personality disorder - cross-sectional comparison with schizophrenia spectrum disorder, major depressive disorder, and anxiety disorders. *Neuropsychiatric disease and treatment, 12*, 2439–2448. http://dx.doi.org/10.2147/NDT.S114671.

Gunderson, J. G. (2009). Borderline personality disorder: ontogeny of a diagnosis. *American Journal of Psychiatry, 166*(5), 530-539. http://dx.doi.org/10.1176/appi.ajp.2009.08121825.

Gunderson, J. G, Stout, R. L., McGlashan, T. H., Shea, M. T., Morey, L. C.; Grilo, C. M., Skodol, A. E. (2011). Ten-year course of borderline personality disorder: Psychopathology and function from the collaborative longitudinal personality disorders study. *Arch Gen Psychiatry, 68*(8), 827–837. http://dx.doi.org/10.1001/archgen psychiatry.2011.37.

Gunderson, J. G., Zanarini, M. C., Choi-Kain, L. W., Mitchell, K. S., Jang, K. L. & Hudson, J. I. (2011). Family Study of Borderline Personality Disorder and Its Sectors of Psychopathology. Arch Gen Psychiatry. 2011 Jul; 68(7): 753–762. http://dx.doi.org/10.1001/archgen psychiatry.2011.65.

Harmon, R.B., Rosner, R. & Owens, H. (1995). Obsessional harassment and erotomania in a criminal court population. *J Forensic Sci, 40*(2), 188-96.PMID: 7602275.

HBO. (1999-2007). *The Sopranos*. Television series.

Herman, J. L. (2015). *Trauma and recovery: The aftermath of violence--from domestic abuse to political terror* (3rd ed., p 135). New York: Basic Books.

Herman, J. L., Perry, J. C. & Van der Kolk, B. A. (1989). Childhood trauma in borderline personality disorder. *Am J Psychiatry, 146*(4), 490–495. http://dx.doi.org/10.1176/ajp.146.4.490.

Hilton, J. L. & von Hippel, W. (1996). Stereotypes. *Annu Rev Psychol, 47*, 237-271. http://dx.doi.org//10.1146/annurev.psych.47.1.237.

Hughes, A. E., Crowell, S. E., Uyeji, L., & Coan, J. A. (2012). A developmental neuroscience of borderline pathology: emotion dysregulation and social baseline theory. *Journal of Abnormal Child Psychology, 40*(1), 21-33. http://dx.doi.org/10.1007/s10802-011-9555-x.

Hyland, P., Karatzias, T., Shevlin, M., Cloitre, M. (2019). Examining the discriminant validity of Complex Posttraumatic Stress Disorder and Borderline Personality Disorder symptoms: Results from a United Kingdom population sample. *Journal of Traumatic Stress, 32*(6), 855-863. http://dx.doi.org/10.1002/jts.22444.

Imagine Entertainment. (1996). *Fear*. Motion picture.

Jowett, S., Karatzias, T., Shevlin, M. & Albert, I. (2020). Differentiating symptom profiles of ICD-11 PTSD, complex PTSD, and borderline personality disorder: A latent class analysis in a multiply traumatized sample. *Personal Disord, 11*(1), 36-45. http://dx.doi.org /10.1037/ per0000346.

Juurlink, T. T., Vukadin, M., Stringer, B., Westerman, M. J., Lamers, F., Anema, J. R.., van Marle, H. J. F. (2019). Barriers and facilitators to employment in borderline personality disorder: A qualitative study among patients, mental health practitioners and insurance physicians. *PLoS One, 14*(7), e0220233. http://dx.doi.org/10.1371/journal. pone.0220233.

Kealy, D. & Ogrodniczuk, J. S. (2010). Marginalization of borderline personality disorder. *J Psychiatr Pract. 16*(3), 145–154. http://dx.doi.org/10.1097/01.pra.0000375710.39713.4d.

Kienlen, K. K., Birmingham, D. L., Solberg, K. B., O'Regan, J. T. & Meloy, J.R. (1997). A comparative study of psychotic and nonpsychotic stalking. *J Am Acad Psychiatry Law, 25*(3), 317-334. PMID: 9323658.

Keuroghlian, A. S., Palmer, B. A., Choi-Kain, L. W., Borba, C. P., Links, P. S., & Gunderson, J. G. (2016). The effect of attending good psychiatric management (GPM) workshops on attitudes toward patients with borderline personality disorder. *Journal of personality disorders, 30*(4), 567–576. http://dx.doi.org/10.1521/pedi_2015_29_206.

Korzekwa, M. I., Dell, P. F., Links, P. S, Thabane, L. & Webb, S. P. (2008). Estimating the prevalence of borderline personality disorder in psychiatric outpatients using a two-phase procedure. *Comprehensive*

Psychiatry 49(4), 380-386. http://dx.doi.org/10.1016/j.comppsych.2008.01.007.

Krause-Utz, A., Winter, D., Niedtfeld, I., & Schmahl, C. (2014). The latest neuroimaging findings in borderline personality disorder. *Current Psychiatry Reports, 16*(438), 45-55. http://dx.doi.org/10.1007/s11920-014-0438-z.

Kreisman, J. J. & Straus, H. (2010). *I Hate You--Don't Leave Me: Understanding the Borderline Personality.* New York, New York: TarcherPerigree/Penguin Random House, LLC.

Kuo, J. R., Khoury, J. E., Metcalfe, R., Fitzpatrick, S. & Goodwill, A. (2015). An examination of the relationship between childhood emotional abuse and borderline personality disorder features: The role of difficulties with emotion regulation. *Child Abuse & Neglect, 39*, 147-155. http://dx.doi.org/j.chiabu.2014.08.008.

Kvaale, E. P., Haslam, N. & Gottdiener, W. H. (2013). The 'side effects' of medicalization: a meta-analytic review of how biogenetic explanations affect stigma. *Clin Psychol Rev, 33*(6), 782-794. http://dx.doi.org/10.1016/j.cpr.2013.06.002.

Kvarstein, E. H. et al. (2015). Changing from a traditional psychodynamic treatment programme to mentalization-based treatment for patients with borderline personality disorder – Does it make a difference? *Psychology and Psychotherapy: Theory, Research and Practice, 88*(1), 71-86. http://dx.doi.org/10.1111/papt.12036.

Laporte, L., Paris, J., Guttman, H., Russell, J. & Correa, J. A. (2012). Using a sibling design to compare childhood adversities in female patients with BPD and their sisters. *Child Maltreat*, 17(4), 318-29. http://dx.doi.org/10.1177/1077559512461173.

Lawn, S. & McMahon, J. (2015). Experiences of care by Australians with a diagnosis of borderline personality disorder. *J Psychiatr Ment Health Nurs. 22*(7):510–521. http://dx.doi.org/10.1111/jpm.12226.

Lequesne, E. R. & Hersh, R. G. (2004). Disclosure of a diagnosis of borderline personality disorder. *J Psychiatr Pract, 10*(3), 170-176. http://dx.doi.org/10.1097/00131746-200405000-00005.

Levy, K. N. (2005). The implications of attachment theory and research for understanding borderline personality disorder. *Development and Psychopathology, 17*(4), 959-986. http://dx.doi.org/10.1017/S0954579405050455.

Levy, K. N., Johnson, B. N., Clouthier, T. L., Scala, J. W., & Temes, C. M. (2015). An attachment theoretical framework for personality disorders. *Canadian Psychology, 56*(2), 197-207. http://dx.doi.org/10.1037/cap0000025.

Lewis, G. & Appleby, L. (1988). Personality disorder: the patients psychiatrists dislike. *Br J Psychiatry, 153*, 44-49. http://dx.doi.org/10.1192/bjp.153.1.44.

Liebman, R. E., & Burnette, M. (2013). It's not you, it's me: An examination of clinician- and client-level influences on countertransference toward borderline personality disorder. *American Journal of Orthopsychiatry, 83*(1), 115–125. http://dx.doi.org/10.1111/ajop.12002.

Lind, M., Vanwoerden, S., Penner, F., & Sharp, C. (2019). Inpatient adolescents with borderline personality disorder features: Identity diffusion and narrative incoherence. *Personality Disorders: Theory, Research, and Treatment, 10*(4), 389–393. http://dx.doi.org/10.1037/per0000338.

Linehan, M. (1993). *Cognitive-behavioral treatment of borderline personality disorder*. New York: The Guilford Press.

Linehan, M. M. & Schmidt, H. III. (1995). The dialectics of effective treatment of borderline personality disorder. In W. T. O'Donohue & L. Krasner (Eds.), *Theories of Behavior Therapy: Exploring Behavior Change* (pp. 553-584). American Psychological Association. http://dx.doi.org/10.1037/10169-020.

Link, B. G. (1982). Mental patient status, work, and income: an examination of the effects of a psychiatric label. *Am Sociol Rev, 47*(2), 202-215. PMID: 7091929.

Link, B. G. (1987). Understanding labelling effects in the area of mental disorders: An assessment of the effects of expectations of rejection. *American Sociological Review*, 52, 96-112. http://dx.doi.org/10.2307/2095395.

Link, B. G., Cullen, F. T., Frank, J. & Wozniak, J. F. (1987). The social rejection of former mental patients: Understanding why labels matter. *American Journal of Sociology, 92*, 1461-1500. http://dx.doi.org/10.1086/228672.

Lucasfilm, Ltd. (2002). *Star Wars Episode II: Attack of the Clones*. Motion picture.

Lucasfilm, Ltd. (2005). *Star Wars Episode III: Revenge of the Sith*. Motion picture.

Major, B. & O'Brien, L. T. (2005). The social psychology of stigma. *Annu Rev Psychol, 56*, 393-421. http://dx.doi.org/10.1146/annurev.psych.56.091103.070137.

The Malpaso Company. (1971). *Play Misty for Me*. Motion picture.

Manning, S. Y. (2011). *Loving Someone with Borderline Personality Disorder.* New York, New York: The Guilford Press.

Markham, D. (2003) Attitudes towards patients with a diagnosis of 'borderline personality disorder': Social rejection and dangerousness. *Journal of Mental Health, 12*(6), 595-612. http://dx.doi.org/10.1080/09638230310001627955

Markowitz, F. E. (1998). The effects of stigma on the psychological well-being and life satisfaction of persons with mental illness. *J Health Soc Behav, 39*(4), 335-347. PMID: 9919855.

Martin, T. & Thomas, S. (2015). Police officers' views of their encounters with people with personality disorder. *J Psychiatr Ment Health Nurs, 22*(2), 125-132. http://dx.doi.org/10.1111/jpm.12099. Epub 2013 Jul 9.

Masland, S. R., Cummings, M. H., Null, K. E., Woynowskie, K. M & Choi-Kain, L. W. (2019). Changes in post-traumatic stress disorder symptoms during residential treatment for borderline personality disorder: a longitudinal cross-lagged study. *Bord Personal Disord Emot Dysregul 6*, 15. http://dx.doi.org/10.1186/s40479-019-0113-4.

Mason, P. T. & Kreger, R. (2010). *Stop Walking on Eggshells -- Taking Your Life Back When Someone You Care About Has Borderline Personality Disorder* (2nd edition). Oakland, CA: New Harbinger Publications, Inc.

McIvor, R. J., Potter, L. & Davies, L. (2008). Stalking behaviour by patients towards psychiatrists in a large mental health organization. *Int J Soc*

Psychiatry, 54(4), 350-357. http://dx.doi.org/10.1177/0020764008090690.

McWilliams, N. (1994). *Psychoanalytic Diagnosis*. New York: The Guilford Press.

Meaney, R., Hasking, P. & Reupert, A. (2016). Borderline Personality Disorder symptoms in college students: The complex interplay between alexithymia, emotional dysregulation and rumination. *PLoS One. 11*(6), e0157294. http://dx.doi.org/10.1371/journal.pone.0157294.

Mehlum, L., Ramleth, R., Tørmoen, A. J., Haga, E., Diep, L. M., Stanley, B. H., Miller, A. L., Larsson, B., Sund, A. M. and Grøholt, B. (2019). Long term effectiveness of dialectical behavior therapy versus enhanced usual care for adolescents with self-harming and suicidal behavior. *Journal of Child Psychology and Psychiatry*, (in press). http://dx.doi.org/10.1111/jcpp.13077.

Meloy, J. R. &, Boyd, C. (2003). Female stalkers and their victims. *J Am Acad Psychiatry Law, 31*(2), 211-219. PMID: 12875500.

Merriam-Webster. (2020). *Stigma*. Available from https://www.merriam-webster.com/dictionary/stigma.

Merza, K., Papp, G. & Szabó, I. K. (2015). The role of childhood traumatization in the development of borderline personality disorder in Hungary. *Eur J Psychiat, 29*(2), Zaragoza abr./jun. 2015. http://dx.doi.org/10.4321/S0213-61632015000200002.

Miller, C. T., & Kaiser, C. R., (2001). A theoretical perspective on coping with stigma. *Journal of Social Issues, 57*(1), 73-92. http://dx.doi.org/10.1111/0022-4537.00202.

Millon, T., Grossman, S., Millon, C., Meagher, S., & Ramnath, R. (2004). The borderline personality disorder. In T. Millon, S. Grossman, C. Meagher & R. Ramnath (Eds.), *Personality disorders in modern life* (2nd ed., pp. 417-516). Hoboken, NJ: John Wiley & Sons, Inc.

Miramax. (2001). *Prozac Nation.* Motion picture.

Mizen, C. S. (2014). Towards a relational affective theory of personality disorder. *Psychoanalytic Psychotherapy, 28*(4), 357-378. http://dx.doi.org/10.1080/02668734.2014.975154.

Morgan Creek Entertainment. (1993). *The Crush*. Motion picture.

Neacsiu, A. D., Lungu, A., Harned, M. S., Rizvi, S. L., & Linehan, M. M. (2014). Impact of dialectical behavior therapy versus community treatment by experts on emotional experience, expression, and acceptance in borderline personality disorder. *Behaviour Research and Therapy, 53*(1), 47-54. https://doi.org/10.1016/j.brat.2013.12.004.

Nehls, N. (1998). Borderline personality disorder: Gender stereotypes, stigma, and limited system of care. *Issues Ment Health Nurs. 19*(2), 97–112. http://dx.doi.org/10.1080/016128498249105.

Netflix. (2016-2018). Love. Television series.

Ociskova, M., Prasko, J., Latalova, K., Sedlackova, Z., Kamaradova, D. Sandoval, A. & Grambal, A. (2017). F*ck your care if you label me! Borderline personality disorder, stigma, and self-stigma. *Activitas Nervosa Superior Rediviva, 58*(3), 16-22. Available from: http://www.rediviva.sav.sk/59i1/16.pdf.

Ogata, S. N., Silk, K. R., Goodrich, S., Lohr, N. E. & Hill, E. M. (1990). Childhood sexual and physical abuse in adult patients with borderline personality disorder. *Am J Psychiatry, 147*(8), 1008–1013. http://dx.doi.org/10.1176/ajp.147.8.1008.

Oldham, J. M, Skodol, A. E., Gallaher, P. E. & Kroll, M. E. (1996). Relationship of borderline symptoms to histories of abuse and neglect: A pilot study. *Psychiatric Quarterly, 67*, 287–295. http://dx.doi.org/10.1007/BF02326372.

O'Neill, A. & Frodl, T. (2012). Brain structure and function in borderline personality disorder. *Brain Structure and Function, 217,* 767-782.

Pagura, J., Stein, M. B., Bolton, J. M., Cox, B. J., Grant, B. & Sareen, J. (2010). Comorbidity of borderline personality disorder and posttraumatic stress disorder in the U.S. population. *J Psychiatr Res, 44*(16), 1190-1198. http://dx.doi.org/10.1016/j.jpsychires.2010.04.016.

Paramount Pictures. (1987). *Fatal Attraction*. Motion picture.

Paramount Vantage. (2007). *Margot at the Wedding.* Motion picture.

Parcesepe, A. M. & Cabassa, L. J. (2013). Public stigma of mental illness in the United States: a systematic literature review. *Adm Policy Ment Health, 40*(5), 384–399. http://dx.doi.org/10.1007/s10488-012-0430-z.

Paris, J. (2007). Why psychiatrists are reluctant to diagnose borderline personality disorder. *Psychiatry (Edgmont), 4*(1), 35–9. PMID: 20805927 PMCID: PMC2922389.

Paris, J. (2015). Borderline personality disorder. In American Psychological Association (Ed.), *A Concise Guide to Personality Disorders* (pp. 73-89). American Psychological Association. http://dx.doi.org/10.1037/14642-007.

Phillips, R. G. & LeDoux, J. E. (1992). Differential contributions of amygdala and hippocampus to cued and contextual fear conditioning. *Behavioral Neuroscience*, *106,* 274-285.

Pier, K. S., Marin, L. K., Wilsnack, J. & Goodman, M. (2016). The neurobiology of borderline personality disorder. *Psychiatric Times*, 33(3). Available from: https://www.psychiatrictimes.com/special-reports/neurobiology-borderline-personality-disorder.

Porter, C., Palmier-Claus, J., Branitsky, A., Mansell, W., Warwick, H. & Varese, F. (2020). Childhood adversity and borderline personality disorder: a meta-analysis. *Acta Psychiatrica Scandinavica, 141*(1), 6-20. http://dx.doi.org/10.1111/acps.13118.

Purcell, R., Pathé, M. & Mullen, P. E. (2001). A Study of Women Who Stalk. *Am J Psychiatry, 158*(2), 2056-2060. http://dx.doi.org/10.1176/appi.ajp.158.12.2056.

Ritsher, J. B., Otilingam, P. G. & Grajales, M. (2003). Internalized stigma of mental illness: psychometric properties of a new measure. *Psychiatry Res, 121*(1), 31-49. http://dx.doi.org/10.1016/j.psychres.2003.08.008.

Ritsher, J. B. & Phelan, J.C. (2004). Internalized stigma predicts erosion of morale among psychiatric outpatients. *Psychiatry Res, 129*(3), 257-265. http://dx.doi.org/10.1016/j.psychres.2004.08.003.

Rosenfield, S. (1997). Labeling mental illness: The effects of received services and perceived stigma on life satisfaction. *American Sociological Review, 62*(4), 660–672. http://dx.doi.org/10.2307/2657432.

Rosenfield, P. J., Stratyner, A., Tufekcioglu, S., Karabell, S., Mckelvey, J. & Litt, L. (2018). Complex PTSD in ICD-11: A case report on a new diagnosis. J *Psychiatr Pract, 24*(5), 364-370. http://dx.doi.org/10.1097/PRA.0000000000000327.

Ruocco, A. C., Amirthavasagam, S., & Zakzanis, K. K. (2012). Amygdala and hippocampal volume reductions as candidate endophenotypes for borderline personality disorder: a meta-analysis of magnetic resonance imaging studies. *Psychiatry Research: Neuroimaging, 201*, 245-252.

Rüsch, N., Angermeyer, M. C. & Corrigan, P. W. (2005). Mental illness stigma: concepts, consequences, and initiatives to reduce stigma. *Eur Psychiatry, 20*(8), 529-39. http://dx.doi.org/10.1016/j.eurpsy.2005.04.004.

Rüsch, N., Hölzer, A., Hermann, C., Schramm, E., Jacob, G. A., Bohus, M., Corrigan, P. W. (2006). Self-stigma in women with borderline personality disorder and women with social phobia. *J Nerv Ment Dis, 194*(10), 766-773. http://dx.doi.org/10.1097/01.nmd.0000239898.48701.dc.

Salzman, J. P, Salzman, C., Wolfson, A. N., Albanese, M., Looper, J., Ostacher M, Schwartz, J., Chinman, G., Land, W. & Miyawaki, E. (1993). Association between borderline personality disorder and history of childhood sexual abuse in adult volunteers. *Compr Psychiatry, 34*(4), 254–257. http://dx.doi.org/10.1016/0010-440X(93)90007-Q.

Sansone, R. A., Levitt, J. L. & Sansone, L. A. (2005). The prevalence of personality disorders among those with eating disorders. *Eat Disord, 13*(1), 7-21. http://dx.doi.org/10.1080/10640260590893593.

Sansone, R. A. & Sansone, L. A. (2010a). Borderline personality and eating disorders: a chaotic crossroads. In M. Maine, D. Bunnell & B. McGilley (eds.), *Special Issues in the Treatment of Eating Disorders: Bridging the Gaps* (pp. 217–232). New York: Elsevier.

Sansone, R. A. & Sansone, L. A. (2010b). Fatal attraction syndrome: Stalking behavior and borderline personality. *Psychiatry (Edgmont), 7*(5), 42–46. PMCID: PMC2882283.

Sansone, R. A. & Sansone, L. A. (2011). Personality Pathology and Its Influence on Eating Disorders. *Innov Clin Neurosci, 8*(3), 14-18. PMCID: PMC3074200.

Sansone, R. A. & Sansone, L. A. (2013a). The relationship between borderline personality and obesity. *Innov Clin Neurosci, 10*(4), 36-40. PMCID: PMC3659037.

Sansone, R. A. & Sansone, L. A. (2013b). Responses of mental health clinicians to patients with borderline personality disorder. *Innov Clin Neurosci, 10*(5-6), 39-43. PMCID: PMC3719460.

Schomerus, G., Schwahn, C., Holzinger, A., Corrigan, P. W., Grabe, H. J., Cartam, M. G. & Angermeyer, M. C. (2012). Evolution of public attitudes about mental illness: a systematic review and meta-analysis. *Acta Psychiatr Scand, 125*(6), 440-452. http://dx.doi.org/10.1111/j.1600-0447.2012.01826.x.

Searchlight Pictures. (2002). *One Hour Photo*. Motion picture.

Searchlight Pictures. (2003). *Thirteen*. Motion picture.

Sheehan, L., Nieweglowski, K. & Corrigan, P. W. (2016). The stigma of personality disorders. *Current Psychiatry Reports 18*(1). http://dx.doi.org/10.1007/s11920-015-0654-1.

Sisti, D., Segal, A. G., Siegel, A., Johnson, R. & Gunderson, J. (2016). Diagnosing, Disclosing, and Documenting Borderline Personality Disorder: A Survey of Psychiatrists' Practices. *J Pers Disord*, 30(6), 848-856. http://dx.doi.org/10.1521/pedi_2015_29_228.

Skoglund, C., Tiger, A., Rück, C., Petrovic, P., Asherson, P., Hellner, C., Kuja-Halkola, R. (2019). Familial risk and heritability of diagnosed borderline personality disorder: a register study of the Swedish population. *Mol Psychiatr*. http://dx.doi.org/10.1038/s41380-019-0442-0.

Soloff, P. H., White, R., Omari, A., Ramaseshan, K., & Diwadkar, V. A. (2015). Affective context interferes with brain responses during cognitive processing in borderline personality disorder: fMRI evidence. *Psychiatric Research: Neuroimaging. 233*(1), 23–35. http://dx.doi.org/10.1016/j.pscychresns.2015.04.006.

Sosic-Vasic, Z., Eberhardt, J., Bosch, J. E., Dommes, L., Labek, K., Buchheim, A., & Viviani, R. (2019). Mirror neuron activations in encoding of psychic pain in borderline personality disorder.

NeuroImage: Clinical, 22. http://dx.doi.org/10.1016/j.nicl.2019.101737.

Stallman, H. M. (2008). Prevalence of psychological distress in university students--implications for service delivery. *Aust Fam Physician, 37*(8), 673-637. PMID: 18704221.

Star Thrower Entertainment 141 & Entertainment Mighty Engine. (2017). *Ingrid Goes West.* Motion picture.

Stone, M. H. (1977). The borderline syndrome: evolution of the term, genetic aspects, and prognosis. *American Journal of Psychotherapy, 31*(3), 345-365. Retrieved from https://search.ebscohost.com/login.aspx?direct=true&db=psyh&AN=1979-01215-001&site=ehost-live.

Stull, L. G., McGrew, J. H., Salyers, M. P., & Ashburn-Nardo, L. (2013). Implicit and explicit stigma of mental illness: Attitudes in an evidence-based practice. *Journal of Nervous and Mental Disease, 201*(12), 1027-1029. http://dx.doi.org/10.1097/NMD.0000000000000056.

Sulzer, S. H., Muenchow, E., Potvin, A., Harris, J., & Gigot, G. (2016). Improving patient-centered communication of the borderline personality disorder diagnosis. *Journal of mental health (Abingdon, England), 25*(1), 5–9. http://dx.doi.org/10.3109/09638237.2015.1022253.

Swenson, C. R. & Choi-Kain, L. W. (2015). Mentalization and dialectical behavior therapy. *American Journal of Psychotherapy, 69*(2), 199-217. Retrieved from https://search.ebscohost.com/login.aspx?direct=true&db=psyh&AN=2015-32680-008&site=ehost-live.

Tebbett-Mock A. A., Saito E., McGee M., Woloszyn P., & Venuti M. (2019). Efficacy of dialectical behavior therapy versus treatment as usual for acute-care inpatient adolescents, *Journal of the American Academy of Child & Adolescent Psychiatry, 59*(1), 149–156. http://dx.doi.org/10.1016/j.jaac.2019.01.020.

Temes, C. M. & Zanarini, M. C. (2018). The longitudinal course of borderline personality disorder. *Psychiatr Clin North Am, 41*(4), 685-694. http://dx.doi.org/10.1016/j.psc.2018.07.002.

The CW. (2015-2019). *Crazy Ex-Girlfriend.* Television series.

The Weinstein Company. (2012). *Silver Linings Playbook.* Motion picture.

Trull, T. (2001). Relationships of borderline features to parental mental illness, childhood abuse, Axis I disorder, and current functioning. *J Pers Dis, 15*(1, 19-32. http://dx.doi.org/10.1521/pedi.15.1.19.18647.

Universal Pictures. (1982). *Frances.* Motion picture.

Usher, B. E. (2016). *Theoretical and empirical perspectives on DBT with borderline personality disorder: removing the stigma* [Unpublished doctoral dissertation]. California School of Professional Psychology, Alliant International University Los Angeles.

Veysey, S. (2014) People with a borderline personality disorder diagnosis describe discriminatory experiences, Kōtuitui. *New Zealand Journal of Social Sciences Online, 9*(1), 20-35, http://dx.doi.org/10.1080/1177083X.2013.871303.

Vermeir, P., Vandijck, D., Degroote, S., Peleman, R., Verhaeghe, R., Mortier, E., Hallaert, G., Van Daele, S., Buylaert, W. & Vogelaers, D. (2015). Communication in healthcare: a narrative review of the literature and practical recommendations. *Int J Clin Pract 69*(11), 1257-67. http://dx.doi.org/10.1111/ijcp.12686.

Virzi, J. (2017). *6 movies that got borderline personality disorder symptoms (mostly) right*. Available from: https://themighty.com/2017/11/movies-borderline-personality-disorder-bpd/.

Walker, P. (2014). *Complex PTSD: From Surviving to Thriving.* USA: Pete Walker. www.pete-walker.com.

Watson, A. C., Corrigan, P. W., Larson, J. E. & Sells, M. (2007). Self-stigma in people with mental illness. *Schizophr Bull, 33*(6), 1312-1318. http://dx.doi.org/10.1093/schbul/sbl076.

Winter, D., Bohus, M. & Lis, S. (2017). Understanding negative self-evaluations in borderline personality disorder-a review of self-related cognitions, emotions, and motives. *Curr Psychiatry Rep, 19*(3), 17. http://dx.doi.org/10.1007/s11920-017-0771-0.

World Health Organization. (2018). *WHO releases new International Classification of Diseases (ICD 11).* Available from: https://www.who.int/news-room/detail/18-06-2018-who-releases-new-international-classification-of-diseases-(icd-11).

Yalom I. D. (1989). *Love's Executioner and Other Tales of Psychotherapy*. New York: Penguin Books.

Zanarini, M. C., Frankenburg, F. R., Reich, D. B., Marino, M. F., Lewis, R. E., Williams, A. A. Khera, G. S. (2000). Biparental failure in the childhood experiences of borderline patients. *J Pers Disord, 14*(3), 264-273. http://dx.doi.org/10.1053/comp.2001.19749.

Zanarini, M. C., Frankenburg, F. R., Khera, G. S. & Bleichmar, J. (2001). Treatment histories of borderline inpatients. *Compr Psychiatry, 42*(2), 144–150. http://dx.doi.org/10.1053/comp.2001.

Zanarini, M. C., Frankenburg, F. R., Reich, D. B., & Fitzmaurice, G. (2012). Attainment and stability of sustained symptomatic remission and recovery among patients with borderline personality disorder and axis II comparison subjects: A 16-year prospective follow-up study. *American Journal of Psychiatry, 169*(5), 476-483. http://dx.doi.org/10.1176/appi.ajp.2011.11101550.

Zivin, K., Eisenberg, D., Gollust, S. E. & Golberstein, E. (2009). Persistence of mental health problems and needs in a college student population. *J Affect Disord, 117*(3), 180-185. http://dx.doi.org/10.1016/j.jad.2009.01.001.

Afterword

The approaches described in this book for understanding, diagnosing and treating Borderline Personality Disorder (BPD) have their origins in widely varying theoretical formulations, expressed in practice through equally disparate methodologies. These range from Object Relations to Cognitive-Behavioral theory, from Dialectical Behavior Therapy to Constructionism, and from Trauma-based models to treatments based on brain imaging demonstrating structural and functional neurological differences in BPD, including the use of psychoactive medications.

Although each of these approaches is very different from the others, they all share several commonalities. Each requires the therapist to develop an understanding of the inner experience of the BPD patient. Each requires that the therapist conveys this understanding to the person with BPD. Each requires that the therapist engages with the person with BPD in a genuine manner, allowing for the development of a therapeutic alliance. Each relies upon the therapeutic alliance not only as a crucible for the BPD person to work through interpersonal issues in real time, but also, as a platform for assisting the BPD person in the acquisition of skills that reduce symptoms and ease interpersonal relationships.

Each of these approaches recognizes that developing an understanding of the individual, establishing rapport, building a therapeutic alliance, working through interpersonal issues in real time, and helping the BPD person develop skill sets for symptom reduction and improved interpersonal functioning requires time. Research data indicate that the time frame for significant, lasting symptom reduction in BPD is between one and two years. The data do not support brief, time-limited therapy models for effective treatment of BPD, creating potential difficulties for fiscally-driven models of mental health care including value-based reimbursement models.

From a broader perspective, the commonalities described above can also be considered elements of a humanistic approach, in which the focus of treatment is on the person and their experience. It is hoped that this book will provide the reader not only with a thorough understanding of the history, evolution, and evidence base for diagnosing and treating BPD, but perhaps more importantly, the perspective that the person diagnosed with BPD is first and foremost a person. Consistent with the treatment of any physical or emotional difficulty, understanding, empathizing with, and appreciating the humanity of that person is the key to good therapeutic outcome in the treatment of BPD.

About the Editor

Charles M. Lepkowsky, PhD, is in private practice in Solvang, California. He is a former chair of the Department of Child and Adolescent Psychiatry at Santa Barbara Cottage Hospital and a past president of the Santa Barbara County Psychological Association. He taught doctoral psychology courses for 14 years, has been on staff at local hospitals for over 30 years, publishes in neurological and psychological journals several times a year, and serves on the editorial boards of several neurological journals. He may be reached at clepkowsky@gmailcom.

INDEX

#

10/10 dopamine transporter (DAT), 74
24 hour rule, 184
5-HT, 74
5-HT receptors, 74
5HTR2A, 74
5HTR2C, 74
5-hydroxytryptomine (5-HT), 74

A

abandonment, 8, 12, 28, 30, 31, 35, 38, 41, 43, 45, 70, 109, 182, 195, 252, 258
abandonment fears, 182, 258
abandonment is internalized, 109
Abdelkarim, Nagui, Esmaiel, & Helal, 107
abuse, 34, 42, 57, 66, 69, 88, 224, 246, 255, 258, 259, 268, 270, 274, 279
abusive relationships, 255
academic performance, 245
access, 103, 116, 121, 164, 176, 186, 189, 190, 194, 196, 199, 233, 245, 248, 252, 255
access to housing, 245
access to means, 186, 189
acting impulsively, 174, 179
acting out, 136, 149
active behavioral change, 9
active self-harm, 75
acts of self-harm, 21
acts of self-mutilation, 25
acute anxiety, 36, 42
acute psychiatric hospital setting, 109
adaptive model, 135, 137
adolescence, 14, 20, 33, 39, 46, 47, 52, 56, 59, 60, 61, 264, 266
adolescent BPD, 46
adolescent populations, 169
adolescents, 10, 16, 34, 35, 46, 47, 55, 60, 61, 81, 107, 123, 125, 127, 128, 169,

170, 187, 200, 202, 203, 204, 252, 261, 264, 271, 273, 278
adrenergic agonists, 121
adulthood, 12, 30, 39, 46, 47, 60, 61, 73, 81, 108, 138, 142, 264
adults, 35, 42, 47, 63, 107, 131, 164, 168, 237, 252
affect tolerance, 145
affective disorder, 5, 49
affective disorder features of BPD, 49
affective disturbance, 72
affective dysregulation, 37, 259
affective experience, 59, 137
affective instability, 12, 25, 26, 36, 38, 44, 49, 88, 259
affective regulation, 228, 231
affective-cognitive schemata, 7
age, iv, 2, 3, 46, 47, 79, 83, 228, 245
aggression, 6, 74, 77, 87, 99, 143, 246, 257
aggressive behavior, 69, 256
aggressiveness, 72, 85
agreeableness, 28
Ahmed, Ras, & Seedat, 78
Ainsworth, Mary, 7
alcohol consumption, 246
alcohol use, 73, 117, 126
alcohol use disorder (AUD), 73, 126
alcoholism, 23
Alexander & French, 152
alexithymia, 37, 246, 273
alloplastic, 137
Alternative DSM-5 Model for Personality Disorders, 26, 61
alternative model, 19, 26
alternative model for personality disorders, 19
Álvarez-Tomás, Ruiz, Guilera and Bados, 34
Amad et al., 42
Amad, Ramos, Thomas, Jardri, & Gorwood, 74, 257
Amad, Ramoz, Peyre, Thomas, & Gorwood, 37
Amad, Ramoz, Thomas, Jadri, & Gorwood, 33
American culture, 245, 247
American Psychiatric Association, vii, viii, 4, 11, 13, 20, 22, 23, 25, 26, 28, 29, 30, 31, 32, 33, 35, 36, 37, 38, 39, 40, 41, 43, 44, 45, 51, 66, 80, 122, 148, 159, 164, 198, 242, 262
American Psychological Association, 16, 17, 239, 265, 271, 275
amygdala, 67, 68, 69, 70, 71, 72, 74, 75, 76, 77, 79, 82, 83, 84, 85, 86, 87, 88, 256, 275, 276
amygdala activation, 75
amygdala volume, 76, 88
anal, 96, 138, 139, 160, 162, 209, 267, 270
anatomy, 89, 138
Anderson, Crowley, Himawan, Holmberg, and Uhlin, 207
Anderson, Lunnen and Ogles, 220, 221
Anderson, Snider, Sellborn, & Krueger, 27
anger, 12, 25, 29, 36, 37, 38, 39, 41, 44, 49, 50, 111, 118, 119, 142, 164, 168, 173, 176, 179, 221, 242, 247, 259
anger dysregulation, 118, 119
anger outbursts, 168
anterior cingulate cortex, 67, 68, 79, 82
anterior cingulate cortex (ACC), 67, 68, 75, 79, 82
antidepressant, 120, 242
antipsychotics, 105, 118, 119
antisocial personality disorder, 30, 45
anxiety, 3, 8, 12, 22, 27, 28, 36, 42, 44, 49, 50, 53, 74, 81, 105, 107, 111, 112, 118, 120, 135, 157, 164, 168, 169, 172, 193, 242, 245, 268
anxiety disorder, 27, 81, 120, 268
anxiety reducing medications, 120
anxiety symptoms, 111
anxiolytic (anti-anxiety) medications, 120

anxiolytics, 120
approach-avoidance behaviors, 34
Aquino Ferreira et al., 42
Aquino Ferreira, Pereira, Benevides, & Melo, 42
Arkowitz & Lilienfeld, 211
Arnoud Arntz, 100
Aron & Poldrack, 74, 257
Aron, Robbins, & Poldrack, 75
arousal, 36, 68, 73, 82, 98, 264
arousal modulation, 68, 73
arrested for harassment or stalking, 169
Asnaani et al., 66
assessment, viii, ix, xi, 27, 48, 59, 61, 102, 154, 184, 186, 188, 190, 191, 206, 271
assessment for safety, 184
assumptions of treatment, 185
attachment anxiety, 8
attachment figures, 7
attachment theory, 7, 9, 16, 97, 271
attendance rates, 113
attention regulation, 73
attention-seeking, 250
attitudes, 145, 165, 201, 244, 251, 253, 260, 269, 277
attribution, 4
atypical antipsychotics, 119
auditory verbal hallucinations (AVH), 105
authorization forms for release of information, 196
autobiographical memories, 70
autonomy, 6, 117, 141, 142
aversive childhood events, 259
Aviram et al., 253
Aviram, Brodsky, & Stanley, 243, 252
avoid abandonment, 109
avoidance, 34, 35, 112, 124, 172, 179, 181, 198, 258
avoidance behavior, 34
avoidant personality disorders, 102
awareness, viii, 134, 135, 137, 139, 142, 144, 148, 149, 150, 152, 153, 154, 155, 156, 157, 158, 174, 177, 178, 194, 244, 253
Axelrod, Perepletchikova, Holtzman, & Sinha, 109, 113
Axis II, 5, 11, 106
Axis II disorders, 106

B

Baer, Peters, Eisenlohr-Moul, Geiger, and Sauer, 41
Ball & Links, 258
Bandelow et al., 258, 259
Bannon, Michelhaugh, Wang, & Sacchetti, 74
Barnicot, Katsakou, Marougka, & Priebe, 243
barriers to employment, 246
basal ganglia, 73, 87
basic autonomy, 6
Bateman & Fonagy, 97, 112
Beauchaine, Hinsaw and Bridge, 39
Beblo et al., 70
Beck, Aaron, 95
Beckstead, Lambert, DuBose, & Linehan, 107
Bedics, Atkins, Comtois, & Linehan, 168
behavior chain analyses (BCA), 173
behavior chains, 174, 194, 196
behavior therapy, 18, 99, 110, 116, 122, 123, 124, 125, 127, 128, 129, 130, 131, 162, 164, 198, 199, 200, 202, 203, 204, 263, 266, 273, 274, 278
behavioral change, 9
behavioral control, 76
behavioral disorders, 95
behavioral dysregulation, 17, 26
behavioral effects of DBT, 79
behavioral impulsivity, 25, 75
behavioral inhibition, 74, 257
behavioral interventions, 102, 228

behavioral manifestations, 6
behavioral theory, 8, 95
behaviors, vii, 2, 4, 13, 22, 23, 24, 34, 35, 45, 66, 97, 103, 109, 110, 112, 119, 143, 159, 163, 164, 165, 166, 167, 169, 170, 171, 172, 173, 174, 177, 178, 179, 181, 182, 184, 185, 186, 188, 192, 193, 194, 196, 198, 223, 224, 227, 229, 231, 242, 244, 245, 246, 251
belief systems, 95, 97, 159, 244
belittling, 251
Belsky et al., 245
Bender et al., 242
benefits of training, 207
benzodiazepines, 120
Berger and Luckmann, 215, 216, 217
Berridge & Kringelbach, 68
better treatment outcomes, 260, 261
bewitchment, 226, 227, 229, 230
bias, 27, 41, 164, 211, 231, 243
bias to the positive, 211
bilateral hippocampus reduction in BPD, 68
binge eating, 12, 33, 34, 172
bingeing and purging, 247
biogenetic explanations, 251, 270
biological correlates, v, 65, 241, 244, 245, 256
biological correlates of BPD, 241, 244, 256
biological correlates of mental illness, 245
biological liability markers for BPD, 74
biological model of psychiatry, 23
biological vulnerabilities, 166
biosocial developmental model of BPD, 9
biosocial model, 9, 15, 36, 39, 267
biosocial theory, 9, 166
biparental abuse or neglect, 259
bipolar disorder, 21, 44, 54, 63, 114, 117, 118, 119
bipolar I disorder, 43, 44
bipolar II disorder, 43, 44
Black et al., 250, 251
black-and-white thinking, 166
blaming, 185
Bloom et al., 110, 112, 113
Bloom, Woodward, Susmaras, & Pantalone, 109, 110
Blum et al., 98
B-MCT, 104
Bodner et al., 250, 253
body awareness, 142
body image, 35, 42
borderline level of organization, 146, 147, 148
Borderline Personality Features Scale for Children (BPFS-C), 245
borderline personality organization, 5, 15, 22, 138, 139
borderline personality traits, 9, 81
borderline personality-related symptoms (BPRS), 8, 15, 267
borderline states, 6, 22, 56, 145
borderline syndrome, 5, 18, 22, 55, 147, 160, 162, 278
Bornovalova et al., 73, 257
Bornovalova, Hicks, Iacono, & McGue, 79
BOSCOT study, 102, 103
bouts of depression, 20
Bowlby, John, 7
BPD in adolescents, 10
BPD in early adolescence, 47
BPD is behaviorally functional, 231
BPD prevalence rate, 249
BPD self-stigma, 241, 255, 260, 261
BPD stigma, 241, 244, 246, 247, 250
BPD suicide attempters, 69
BPD symptoms, 5, 6, 79, 99, 102, 103, 111, 113, 116, 169, 243, 249
BPD symptoms tend to decline with age, 79
BPD therapist stigma, 241
brain, 4, 13, 23, 46, 47, 52, 54, 55, 65, 67, 68, 69, 70, 71, 72, 74, 75, 76, 77, 78, 79, 82, 84, 85, 87, 89, 91, 114, 121, 131, 225, 256, 277, 281
brain abnormalities, 89

brain differences, 76, 78, 79
brain function, 82, 84, 114, 121
brain maturation, 47
brain structural and functional differences, 77
brain structure, 4, 65, 67, 69, 70, 76, 77, 79, 85, 86, 274
brain structure and functioning, 77
brain structure studies, 69, 70
Brambilla et al., 69
Brambilla, Barale, Caverzasi, & Soares, 76
Brambilla, Soloff, Sala, Nicoletti, Keshavan, & Soares, 68
breach in confidentiality, 188
Bremner et al., 77
Broadbear et al., 116, 117
Brodmann areas (BAs), 68, 69
Brooks, Baltazar, & Munjack, 27
Brown, Manuck, Flory, & Hariri, 75, 257
Brown, Marquis and Guiffrida, 178
Buber, Martin, 235
Bui, Rodgers, Chabrol, Birmes, & Schmitt, 249
bulimia, 34, 247
bulimia nervosa, 34, 247
Burr, 217, 222, 227, 236
bursts of rage, 8
Bush, Luu, & Posner, 68
Buspirone, 120
Butler, Chapman, Foreman, and Beck, 96
Byrnes, Fava, Feinman, & Harari, 170

C

Calvo, Valero, Saez-Francas, Gutierrez, Casas, & Ferrer, 27
Cantor, Smith, French, & Messich, 24
capacity to self-soothe, 145
carbamazepine, 119
caregiver-child interaction, 141
caring attitudes toward patients, 251
Carpenter, Tomko, Trull, & Boomsma, 37
case management model, 99
case managers, 115
case studies, 143, 165
Casey et al., 46
Casey, Jones, & Hare, 46, 47
Catthoor, Feenstra, Hutsebaut, Schrijvers, & Sabbe, 252
causal relationship, 262
CBT plus TAU, 102
central nervous system, 74
Chapman et al., 181
Chapman, Rosenthal, Dixon-Gordon, Turner, & Kuppens, 181
child maltreatment, 56
childcare, 114
childhood, 7, 14, 15, 20, 22, 33, 37, 39, 42, 56, 57, 60, 61, 66, 69, 76, 77, 88, 90, 101, 114, 134, 145, 225, 245, 257, 258, 259, 262, 265, 266, 267, 268, 270, 273, 274, 275, 276, 279, 280
childhood abuse, 66, 69, 88, 246, 258, 279
childhood abuse and/or neglect, 258
childhood emotional abuse, 57, 259, 270
childhood history, 259
childhood history of neglect, 259
childhood interpersonal trauma, 259
childhood neglect, 114
childhood sexual abuse (CSA), 42, 114, 259, 267, 276
childhood trauma, 61, 77, 90, 258, 262, 268, 273
children, 42, 47, 53, 141, 245, 250, 263
Children in the Community Study (CIC), 47
Choi-Kain et al., 95, 99, 107, 260
Choi-Kain, Finch, Masland, Jenkins, & Unruh, 165
Choi-Kain, Glasserman, & Finch, 115
chronic exposure, 257
chronic fears of abandonment, 8
chronic feelings of anger, 29
chronic feelings of emptiness, 12, 26, 37, 43

chronic feelings of inadequacy, 20, 29, 31
chronic invalidation, 165
chronically suicidal adult patients, 166
cingulate, 69, 77, 82, 83, 85
cingulate gyrus, 69
Clark, Fox, & Long, 260
Clarke, Taylor, Bolderston, Lancaster, & Remington, 260
Clarkin et al., 24, 25, 45
Clarkin, Widiger, Francis, Hurt, & Gilmore, 24
client empowerment, 226
clients, 94, 97, 107, 112, 123, 171, 179, 181, 207, 209, 213, 216, 218, 220, 223, 225, 226, 227, 228, 229, 230, 231, 232, 234, 235, 266
clients in Egypt, 107
clinical presentation, 50
clinical psychology, 207, 208
clinical trial, 96, 102, 106, 200, 202, 204, 211, 219, 236
clinical trials, 96, 102, 211, 219
clinician burnout, 164, 194
clinician pessimism, 251
clinician stigma, 243, 253, 259, 261
clinician training, 261
close relationships, 30, 31
cluster B personality disorders, 45
cluster C, 12, 50, 71
clusters, 21, 24, 25, 26, 28, 29, 40, 59, 73, 258
clusters of BPD features, 25
clusters of personality traits, 28
clusters of symptoms, 21, 24, 26, 29
Cochrane Collaborative Review, 168
coding of rewards, 68
cognitive behavioral therapy (CBT), 93, 94, 95, 96, 98, 100, 101, 102, 103, 104, 105, 112, 116, 121, 126, 127, 129, 219, 220
cognitive capacities, 98
cognitive control, 32, 44, 46, 61, 68, 73, 75
cognitive disturbance, 66, 72
cognitive function, 245
cognitive map, 49
cognitive perspective, 10
cognitive process, 42, 52, 98, 106, 126, 131, 260, 277
cognitive processing, 42, 106, 126, 131, 260, 277
cognitive processing differences in BPD, 260
cognitive reaction, 154
cognitive rehabilitation, 105, 106, 130
cognitive slippage, 41
cognitive theory, 8, 95
cognitive therapies, 100, 125, 219, 220
cognitive-behavioral model, 9
cognitive-behavioral strategies, 166, 167
Cohen, Crawford, Johnson, & Kasen, 47
cohesive sense of identity, 150
collaborative longitudinal personality disorders study (CLPS), 34, 49, 56, 57, 90, 126, 268
college students, 246, 273
coming out, 261
common factors, 210, 212, 232, 235, 236
communication, 41, 148, 171, 172, 181, 188, 193, 196, 232, 278
communication skills, 193
communication strategies, 171, 194
comorbid, 27, 35, 43, 48, 59, 69, 76, 77, 79, 105, 117, 120, 126, 130, 164, 168, 170, 242, 258
comorbid anxiety disorders, 27, 120
comorbid depression, 43, 168
comorbid eating disorders, 120
comorbid issues, 164
comorbid MDD, 76, 77
comorbid personality disorder, 105
comorbid post traumatic stress disorder (PTSD), 67, 69, 76, 104, 201, 219, 242, 256, 257, 258, 260, 269, 275, 279
comorbid psychiatric disorders, 79

comorbid schizotypal personality disorder, 69
comorbidity, 25, 33, 59, 76, 94, 104, 112, 116, 117, 129, 243, 274
comorbidity for BPD and PTSD, 104
compassion, 165, 194, 234, 236, 237
competencies, 246
complementary countertransference, 145, 148
completed suicide rate, 109
complex post-traumatic stress disorder (CPTSD), 242, 244, 257, 258, 259, 264, 266
complex trauma, 165
complexity, 158, 164, 193, 242
compliance, 111, 112, 115, 120
compromised functioning, 77
conceptualization, viii, ix, xi, 1, 2, 6, 23, 99, 130, 133, 149, 212
conduct disorder, 245
confidentiality, 165, 187
confirmatory factor analysis, 25, 59
conflict, 108, 120, 148, 149, 156, 166, 182, 183, 228, 230
conflict resolution, 108
conflicted internal working models of relationships, 99
Congdon & Canli, 74, 257
connectivity, 46, 71, 72, 77, 79, 84, 85, 86, 90, 203
conscience, 136
conscientiousness, 28
conscious, 3, 4, 135, 136, 137, 139, 144, 152, 186, 229, 234, 254
conscious awareness, 137
conscious mind, 135, 137
constructed reality, 217, 226, 230, 236
constructionism, 206, 214, 215, 217, 218, 221, 224, 226, 227, 233, 235, 281
constructionist, vi, vii, ix, 205, 207, 215, 216, 217, 218, 222, 223, 227, 231, 232, 233, 234, 235
constructionist perspective, ix, 205, 207, 223, 227, 235
consultation, vii, 107, 127, 129, 132, 169, 171, 184, 191, 192, 194, 197, 198
consultation team, 129, 169, 171, 184, 191, 194, 197, 198
consumer operated services, 261
contextual model, 205, 206, 210, 214, 216, 217, 218, 219, 220, 221, 226, 230, 232, 235, 238, 239
contextual model group, 206, 210, 221, 232
continuum of personality traits, 27
contraception use, 119
contradictory amygdala results, 77
contradictory findings, 76
control condition, 104
control group, 72, 74, 75, 76, 180
controlled studies, 102, 105
controlled trials, 105, 125, 168
core pathophysiological processes, 78
corrective experiences, 152, 153
correlation analyses, 78
Corrigan & Calabrese, 253
Corrigan & Kleinlein, 245, 252
Corrigan, Larson, & Rüsch, 244, 253, 254, 261
Corrigan, Morris, Michaels, Rafaczm, & Rüsch, 245
cortex, 46, 68, 71, 72, 73, 83
corticolimbic system, 67
cost, 102, 112, 121, 170, 197, 229
cost effectiveness, 121, 197
counseling, 120, 124, 129, 179, 198, 203, 209
counselors, 97, 115
countertransference, 145, 161, 162, 251, 254, 271
Crawford et al., 119
Crick, Murray-Close, & Woods, 245
crisis, 11, 34, 49, 109, 110, 112, 129, 160, 164, 179, 184, 194, 196, 197
crisis management, 164, 196

crisis moments, 179
Cristea et al., 168, 221, 260
criterion variance, 24
critical links, 176
Crocker, Major, & Steele, 245
cross-sectional, 78, 268
cross-sectional studies, 78
Crowell et al., 39
Crowell, Beauchaine and Linehan, 9, 39
cues, 84, 166, 180, 228, 254
culture, viii, 2, 107, 166, 212, 213, 214, 215, 216, 217, 222, 226, 232, 233, 253
current limit, 84
Cuthbert et al., 37
cutting, 176, 186, 187
cytoarchitecture, 68

D

D.W. Winnicott, 142
D4 receptors, 74
damaging relationships, 181
dangerous stalkers, 249
dangerousness, 245, 272
Darios, Zakzanis and Ruocco, 37
Davidson & Parker, 219
Davidson et al., 103
Davidson, Abercrombie, Nitschke, & Putnam, 69
Davidson, Tyrer, Norrie, Palmer, and Tyrer, 102
Davis & Whalen, 67, 69
day hospital program, 113
day hospitalization, 113, 114
DBT assumptions, 185
DBT skills group, 177
deactivating the attachment system, 111
deaf clients, 107
decision-making authority, 245
decision-making process, 145
decision-making processes, 145
declarative memory, 67
deconstructing BPD, 223
deconstruction of the concept of techniques, 231
DeCou, Comtois, and Landes, 168
decrease in libido, 119
deep shame, 255
defense mechanism, 135, 136, 144, 146, 150, 154, 156, 157, 158
deficiency, 23
delusion, 17
denial, 5, 115, 149, 150, 156, 157
departures from reality, 149
depression, 20, 33, 35, 41, 43, 49, 50, 55, 59, 63, 74, 77, 81, 82, 83, 89, 90, 105, 107, 112, 118, 164, 168, 169, 197, 221, 242, 245, 264
depressive symptoms, 111
depressivity, 28
depth, ix, 133, 158, 167, 188
derealization, 21
derogatory language, 251
DeShong, Grant and Mullins-Sweatt, 12
despair, 20, 34, 36
detrimental behaviors, 177
devaluation, 12, 28, 31, 149, 150, 156, 157, 158, 253
developmental process, 233
developmental psychopathology, 7, 9, 14, 266
developmental psychopathology theory, 7
developmental stage theory, 6
Diagnostic and Statistical Manual of Mental Disorders (DSM), vii, viii, 4, 11, 12, 19, 22, 23, 24, 25, 26, 27, 28, 29, 32, 37, 39, 43, 44, 45, 47, 51, 54, 57, 58, 59, 62, 63, 108, 148, 257
diagnostic categorization, 12
diagnostic criteria, viii, xi, 5, 10, 19, 21, 23, 24, 25, 29, 32, 42, 43, 44, 50, 102, 105, 109, 110, 178, 206, 231, 258

diagnostic criteria for BPD, 19, 21, 43, 110, 178
diagnostic efficiency, 24
diagnostic features, 26, 27
diagnostic groupings, 23
diagnostic overlap, 25, 45
diagnostic sensitivity, 23
diagnostic tools, 80
diagnostic-centric, 206
dialectical behavior therapy (DBT), vi, vii, 9, 18, 75, 79, 94, 106, 107, 110, 111, 113, 116, 121, 122, 123, 124, 125, 127, 128, 129, 130, 131, 162, 163, 164, 165, 166, 167, 168, 169, 171, 172, 173, 174, 175, 176, 177, 178, 179, 180, 181, 182, 183, 184, 185, 186, 187, 192, 193, 194, 195, 196, 197, 198, 199, 200, 201, 202, 203, 204, 218, 221, 231, 260, 263, 266, 273, 274, 278, 279, 281
dialectical behavior therapy for adolescents (DBT-A), 107, 127, 128, 169, 177, 182, 183, 200, 202
dialectical strategies, 166
dialectics, 16, 166, 271
diary card, 172, 173, 174, 196
differential diagnosis, viii, ix, 27, 43, 58
differential diagnosis of borderline personality disorder, 58
differentiation, 45, 85, 116, 142
difficulties with emotional regulation, 259
difficulty thinking clearly, 164
Dimeff & Linehan, 194, 244, 260
dimensional model, 27, 29
dimensional model for personality disorder diagnoses, 27
dimensional model of personality organization, 27
discrimination, 242, 244, 250, 252, 253, 254
disgust, 37, 73, 254
disinhibited fear responses, 69
disinhibition, 29
disorder, 2, 4, 6, 11, 23, 27, 33, 42, 43, 44, 45, 47, 48, 59, 63, 66, 67, 69, 73, 76, 77, 78, 80, 81, 83, 87, 94, 96, 98, 99, 101, 102, 105, 106, 108, 110, 111, 114, 116, 120, 124, 126, 127, 148, 164, 168, 203, 220, 242, 245, 247, 257, 262, 264, 268, 271, 274, 275, 279
disposition, 27
disputing the diagnosis, 231
dissociation, 21, 42, 61, 84, 149, 160, 231
dissociation and ego state therapy, 231
dissociations, 66
dissociative experiences, 111
dissociative states, 28, 72
dissociative symptoms, 42, 69
distorted self-image, 66
distortions, 20, 30, 31, 38, 41, 69
distraction, 84, 180, 191, 194
distress, 97, 107, 108, 120, 130, 131, 136, 176, 179, 186, 187, 188, 190, 194, 201, 246, 265
distress tolerance, 107, 120, 176, 177, 179, 188, 201
disturbances in self-representation, 10
disturbances of self-organization (DSO), 258
disturbed relatedness, 26
disturbed relationships, 26, 72, 259
Ditty, Landes, Doyle & Beidas, 194
divalproex sodium, 119
Diwadkar et al., 77
Dixon-Gordon, Turner, Rosenthal and Chapman, 181
dodo bird effect, 210
domains of personality traits, 27
domestic violence, 169, 200
dopamine, 46, 61, 74, 81, 257, 263
dopamine D4 receptor (DRD4), 74
dorsal anterior cingulate, 71
dorsal insula, 71, 73
dorsal lateral prefrontal cortex, 46

dorsolateral prefrontal cortex (DLPFC), 67, 68, 75
double-blind, parallel, placebo controlled study, 119
down regulating, 72
Drapalski et al., 253
Driesen, 258
drives, 2, 3, 4, 10, 43, 134, 144
drop out of treatment, 94, 243
drug use disorder (DUD), 73, 76
DSM III, 22
DSM-5, 11, 12, 19, 26, 27, 28, 29, 32, 37, 39, 43, 44, 45, 47, 51, 54, 57, 108, 257
DSM-5 Alternative Model for Personality Disorders, 28, 29
DSM-5 diagnostic criteria, 19, 29, 44
DSM-I, 4, 11, 12, 22, 23, 24, 25, 26, 57, 59, 62, 63, 148
DSM-II, 4, 11, 22, 23, 24, 25, 26, 148
DSM-III, 5, 11, 23, 24, 25, 26, 148
DSM-III diagnostic criteria for BPD, 25
DSM-III-R, 25
DSM-IV, 11, 12, 25, 57, 59, 62, 63
DSM-IV Diagnostic Interview for DSM-IV Personality Disorders, 26
Duncan, Miller, Wampold, & Hubble, 206, 223
dynamic forces, 2
dysfunctional strategies, 226
dysphoria, 12, 36, 39, 43, 44, 118
dysregulation, 9, 17, 26, 61

E

early academic and social functioning, 245
early adulthood, 12, 30, 39, 46, 47
early biological vulnerabilities, 9
early life trauma, 66
early trauma, 8, 263
easily bored, 38
eating disorders, 117, 120, 129, 164, 168, 170, 193, 242, 247, 276
education, 93, 98, 100, 130, 206, 214, 246, 247, 254
educational websites, 255
effect of psychotherapy on the brain, 75
effects of Psychotherapy on BPD, 75
efficacy, 21, 95, 98, 104, 110, 111, 112, 113, 116, 117, 118, 119, 121, 125, 128, 130, 144, 168, 169, 197, 199, 202, 204, 219, 236, 237, 253, 254, 256, 265, 278
efficacy of antidepressants in the treatment of BPD, 118
efficacy of CBT, 96
efficacy of inpatient treatment, 112
Egan, Haley, & Rees, 260
ego, 1, 3, 4, 5, 6, 10, 55, 134, 135, 136, 137, 138, 144, 145, 147, 149, 150, 153, 154, 156, 158, 160, 162, 216, 222, 228, 239
ego defense mechanisms, 1, 3, 136
ego integration, 6
ego psychologist, 5
ego psychology, 1, 4, 134, 136, 160
ego state therapy, 228
ego states, 144, 145, 216, 228
ego strength, 145, 154, 156, 158
electroconvulsive therapy, 110
elevated levels of alexithymia, 37
Ellis, Albert, 95
Ellison, Rosenstein, Morgan, & Zimmerman, 20
Elsner et al., 38
Elsner, Broadbear and Rao, 38
emergency, 31, 35, 102, 103, 168, 190, 192, 194, 196, 197, 247
emergency protocol, 190
emergency psychiatric visits, 102
emergency room contact, 102
emergency room visits, 168, 192, 197
emergency services, 102, 103
Emil Kraepelin, 146

emotion, 10, 15, 41, 45, 54, 56, 57, 82, 83, 86, 87, 91, 95, 101, 113, 125, 155, 163, 164, 181, 183, 188, 197, 198, 201, 203, 242, 267, 268, 270
emotion dysregulation, 15, 60, 132, 163, 164, 180, 183, 197, 203, 242, 269
emotion regulation, 10, 15, 54, 56, 57, 83, 86, 113, 122, 177, 180, 181, 188, 198, 199, 200, 201, 267, 270
emotion regulation skills, 180, 181
emotional abuse, 259
emotional and physical abuse and neglect, 39
emotional cascade model, 13, 14, 266
emotional disorder, 11
emotional distress, 38, 47, 73, 149, 187, 246
emotional dyscontrol, 39
emotional dysregulation, 8, 9, 12, 20, 39, 46, 58, 66, 82, 101, 150, 193, 242, 258, 273
emotional experience, 4, 129, 149, 150, 157, 180, 193, 203, 274
emotional fixation, 250
emotional hypersensitivity, 72
emotional information, 68
emotional intensity, 180
emotional lability, 9, 28, 34, 74, 180, 257
emotional loading, 71
emotional problems, 95, 245
emotional reactions, 32, 72, 166
emotional regulation, 68, 73, 76, 79, 97, 107, 246
emotional regulation skills, 79
emotional regulatory processes, 80
emotional responses, 37, 39, 68
emotional state, 34, 36, 69, 77, 99, 158, 179
emotional states, 77, 179
emotional stimuli, 177, 180
emotional vulnerability, 9, 14, 31, 39, 194, 266
empathy, 28, 34, 116, 144, 154, 156
empirical studies, 96
empirically supported principles of change, 151, 159
employment, 32, 241, 243, 244, 246, 269
empowerment, 226, 261
encoding, 60, 89, 277
endophenotypes, 88, 276
energy, 44, 138, 140, 147, 193
Engler & Fulton, 228
enhanced usual care (EUC), 170, 202, 273
Ensink et al., 10
Ensink, Biberdzic, Normandin, & Clarkin, 6
environment, 3, 20, 37, 39, 53, 55, 89, 97, 104, 114, 137, 138, 139, 151, 166, 167, 192, 193, 229, 256
environmental factors, 9, 37, 44, 108, 114, 166, 257
environmental influences, 73, 81, 264
environmental risk factors, 9
environmental stress, 43
enzyme production, 257
episode of deliberate self-harm, 102
episodes of self-harm, 102
Erikson, Erik, 6
erratic and impulsive behavior, 109
erratic and unstable behavior patterns, 108
Esquivillas et al., 34
establishing and maintaining strong therapeutic alliance, 152
etiology, viii, 1, 5, 8, 66, 67, 98, 143, 146, 255
Etkin, Egner, & Kalisch, 79
evidence, 29, 37, 41, 47, 50, 66, 74, 76, 78, 79, 96, 105, 107, 108, 110, 111, 112, 113, 118, 123, 126, 127, 131, 145, 148, 149, 164, 165, 168, 193, 206, 207, 208, 209, 218, 219, 220, 221, 239, 241, 245, 252, 253, 254, 256, 258, 259, 260, 264, 265, 277, 278, 282
evidence regarding DBT, 168
evidence-based approach, 29
evidence-based practices, 218, 254, 265

evidence-based psychotherapeutic practices, 254
evidence-based treatments (EBT), 95, 96, 108, 110, 165, 219, 256, 260, 261
evidenced based therapy, 95
evidenced-based treatment, 79
evolution, vii, viii, 4, 18, 19, 50, 128, 134, 162, 202, 206, 261, 278, 282
exaggeration, 215, 249
excessive spending, 34
existential interventions, 231
experiential imagery, 100
experimental design, 221
expert, iv, 145
exposure, 41, 180, 200, 201, 219, 255, 257
external other/object, 140
externalization, 115, 246

F

facial expression, 37, 41
facilitating awareness, 152
factor structure, 25
Fairbairn, W.R.D., 141
family environment, 33
family history, 263
family influence, 9
family interventions, 112
family members, 33, 43, 45, 73, 182, 256
family system, 228
family therapy, 100
family/social supports, 115
Farrell and Shaw, 104
fast-acting anxiolytic medications, 120
fatal attraction, 248, 266, 274, 276
fear, 25, 30, 31, 32, 36, 44, 67, 69, 84, 87, 135, 157, 164, 182, 188, 193, 242, 256, 275
fear of abandonment, 25, 30, 164, 182, 188, 242
fear response, 67, 69, 256
fear responses, 67, 69, 256
feelings, 8, 12, 20, 22, 26, 28, 29, 31, 34, 37, 41, 43, 44, 49, 86, 97, 109, 115, 120, 164, 166, 179, 214, 227, 242, 252, 254, 255, 258
feelings of emptiness, 8, 28, 38, 164, 242, 258
feelings of inadequacy, 252
Feigenbaum et al., 168
feminist psychological perspectives, 7
feminist psychology, 7
film, 247, 248, 249
first generation, 118, 119
first generation antidepressants, 118
first generation of antipsychotics, 119
five-factor model (FFM), 27
Fleischhaker et al., 170
Flückiger, Del Re, Wampold, Symonds, & Horvath, 165
fluctuating sense of self, 164, 242
fluid, 32, 213, 217, 222, 223, 226, 232
focus on acceptance alone, 107
forensic institutions, 168
forensic studies, 249
Fowler, Madan, Allen, Oldman, & Frueh, 21
fragile, 21, 251, 254
Francois et al., 119, 120
Francois, Roth, and Klingman, 118
Freud, Sigmund, 1, 2, 3, 4, 5, 14, 15, 17, 134, 135, 136, 137, 138, 139, 141, 146, 148, 149, 152, 160
Freudian model, 142, 150
Fromm, Erich, 143
Fromm-Reichmann, Frieda, 143
frontal cortex, 69, 72, 80
frontal eye fields, 71
frontolimbic neural links, 12
frustration tolerance, 113
Fruzetti & Levensky, 169
functional brain imaging, 65, 70, 256

functional brain imaging studies, 65, 70, 256
functional brain imaging studies in BPD, 65
functional changes, 75
functional connectivity, 71, 72, 79, 85, 86, 203
functional connectivity studies, 71
functional MRI (fMRI), 70, 72, 81, 82, 83, 86, 91, 131, 277

G

Gabbard & Ball, 114, 118, 121
Gaher et al., 181
Gaher, Hofmann, Simons, & Hunsaker, 180
gains in the activation of bilateral middle/inferior frontal gyri, 75
gains in the activation of specific brain regions, 75
Gallop, Lancee, & Garfinkel, 251
Geisen-Bloo et al, 100
gender, 8, 15, 77, 79, 111, 228, 267, 274
gender differences, 8, 79
gender-specific, 15, 77, 267
general psychiatric management (GPM), 99, 165, 201, 260, 269
genetic component, 73, 256
genetic model, 135, 138
genetic polymorphisms, 257
genetic predisposition, 37, 39, 42, 257
genetic studies, 65, 73, 74, 256
genetic studies and BPD, 65
genetic vulnerability, 33, 39
genetics, 51, 60, 66, 80, 81, 85, 114, 256, 259, 262
genital, 138
Gergen, Kenneth, 234
Germán, et al., 107
gestures, 12, 35, 193
Ghiasi, Mohammadi, and Zarrinfar, 10
Gianoli, Jane, O'Brien, & Ralevski, 117
Gill and Warburton, 9
global assessment of functioning (GAF), 48, 50
goal directed behavior, 68, 167
Godbout et al., 8
Godbout, Daspe, Runtz, Cyr and Briere, 8
good enough parenting, 142
good psychiatric management, 201, 260, 269
Goodman & Yehuda, 258, 259
Goodman et al., 66, 75, 79
graduate education, 206
graduate program, 207
graduate students, 194, 207, 208
Grambal et al., 253
gray matter, 68, 69, 75
Grinker, Werble, & Drye, 147
group identity, 261
group schema therapy, 104, 125, 129
group therapy, 97, 99, 100, 104, 132, 170, 206, 243
group treatment, 98
Groves, Backer, van den Bosch & Miller, 170
guidelines, 115, 116, 117, 165
Guile et al., 47
Guile, Boissel, Alaux-Cantin, & Garny de La Riviére, 47
Guinea et al., 35
Gunderson & Lyons-Ruth, 21, 30, 37
Gunderson & Phillips, 43
Gunderson and Singer, 22
Gunderson et al., 50, 73, 79, 94, 243, 256

H

hallucinations, 7, 41, 105, 147
Hankin & Adela, 35
harm to self or others, 103, 109
harmful childhood environments, 39
Harned et al, 168

Harned, Korslund, & Linehan, 168
Harry Stack Sullivan, 3, 143
Hart, Radua, Nakao, Mataix-Cols, & Rubia, 78
Haw & Stubbs, 117, 120
Haw and Stubbs, 116
Hazlett et al., 69, 77
health, vii, viii, ix, 11, 13, 20, 21, 28, 29, 51, 55, 87, 94, 96, 103, 105, 109, 110, 112, 114, 115, 122, 125, 126, 127, 128, 194, 199, 200, 203, 212, 214, 215, 216, 219, 238, 241, 242, 243, 244, 245, 246, 247, 250, 251, 252, 253, 254, 257, 260, 262, 263, 264, 266, 270, 272, 274, 277, 278, 280, 282
health care, 112, 241, 242, 243, 244, 251, 254
health care professionals, 243, 251
health care providers, 115, 241, 242, 244, 250, 251, 254
health care system, 112, 251
health practitioners, vii, 109, 110, 114, 252
health problem, 105, 126, 212, 247, 257, 280
health promotion, 266
health services, 247, 252
Heard & Linehan, 9
heart attack, 193
heart rate, 181
heightened activity in limbic regions, 71
helplessness, 20, 34, 49, 50
Herbert et al., 219
heritability, 73, 81, 257, 277
Herman, Perry & Van der Kolk, 258
Herpertz et al., 70
heterogeneity, 66
heterogeneous symptoms, 23
higher level of care, 192
higher order thinking, 145
high-risk individuals, 165
Hill and Knox, 207, 209
Hilton & von Hippel, 244
hippocampal volume, 69, 74, 76, 81, 88, 89, 90, 276
hippocampus, 67, 68, 69, 72, 74, 76, 86, 87, 88, 256, 275
hippocampus volume, 76
hippocampus-orbitomedial prefrontal cortex circuit, 70
Hiraoka, Crouch, Reo, Wagner, Milner, & Skowronski, 42
history, vii, viii, ix, 14, 33, 35, 43, 45, 77, 85, 93, 97, 119, 120, 158, 165, 186, 188, 206, 207, 216, 242, 258, 276, 282
history of trauma, 33, 120
histrionic personality disorder, 30
Hoch and Polatin, 147
Hofmann et al, 96
Hofmann, Asnaani, Vonk, Sawyer, and Fang, 95
Holder, Holliday, Pal, and Suris, 104
hopelessness, 29, 38, 49, 50, 168, 255
Horga, Kaur, & Peterson, 67, 77, 78, 79
hormone focused therapies, 121
Horney, Karen, 143
hospital admissions, 168
hospital emergency departments, 247
hospital setting, 109, 192
hospital treatment, 108, 109, 113, 114
hospitalization, 44, 108, 109, 110, 112, 113, 114, 123, 128, 192, 243
household expression, 247
Hughes, Crowell, Uyeji and Coan, 12
Hulvershorn, Cullen, & Anand, 78
human, 3, 4, 8, 81, 83, 88, 91, 97, 134, 135, 137, 146, 214, 234, 263
human experience, 137
Hunnicutt Hollenbaugh & Lenz, 107
hypersensitivity, 22, 37, 55, 72, 100, 180
hypervigilance, 20, 258
hypothalamus, 90
hypothesis, 106, 111

I

ICD-11, 257, 264, 269, 275
Id, 135, 136, 144, 160
idealization, 12, 28, 31, 149, 150, 156, 158
idealization and devaluation, 12, 28, 31
idealizing, 224
identification, viii, 5, 32, 146, 149, 150, 156, 157, 158, 244
identity, 5, 6, 10, 12, 16, 24, 26, 28, 32, 33, 38, 39, 43, 50, 99, 140, 148, 149, 150, 151, 153, 160, 224, 227, 233, 254, 259, 261, 267, 271
identity confusion, 5, 151
identity development, 6, 149
identity diffusion, 6, 10, 16, 99, 271
identity disturbance, 12, 24, 26, 32, 38, 43, 259
identity integration, 6, 10, 148, 150
identity integration disruption, 6
imaging equipment, 121
imbalanced sense of self and other, 154
immediate gratification, 135
impaired brain development, 226
impaired inhibitory control, 74
impairment in emotional interoception, 37
improve outcomes, 115, 212, 214
improvements, vii, 72, 75, 98, 111, 113, 119, 211, 221, 260
improvements in brain structures, 76
impulse control, 66, 74, 91, 178
impulse-driven behavior, 46
impulsive, 21, 26, 30, 33, 34, 40, 44, 46, 49, 50, 69, 109, 119, 163, 164, 169, 170, 172, 179, 189, 242, 243, 249, 256
impulsive acting-out risk-taking behavior, 26
impulsive acts, 29, 30, 49, 50
impulsive acts of self-harm, 49
impulsive behavior, 109, 119, 163, 164, 169, 170, 172, 179, 242, 243
impulsive emotionally-driven decision-making, 40
impulsive or aggressive behaviors, 69
impulsive, sensation-seeking proclivities, 46
impulsivity, 9, 12, 25, 26, 28, 33, 39, 71, 72, 75, 82, 97, 108, 109, 114, 119, 120, 168, 178, 197, 245, 264
inadequate training, 252
inadequate vocational support, 246
inappropriate anger, 25
inappropriate, intense anger, 12, 38
incapable, 34, 36, 245
incompetence, 245
inconsistent personality/emotional organization, 153
increased impulsivity, 108
increased risk factor for completing suicide, 35
increased white matter volume in BAs 24 and 31, 69
in-depth assessment, 188
individual differences, 66, 82, 264
individual therapy, 99, 100, 107, 169, 171, 172, 177, 183, 206, 243
individual therapy protocols, 206
individuals, 6, 11, 20, 21, 26, 28, 29, 30, 31, 32, 33, 34, 35, 36, 37, 38, 39, 40, 41, 42, 43, 49, 50, 67, 68, 70, 71, 78, 79, 105, 127, 130, 164, 165, 166, 167, 168, 177, 178, 179, 181, 182, 186, 188, 189, 195, 197, 202, 215, 224, 229, 251, 254, 258
individuation, 28, 31, 142, 145
industrialization, 3
ineffective behaviors, 172, 173, 184, 185
ineffective responses, 171, 174
ineffective strategies, 228
ineffective treatment models, 94
infant attachment, 7
inferior frontal gyrus, 75
inferior parietal lobe, 71
information variance, 24
informed decision-making model, 117

inhibition, 68, 74, 75, 80, 83, 257, 262
inhibitory regulation, 256
initial onset of symptoms, 20
initiation, 67, 113, 114, 229
injury, iv, 21, 35, 52, 56, 61, 72, 73, 86, 90, 109, 114, 122, 138, 168, 170, 184, 186
inner experience, 150, 281
inner world, 155
inpatient and outpatient treatment, 94
inpatient hospital treatment, 112
inpatient hospitalization, 112, 113, 114
in-patient psychiatric services, 102
inpatient psychiatric stays, 107
inpatient treatment, 110, 111, 112, 113, 114, 123, 131
inpatient units, 168
insula, 70, 73
integrated self, 158
integration, 4, 6, 9, 10, 39, 42, 46, 148, 150, 151, 153, 161, 260
integrity, 67, 233
intense anxiety, 28
intense emotional states, 99
intense inner pain, 26
intensive outpatient programming (IOP), 110, 113, 114
interception, 73
interdependence, 141
internal drives, 2
internal family systems, 228
internal other/object, 140
internal self, 153
internal working models, 99
internalized as good or bad object representations, 6
internalized objects, 143
interpersonal boundaries, 246
interpersonal contact, 138
interpersonal difficulties, 163, 164, 242, 243, 258
interpersonal dynamics, 99
interpersonal effectiveness, 107, 177, 181, 182, 183
interpersonal events, 4
interpersonal hypersensitivity, 37, 55, 100
interpersonal interaction impairment, 12
interpersonal interactions, 1, 2, 4, 97
interpersonal problems, 165, 195
interpersonal psychoanalysis, 3
interpersonal relations, 8, 12, 22, 25, 31, 32, 66, 97, 99, 108, 109, 115, 120, 178, 182, 281
interpersonal relationship conflict, 120
interpersonal relationship difficulties, 108
interpersonal relationships, 8, 12, 22, 25, 31, 32, 66, 97, 108, 109, 115, 182, 281
interpersonal sensitivity, 28
interpersonal skills, 236
interpersonal strategies, 195
interpersonally sensitive, 251
interrater reliability of coefficients, 25
intervention, 9, 11, 27, 103, 105, 113, 129, 164, 189, 191, 203, 211, 213, 221, 225, 230, 244, 260
intimacy, 28, 30, 113
intolerance for being alone, 8
intrapersonal dynamics, 134
introjected, 144, 158
introjection, 145, 149
invalidating parenting, 9
invalidating social environment, 9
irresponsible spending, 178
irritability, 12, 29, 36
isolating, 167, 172
issues, 53, 61, 101, 108, 164, 195, 217, 219, 233, 242, 245, 281

J

Jowett, Karatzias, Shevlin, & Albert, 258
judging, 185
Juliet Mitchell, 7

Juurlink et al., 244, 246

K

Kahlbaum, Karl, 3
Kamphause et al., 72
Kamphausen et al., 71
kappa (k) values, 23
Kate Davidson et al, 102
Kealy & Ogrodniczuk, 252
Kellogg & Young, 100
Keuroghlian et al., 165, 260
Kiselica, Webber, & Bornovalova, 179
Klein, Fairbairn, Winnicott, Kernberg, 133
Klein, Melanie, 141
Klonsky & Muehlenkamp, 35
Klonsky and Mueuhlenkamp, 35
Koenigsberg et al., 70
Kohut & Wolf, 6
Kohut, Heinz, 5, 143
Korzekwa, Dell, Links, Thabane, & Webb, 243
Krause & Schmahl, 76
Krause-Utz et al., 70, 71, 73
Krause-Utz, Frost, Winter, & Elginga, 68
Krause-Utz, Winter, Liedtfeld, & Schmahl, 67
Kredlow et al., 104
Kreisman & Straus, 248
Kröger et al., 107, 110, 111, 112
Kröger, Harbeck, Armbrust, & Kliem, 106
Krueger & Hopwood, 27
Krueger, Derringer, Markon, Watson, & Skodol, 27
Kuo et al., 259
Kuo, Fitzpatrick, Metcalfe, & McMain, 180
Kuo, Khoury, Metcalfe, Fitzpatrick, & Goodwill, 259
Kvaale, Haslam, & Gottdiener, 251
Kvarstein, Pederson, Urnes, Hummelen, Wilberg, & Karterud, 10

L

lack of identity integration, 153
lack of research based evidence, 118
lack of structure, 246
lack of training effects, 207, 208
Laing, R. D., 7
Lambert & Ogles, 209, 212
Lamotrigine, 119, 124
Laporte et al., 258
Laporte, Paris, Guttman, Russell, & Correa, 246
large cost of hospitalization, 112
large sample size, 111
Latina clients, 107
law enforcement, 247
Lawn & McMahon, 252
lay population, 244
learning, 61, 138, 177, 179, 180, 193
Lee, Cameron & Jenner, 168
Lee, Soares, Beique, 77
left amygdala, 72
left cuneus, 71
left frontopolar cortex (FPC), 71
left hippocampus, 72
left inferior parietal lobule, 71
left insula, 71
left orbitofrontal cortex, 72
left temporal fusiform, 72
legal system, 247
Leichsenring, Leibing, Kruse, New, & Leweke, 66, 112
Lenz & Del Conte, 107
Lequesne & Hersh, 255
levels of organization, 146, 148
Levy, Johnson and Clouthier et al., 8
Lewis & Appleby, 250
libidinal drive, 6
Lieb, Zanarini, Schmahl, Linehan, & Bohus, 66, 76
Liebman & Burnette, 251, 254

life course, 20, 33
life experiences, 21
life goal achievement, 254
life satisfaction, 272, 275
lifespan, 34, 49, 135, 245
life-threatening behaviors, 170, 171
life-threatening information, 171
lifetime, 26, 34, 52, 110, 243, 256
lifetime hospitalization, 110
likelihood of birth defects, 119
limbic, 46, 69, 72, 73, 77, 86
limbic activity, 77
limbic circuits, 69
limited re-parenting, 100
limit-setting, 34, 195
Lind, Vanwoerden, Penner, and Sharp, 11
Linehan & Schmidt, 9
Linehan & Wilks, 108, 178, 180
Linehan et al., 169, 177
Linehan Risk Assessment and Management Protocol (LRAMP), 189
Linehan, Armstrong, Suarez, Allmon, & Heard, 168
Linehan, Heard, & Armstrong, 168
Linehan, Marsha, 107, 163, 166, 185, 260
Link, Cullen, & Frank, 253
Lis and Myhr, 105
Lis et al., 76, 77
Lis, Greenfield, Henry, Guile, & Dougherty, 76
lithium carbonate, 119
London, 3, 14, 16, 17, 102, 160, 161
loneliness, 8, 50, 188, 235
long term efficacy, 113
longitudinal course of borderline personality disorder, 61, 278
longitudinal study, 56, 94, 201, 245, 265
longitudinal twin sample, 73
longitudinal twin studies, 256
loss of inhibitory regulations, 69
low self-esteem, 253, 254
low self-worth, 29, 30
Luborsky, Singer, and Luborsky, 209
Lynch et al., 107, 108, 178
Lynch, Chapman, Rosenthal, Kuo, & Linehan, 107, 178

M

magnetic resonance, 55, 80, 83, 88, 89, 276
magnetic resonance imaging (MRI), 55, 67, 78, 80, 81, 83, 84, 88, 89, 276
Mahler, Margaret, 142
mainstream American culture, 247
Major & O'Brien, 244
major depressive disorder (MDD), 21, 73, 76, 84, 94, 117, 242, 268
maladaptive behaviors, 13, 181, 231
maladaptive cognitions, 95
maladaptive coping behaviors, 180
maladaptive thought processes, 95
Malouff, 207, 237
management, 98, 99, 113, 116, 128, 141, 156, 170, 201, 228, 260, 264, 267, 269
Mancke et al., 75, 76
Mancke, Herpertz, Hirjak, Knies, & Bertsch, 76
manipulative, vii, 248, 250, 251, 252
manualized, 99, 107, 113, 170, 206, 207, 221
manualized approach, 113
manualized group therapy models, 206
manualized treatment program, 207
Martin & Thomas, 247
Martín-Blanco et al., 116, 117, 120
Masland, Cummings, Null, Woynowskie, & Choi-Kain, 260
Mason & Kreger, 248
Masterson, James, 143
matched control study, 113, 122
maternal separation, 66
Matusiewicz, Hopwood, and Lejuez, 102
McCauley et al., 169

McClean Study of Adult Development (MSAD), 34, 48, 50
McGlashan et al., 49
McMain et al., 95
McMain, Newman, Segal, and DeRubeis, 95
media, viii, 247, 249, 250, 255
media portrayals of BPD, 247, 248
medial prefrontal cortex, 71, 82
medial temporal cortex, 68
medial temporal lobe, 71
medical, xi, 125, 186, 187, 206, 215, 221, 235, 249
medical model, 206, 215, 219, 221, 235
medication, 72, 77, 83, 105, 110, 115, 116, 118, 119, 120, 121, 124, 192, 242
medication compliance, 115, 120
medication efficacy with BPD, 116
medication treatment guidelines, 115
Meehan et al., 41
Meehan, Clarkin, & Lenzenweger, 29, 41
Mehlum et al., 169, 261
memory consolidation, 67
memory function, 87
mental breakdown, 249
mental disorder, 4, 51, 80, 122, 159, 198, 271
mental health, vii, viii, ix, 13, 20, 21, 27, 29, 51, 94, 103, 110, 112, 115, 126, 127, 194, 212, 214, 215, 216, 219, 226, 238, 242, 243, 245, 246, 247, 250, 251, 252, 253, 254, 260, 262, 263, 269, 272, 277, 278, 280, 282
mental health crisis, 110
mental health diagnoses, 226, 243, 245, 251, 252, 253, 254
mental health practitioners, vii, viii, 109, 110, 114, 250, 252, 269
mental health professionals, viii, ix, 21, 27, 29, 115
mental illness, 4, 95, 105, 127, 136, 245, 253, 256, 265, 266, 272, 274, 275, 277, 278, 279
mental representation, 140, 145, 158
mental representations, 138, 145, 158
mentalization based therapy, 116
mentalization-based treatment (MBT), 9, 16, 96, 98, 113, 122, 270
Merza, Papp, & Szabó, 258, 259
meta-analyses, 96, 124, 126, 205, 208, 210, 219
meta-analysis, 42, 47, 51, 58, 61, 62, 68, 86, 87, 88, 89, 168, 199, 200, 243, 250, 258, 263, 265, 276, 277
metabolic rates, 77
meta-cognitive training, 104
metaphor, 156, 216, 217, 232
middle/superior temporal gyrus, 72
military sexual trauma-related PTSD, 105
Miller & Hubble, 206
Miller & Kaiser, 242
Miller, Hubble, & Duncan, 206
Miller, Scott, 218, 223
Millon et al., 2
mindful preparation, 196, 198
mindfulness, 9, 107, 177, 178, 179, 194, 196, 198, 200, 237
mindfulness skills, 178, 179
Minzenberg, Fan, New, Tang, & Siever, 70
mirroring, 151, 153
Mistry, Escott-Price, Florio, Smith, & Zammit, 42
Mitchell & Black, 2, 4
Mizen, 11, 17, 273
models, vii, viii, ix, 8, 15, 37, 57, 58, 66, 94, 95, 117, 121, 134, 135, 137, 138, 142, 144, 159, 169, 188, 197, 206, 215, 221, 228, 236, 239, 267, 281, 282
molecular genetic research, 65, 74, 257
Molecular Genetic Research in BPD, 74, 257
molecular genetics, 256

monoamine oxidase inhibitors (MAOIs), 118
mood change, 119
mood disorder, 43, 44, 89
mood instability, 20, 28
mood stabilizers, 118
mood stabilizing medication, 242
mood swings, 2, 43, 44
Morey & Skodol, 27
mother-father-infant bonding, 142
mother-infant dyad, 142
motivation, 10, 68, 152, 153, 188
motor inhibitory control, 75
movement control, 73
MRI techniques, 67, 78
MSAD study, 48, 50
multi-axial diagnostic system, 5
multiple factors, 66, 259

N

narcissistic personality disorder, 7, 11, 30, 45
National Institute for Clinical Excellence (NICE), 116
Native American and Alaskan Native clients, 107
natural consequence, 174
Navarro-Haro et al., 107
Neacsiu, Lungu, Harned, Rizvi, & Linehan, 107, 181, 261
Neacsiu, Ward-Ciesielski, & Linehan, 106, 178
need of restraints, 170
negative affect, 34, 39, 41
negative clinician assumptions, 250
negative clinician attributions, 243
negative consequences, 176, 186, 244
negative countertransference, 251, 254
negative effect on the therapist, 223
negative emotions, 71, 180
negative experiences, 255
negative outcomes, 28
negative self-concept, 242, 254, 258
negative self-reference, 28
negative social interactions, 70
neglect, 39, 114, 246, 258, 259, 274
Nenadic et al., 104
Nenadic, Lamberth, and Reiss, 104
Neofreudian, 139
neurobiological alterations, 66
neurobiological correlates, 65, 261
neurobiological underpinnings of BPD, 66, 78, 260
neurobiology, 42, 58, 83, 87, 275
neurocognitive deficits, 69
neuroimaging, 65, 67, 76, 77, 78, 79, 80, 84, 85, 88, 89, 90, 131, 203, 256, 258, 270, 276, 277
neuroimaging in BPD, 67
neuroimaging studies, 65, 67, 76, 77, 78, 79, 80, 88, 89, 90, 258
neuroimaging, borderline personality disorder, genetic and molecular genetic research, 65
neurological causes, 79
neurological correlates, viii, 79
neuron-specific enzyme, 74
neuropathology of BPD, 80
neuropsychological deficits, 258
neuroscience, 15, 46, 47, 81, 268
neuroses, 2, 3, 17, 18, 61, 89, 131, 162, 215
neurosis, 2, 3, 4, 5, 7, 12, 22, 66
neurotic, 2, 3, 5, 6, 7, 12, 146, 147, 148, 149
neurotic ego defenses, 3
neurotic level of organization, 148
neurotic symptoms, 3, 6
neurotic-borderline-psychotic (NBP), 146, 148
neuroticism, 7, 13, 14, 28, 266
neurotic-psychotic continuum, 147
neurotransmission, 61, 74
neurotransmitter, 67, 257

neurotransmitter receptor polymorphism, 257
New et al., 72
Niedtfeld et al, 70, 73
nine diagnostic features, 30
Nock, 73, 86
Nokar et al., 35
non-sedating anxiolytic medication, 120
non-suicidal self-injury (NSSI), 35, 61, 72, 73, 90, 109, 114, 115, 119, 122, 164, 168, 170, 186, 187, 188, 196, 242
numbness, 21
Nunes, Wenzel, Borges, Porto, Caminha, de Oliveira, 68
nurses, 250, 251
nursing, 251, 267

O

obesity, 247, 277
object constancy phase, 142
object relations, v, vii, 1, 5, 6, 8, 56, 133, 134, 139, 140, 141, 142, 143, 144, 145, 146, 151, 153, 154, 155, 156, 158, 159, 160, 161, 281
object relations theory, v, 1, 8, 56, 133, 134, 139, 141, 142, 143, 144, 151, 153, 159, 160, 161
objective reality, 144
observable behavior, 13
observed behavior, 39
observing ego, 136, 145, 149, 151, 152, 156, 158
Ochsner & Gross, 67
Ochsner, Bunge, Gross, & Gabrieli, 79
Ociskova et al., 252
Ogata et al., 259
Ogata, Silk, Goodrich, Lohr, & Hill, 258
Okiishi et al., 209
Oldham et al., 259
Oldham, Skodol, Gallaher, & Kroll, 258
omega-3 fatty acids, 121
omnipotent control, 149, 156, 157, 158
online support groups, 255
onset during early adulthood, 108
opioid antagonists, 121
opportunities, 167, 195, 227, 232, 244, 245, 254
optimism, 3, 203, 230, 261
oral, 138
orbital frontal insula, 71
orbitofrontal cortex (OFC), 68, 71, 72, 83
organize, 138, 147, 149, 150, 151, 154
Ormont, Hunt, & Corman, 136
ortibofrontal cortex, 68
Otilingam & Graiales, 253
Otto Kernberg, 5, 6, 99, 142, 147
outcome research, 13, 95, 121, 159, 206, 210, 211, 213
outpatient, 27, 54, 94, 104, 110, 113, 132, 168, 177, 192, 193, 243
outpatient clinics, 168, 243
outside of cultural and societal expectations, 108
overlap, 25, 45, 150, 258, 259, 261
overlap with CPTSD, 261
overrepresentation of women, 20
oxytocin, 121

P

Packard & Knowlton, 73
Pagura et al., 258
pain, 21, 26, 33, 35, 38, 39, 41, 60, 86, 89, 116, 137, 179, 185, 187, 190, 222, 277
panic attacks, 193, 250
panic disorder, 53
panic symptoms, 193
Paolini et al., 116, 118, 119, 120
Paolini, Mezzetti, Pierri, & Moretti, 116
paradigm, 206, 235
parahippocampal gyri, 72

parahippocampus gyrus, 72
para-limbic, 73
paranoid ideation, 44, 45
parasuicidal behavior, 107
Parcesepe & Cabassa, 245
parent-infant dyad, 141
parenting, 9, 10, 100, 142
parents, 6, 33, 39, 182
parietal lobe, 71
Paris & Zweig-Frank, 36, 44
part object, 151
part other/object, 141
part self, 151
partial hospitalization programming (PHP), 110, 113, 114
participants, 49, 71, 79, 102, 103, 104, 105, 111, 113, 116, 117, 119, 177, 181
part-self, 143
Pascual et al., 105
pathology, 15, 57, 58, 96, 127, 128, 139, 143, 148, 227, 232, 259, 268
patient comorbidity, 116
patient self-report, 27
patient-centered decision-making model, 117
patient-clinician relationship, 115
patriarchal perspective, 7
patterns of neural activation, 77
Pennay et al., 168
perceived slights and insults, 29
perceptual distortions, 69
perfect agent model, 117
perpetrators of domestic violence, 169
personal accomplishment, 33
personal development, 40
personal life, 177
personal relations, 114
personal relationship, 114
personality, viii, 1, 5, 6, 7, 8, 9, 10, 11, 14, 15, 16, 17, 19, 20, 21, 22, 24, 26, 27, 28, 29, 30, 33, 35, 38, 40, 42, 44, 45, 46, 47, 48, 50, 51, 52, 53, 54, 55, 56, 57, 58, 59, 60, 61, 62, 63, 69, 71, 81, 83, 85, 87, 90, 91, 94, 98, 99, 100, 102, 104, 105, 106, 108, 114, 124, 125, 126, 127, 128, 129, 130, 131, 134, 136, 138, 139, 143, 146, 147, 148, 149, 153, 157, 160, 161, 164, 185, 198, 199, 201, 222, 226, 228, 242, 247, 250, 252, 262, 263, 264, 265, 266, 267, 268, 269, 271, 272, 273, 274, 275, 276, 277, 279
personality disintegration, 28, 30
personality disorder (PD), vii, viii, ix, 2, 4, 5, 7, 8, 10, 11, 14, 15, 16, 17, 19, 20, 22, 25, 26, 27, 29, 40, 42, 45, 47, 48, 50, 52, 53, 54, 55, 56, 57, 58, 59, 60, 61, 62, 63, 66, 69, 70, 71, 75, 80, 83, 86, 91, 94, 98, 99, 101, 102, 104, 105, 106, 108, 114, 122, 124, 125, 129, 130, 131, 133, 134, 143, 148, 157, 164, 179, 198, 201, 204, 205, 206, 218, 222, 226, 229, 242, 247, 248, 250, 251, 252, 255, 258, 263, 264, 266, 269, 271, 272, 273, 275, 276, 277, 281
personality factors, 27
personality inventories, 27
personality inventory for DSM-5 (PID-5), 27, 54
personality structure, 1, 38, 136, 161
personality traits, 9, 26, 27, 28, 29, 46, 50, 62, 81
person-centered orientations, 111
phallic, 138
pharmacological intervention, 27
pharmacological treatment, 79, 80, 116, 130
pharmacological treatment for BPD, 80
phenotypes for BPD, 26
Phillips & LeDoux, 69, 256
Phillips, Drevets, Rauch, & Lane, 67
phone coaching, 169, 171, 176, 183, 184, 187, 195, 197
phone coaching call, 184
PHP/IOP, 110, 113
physical abuse, 39, 41, 56, 246, 274

physical health, 164, 241, 242
physical health issues, 164, 242
physical inactivity, 246
physical mobility, 142
physician empathy, 116
physicians, 269
physiological arousal, 36
Pier, Marin, Wilsnack, & Goodman, 67, 68, 71, 73, 74, 77, 257
pilot study, 104, 129, 274
placebo, 119, 211, 220
placebologists, 212
polypharmacy, 116
polysubstance abuse, 34
polythetic categorical system, 26
polythetic diagnostic nomenclature, 23
polythetic diagnostic system, 21
polythetic system, 24
Pompili, Girardi, Roberto, & Tatarelli, 20
Pompili, Girardi, Ruberto, & Ruberto, 20
poor BPD treatment outcomes, 243
poor community understanding, 245
poor impulse controls, 29
population, 20, 25, 33, 36, 47, 67, 69, 70, 77, 79, 104, 109, 111, 112, 113, 114, 115, 117, 119, 164, 244, 246, 268, 269, 274, 277, 280
population prevalence, 114
Porter et al., 258
portico-cortical (superior longitudinal fasciculus), 69
portico-subcortical bundles, 69
positive attitudes, 260
positive emotions, 181
positive hit rate, 24
positron emission tomography, 67
post traumatic stress disorder, 80, 88
posterior cingulate cortex, 71
postmodernism, 215
posttraumatic stress, 42, 120, 126, 127, 164, 168, 269, 274
post-traumatic stress disorder (PTSD), 67, 69, 76, 85, 104, 201, 219, 242, 256, 257, 258, 260, 269, 272, 275, 279
potential overdose, 120
potentially self-damaging, 12, 33
preconscious, 136, 137
precuneus, 73
predictors of BPD, 256
prefrontal cortex, 46, 68, 70, 71, 72, 73, 75, 82, 88, 90
prejudgment, 244
prejudice, 242, 244, 250, 254, 266
preparation, iv, 36, 198
prevalence of BPD, 20, 73, 243, 247, 256
prevalence rate, 35, 40, 47, 249, 256
prevalence rate of BPD in family members, 256
prevalence rates, 47
preverbal ideas, 137
primitive defense mechanisms, 99, 149, 150, 158
primitive defenses, 149, 150, 154, 156
primitive ego defenses, 5
primitive idealization, 149, 150, 156, 157, 158
principles, 101, 151, 153, 159, 160, 232
Prochaska, Norcross, & DiClemente, 152
prodromal, 20, 46
prognosis, 11, 18, 48, 105, 162, 165, 217, 225, 226, 278
projection, 22, 115, 149, 157
projective identification, 5, 149, 150, 156, 157, 158
promiscuity, 178
promoting hope for change, 152
pseudoneurotic schizophrenia, 147
pseudoscience, 219, 220
psyche, 3, 134, 135, 136, 138, 139, 141, 145, 146, 147, 149, 150, 225
psychiatric conditions, 37, 78
psychiatric crisis services, 168
psychiatric diagnosis, 60, 94, 250

psychiatric disorder, 77, 78, 79, 105, 111, 117
psychiatric disorders, 79, 105, 117
psychiatric hospital settings, 108
psychiatric hospitalization, 168, 243, 255
psychiatric hospitals, 109, 110, 243
psychiatric nurses, 250, 251
psychiatric symptom, 109, 253
psychiatric treatment centers, 99
psychiatrists, 110, 147, 249, 250, 251, 271, 272, 275, 277
psychiatry, 18, 23, 126, 161, 162, 202
psychoactive medications, 243, 281
psychoanalytic, vii, 2, 3, 5, 7, 8, 11, 13, 14, 17, 18, 21, 22, 23, 56, 61, 89, 127, 131, 133, 134, 135, 148, 159, 160, 161, 162, 273
psychoanalytic theoreticians, 23
psychoanalytic theory, 7, 11, 22, 133, 134, 135
psychoanalytically oriented psychotherapy, 99
psychodynamic, 2, 5, 8, 10, 16, 111, 134, 160, 161, 168, 170, 218, 221, 231, 270
psychodynamic perspective, 134
psychodynamic treatment models, 221
psychoeducational intervention, 106
psychoeducational interventions, 106
psychoendocrinological, 258
psychogenic, 4
psychogenic origin, 4
psychological birth, 17, 142
psychological borderland, 147
psychological distress, 103, 278
psychological problems, 96
psychological stress, 179
psychological well-being, 272
psychologists, 17, 97, 130, 207, 220, 250, 251, 260, 266
psychology, viii, ix, 1, 2, 3, 4, 7, 8, 134, 136, 160, 179, 194, 207, 215, 237, 262
psychometric properties, 275
psychopathology, 8, 15, 55, 83, 94, 148, 215, 221, 222, 223, 232
psychopharmacological interventions, 100
psychopharmacological treatment, 114, 115
psychopharmacology, 81, 94, 114, 115, 121, 126, 128
psychoses, 2, 3, 4, 6
psychosexual, 138, 139, 141
psychosexual development, 139
psychosexual stages, 138
psychosis, 2, 3, 4, 7, 12, 22, 23, 40, 66, 105, 109, 119, 149, 245
psychosocial functioning, 50, 106, 130
psychosocial stress, 66
psychotherapists, xi, 94, 209, 212, 214, 223, 251
psychotherapy, vii, 14, 15, 16, 17, 18, 31, 65, 75, 85, 96, 99, 101, 113, 116, 117, 120, 121, 122, 125, 126, 127, 128, 129, 131, 132, 134, 143, 151, 159, 160, 161, 162, 168, 197, 198, 200, 202, 204, 205, 206, 207, 208, 209, 210, 211, 212, 214, 215, 216, 218, 219, 221, 223, 226, 228, 233, 236, 237, 238, 239, 263, 267, 270, 273, 278, 280
psychotic, 2, 3, 5, 6, 7, 12, 22, 40, 146, 147, 148, 149, 150, 192, 269
psychotic level, 146, 149
psychotic symptoms, 41
psychotropic medication, 72, 77, 116, 243
psychotropic medications, 77, 117, 243
public awareness of BPD, 247
public health, 95
public stigma, 244, 245, 265, 274
putamen, 71, 73

Q

quality of life, 119, 121, 172, 186, 253
quasi-psychotic cognitions, 49
Quattrini et al., 69, 180

R

Racker, Henirich, 145
radical acceptance, 9, 179
radical acceptance of life, 179
rage, 20
randomized clinical study, 102
randomized controlled trials, 105, 125, 168
rapprochement phase, 142
rate of completed suicide, 36
rate of suicid, 20, 35
Rathus & Miller, 169, 183
rational affective theory, 11
reactions, 4, 8, 22, 28, 43, 145, 166, 180, 182, 251, 254
reactivity, 2, 12, 36, 72, 166, 180, 201
reading, 41, 176, 180, 215
reality, 5, 6, 7, 22, 40, 41, 44, 69, 97, 99, 135, 137, 138, 144, 146, 147, 148, 149, 150, 153, 154, 179, 185, 209, 213, 215, 216, 217, 220, 222, 224, 225, 226, 230, 232, 235, 236, 238
reality testing, 6, 22, 41, 148, 153
reasoning, 32, 46, 112, 137
reckless driving, 12, 33, 34
recognition, 8, 10, 11, 37, 54, 57, 235, 244
recommendations, iv, 66, 116, 126, 279
recovery, 48, 62, 63, 106, 132, 253, 268, 280
reduced cingulate gray matter, 69
reduced gray matter concentration, 68
refusal to treat people with BPD, 250
regressions and countertransference, 49
regular treatment attendance, 112
regulation of impulses and emotions, 68
rehabilitation, 105, 106, 130
Reich & Stone, 5
rejection, 7, 30, 32, 38, 43, 44, 45, 70, 109, 115, 155, 181, 195, 252, 271, 272
relapse rates, 49
relationship tolerance, 113
reliability, 23, 25, 27, 60
reliability coefficients, 23, 25
relief, 35, 47, 118, 119, 121, 156, 181, 182, 187
remission, 42, 48, 49, 50, 62, 106, 132, 170, 256, 261, 280
re-parenting, 100
repeated hospitalizations, 36
representation, 140, 157
researchers, 26, 44, 46, 70, 98, 100, 106, 107, 110, 113, 181, 211
residential treatment, 75, 124, 243, 272
resistance, 3, 124, 255
resistance to psychotherapists, 255
resistance to seeking treatment, 255
resolution, 30, 182, 261
resources, 100, 112, 147, 242, 247
response, 7, 10, 13, 29, 37, 39, 68, 72, 75, 80, 84, 86, 105, 127, 156, 157, 174, 177, 178, 179, 180, 210, 229, 251, 262
response inhibition, 68, 75, 80, 262
responsibility, iv, 3, 113
retrospective, 27, 40, 47, 130, 246, 249
retrospective self-reports, 246
retrospective study, 40, 47, 249
rewards, 61, 68, 88, 229, 248
right amygdala, 72
right middle temporal cortex, 71
right parahippocampal gyrus, 72
risk, vii, 9, 10, 21, 26, 27, 28, 29, 30, 34, 35, 36, 37, 42, 46, 47, 50, 55, 56, 59, 61, 63, 66, 114, 119, 136, 163, 164, 165, 170, 178, 189, 190, 192, 193, 194, 196, 202, 243, 246, 263, 277
risk assessment, 164, 170, 189, 190, 194, 196
risk factors, 9, 27, 35, 42, 47, 56, 66, 192, 263
risk for pregnancy, 119
risk-taking, 26, 34, 36, 55, 61, 178
risk-taking behavior, 29, 36, 178
risk-taking in sexual encounters, 34

risky behaviors, 178
Ritsher & Phelan, 253
Ritsher & Rosenfield, 253
Rizvi, Steffle, & Carson-Wong, 106
Rosell & Siever, 72
Rosenfeld et al., 169
ruminative thoughts, 41
Ruocco et al., 75
Ruocco, Amirthavasagam, & Zakzanis, 74, 256
Ruocco, Amirthavasagam, Choi-Kain, & McMain, 71
Rüsch et al., 253
Rusch, Guastello, and Mason, 25

S

safety, 31, 34, 35, 97, 108, 109, 114, 115, 117, 119, 121, 140, 142, 171, 173, 174, 183, 184, 189, 191, 192, 196
salience network, 71
Salzman et al., 259
Sanislow et al., 25
Sansone & Sansone, 247, 249, 251, 252, 253
Sansone, Levitt & Sansone, 247
Sarhan, et al., 35
Sauer-Zavala, Bentley, & Wilner, 242
schema, 104, 125, 126, 129, 132
schema cognitive behavioral group therapy (SCBT-g), 104
schema therapy institute, 100
schema-focused therapy (SFT), 100
schemas, 95, 101, 132
Schilling, Moritz, Kriston, Krieger, and Nagel, 104
schizophrenia, 5, 23, 60, 82, 114, 119, 147, 160, 268
schizophrenic patients, 251
schizotypal personality disorder, 22, 45, 69
Schmahl & Bremner, 77
Schmahl et al, 68, 69, 76, 77, 78
Schmahl, Vermetten, Elzinga, & Bremner, 68
Schomerus et al., 245
school, 32, 194, 209, 210, 226, 228, 233, 245
Schore, 226, 238
Schulze et al., 70
science, 10, 83, 216, 238
scratching, 186, 187
second generation antidepressants, 118
second generation antipsychotics, 119
secondary education, 246
Seidler & Wagner, 219
Selby, Anestis and Joiner, 13
selective serotine reuptake inhibitors (SSRIs), 118
self, viii, 5, 6, 7, 10, 11, 12, 16, 21, 25, 26, 27, 28, 29, 30, 31, 32, 33, 34, 35, 36, 38, 39, 40, 41, 42, 44, 45, 46, 50, 52, 53, 55, 56, 58, 66, 70, 71, 73, 75, 86, 88, 95, 97, 101, 102, 103, 105, 108, 109, 110, 113, 114, 117, 120, 136, 138, 139, 140, 141,143, 146, 149, 150, 151, 152, 153, 156, 157, 158, 160, 161, 164, 167, 168, 169, 171, 173, 174, 176, 178, 179, 180, 181, 182, 184, 186, 187, 188, 193, 195, 196, 197, 198, 200, 201, 202, 204, 216, 222, 224, 227, 228, 231, 234, 237, 241, 242, 243, 244, 246, 247, 251, 252, 253, 254, 255, 259, 260, 261, 264, 265, 268, 273, 274, 276, 279
self exists between people, 231
self-applied stereotypes, 254
self-concept, 242, 254, 258
self-control, 97, 120
self-destructive, 25, 33, 35, 70, 101, 228, 231, 251, 254, 255
self-destructive behavior, 33, 70, 101, 231, 255
self-destructive behaviors, 33, 70, 101, 231, 255

self-directed behaviors, 34
self-directed violence, 168
self-disgust, 254
self-disorders, 6
self-efficacy, 117, 253, 254
self-enhancement, 254
self-esteem, 188, 253, 254
self-evaluations, 279
self-fulfilling prophecy, 243, 251, 252
self-harm, 25, 29, 34, 36, 53, 66, 70, 73, 75, 88, 103, 109, 110, 113, 114, 167, 168, 169, 171, 173, 174, 176, 179, 184, 187, 197, 202, 224, 243, 246, 252
self-harm behavior, 34, 75, 109, 110, 170, 171, 174, 184
self-harming behavior, 66, 70, 73, 109, 114, 202
self-help groups, 243
self-help literature, 248
self-identify, 244
self-identity, 28, 33, 38, 50
self-image, 12, 28, 30, 32, 34, 40, 43, 45, 66, 108, 109, 113, 178, 241, 246
self-injurious behavior, 55, 58, 186, 200, 246
self-injury, 21, 35, 52, 56, 86, 170, 184
self-interactions, 6
self-mutilating behavior, 12, 33, 35
self-mutilation, 25, 26, 50, 102
self-object, 6
self-organization, 258
self-other/object confusion, 140
self-psychologist, 5
self-referential processing, 73
self-reflect, 136, 151
self-reflective, 136
self-regulation, 120
self-report measures, 27, 259
self-reported physical health, 105
self-reports, 246
self-representation, 140
self-soothe, 180
self-stigma, 244, 253, 254, 255, 260, 261, 265, 268, 274, 276, 279
self-verification, 254
self-worth, 29, 30, 32, 45
sensitivity, 23, 24, 28, 30, 38, 41, 45, 166
separation and individuation, 31, 142, 145
separation insecurity, 28
separation-individuation theory, 142
serotonin, 74, 118, 257
serotonin metabolism, 257
serotonin synthesis, 74
serotonin-norepinephrine reuptake inhibitors (SNRIs), 118
Sescousse, Caldu, Segura, & Dreher, 68
setting boundaries, 181
severe dissociative symptoms, 25, 44
severe mental illness (SMI), 105, 127
sexual abuse, 41, 42, 52, 259
sexual activity, 119
sexual development, 10
sexual identity, 233
Shah & Zanarini, 33
shame, 173, 242, 254, 255
shamed child, 145
shared decision-making model, 117
Sharp et al., 47
Sharp, Vanwoerdden, & Wall, 47
Sheehan, Nieweglowski, & Corrigan, 164, 243
Shin, Goldstein, & Pick, 41
showing, 49, 111, 230, 259
side effects that affect motor control, 119
Sisti et al., 251
Sisti, Segal, Siegel, Johnson, & Gunderson, 254
skill acquisition, 208
skills group, 169, 171, 176, 177, 182, 183
skills training, 98, 107, 128, 131, 164, 169, 177, 185, 192, 197, 202, 264
Skodol et al., 26
Skoglund et al., 257
Sloan, Berke, & Shipherd, 107

Slotema et al., 105
slower return to baseline in amygdala activation, 71
Soares & Mann, 76
social adjustment, 221
social change, 265
social construct, 205, 206, 234, 237
social constructionism, 206, 222, 236
social control, 215
social disapproval, 70
social distance, 260
social environment, 9
social group, 30, 32, 214
social interaction, 44, 70
social justice, 199
social life, 222
social perception, 9
social phobia, 53, 253, 276
social psychology, 4, 265, 266, 272
social relations, 227
social relationships, 227
social situations, 32, 70, 179, 223
social skills, 227, 229
social stigmatization, 242
social support, 115
social workers, 250, 251
society, 2, 136, 255
soft bipolarity, 44
Soloff et al., 69, 70, 76
Soloff, Nutche, Goradia, & Diwadkar, 68
Soloff, White, Omari, Ramaseshan, & Diwadkar, 260
solution, 176, 182, 183, 191
solution analysis, 176, 191
somatogenic, 4
Sosic-Vasic et al., 70, 256
specialized psychotherapeutic treatment (OPT), 113
specialized psychotherapy, 116
specific factors, 210, 211, 218, 233, 235
specificity, 23, 25, 27
spending, 12, 33, 34, 108, 121, 178
spending more time in therapy, 108, 121
Spitzer & Fleiss, 23
Spitzer et al., 23
Spitzer, Endicott, & Gibbon, 22
splitting, 5, 6, 10, 149, 150, 153, 156, 157, 158, 182
splitting mechanism, 150
stability, 31, 62, 113, 120, 132, 138, 150, 220, 222, 224, 280
stability of self-image, 113
stable self-representations, 151
stalkers, 249, 273
stalking, 203, 248, 269, 272, 276
standard DBT, 168, 169, 171, 177, 183, 184, 197
Stanfield et al., 78
Steele & Siever, 66
Steffens et al., 77
Steinberg & Morris, 46
Stephan et al., 116, 117
Stephan, Krawitz, & Jackson, 116
Stepp, Keenan, Hipwell, & Krueger, 20
stereotypes, 244, 252, 253, 254, 274
stereotyping, 242, 243, 244, 250
stigma, vi, 164, 166, 204, 241, 242, 243, 244, 245, 246, 247, 248, 252, 253, 254, 255, 257, 259, 260, 261, 264, 265, 266, 267, 268, 270, 272, 273, 274, 275, 276, 277, 278, 279
stigmatization, viii, 242, 246, 252
stigmatized, 242, 245, 253
stigmatizing, 47, 243, 244, 248, 249, 250, 252, 254
stigmatizing diagnosis, 254
stigmatizing practices, 252
Stoffers & Lieb, 117, 121
Stoffers et al., 168
Stoffers, Rucker, Timmer, Huband, and Lieb, 221
strengthening healthy relationships, 181
stress, 12, 25, 26, 28, 29, 40, 67, 70, 72, 193, 194, 196, 222, 242, 246, 256, 257

stressful events, 41, 70
stressors, 39, 66, 114, 151, 192, 194
stress-related paranoid ideation, 26
striatal, 46
structural alterations in BPD, 68
structural and functional changes, 75
structural and functional differences, 76
structural and functional neurological differences, 79, 281
structural changes, 100
structural differences, 69
structural or functional differences, 76
structured clinical management (SCM), 99
structured treatment protocol, 115
Strupp and Hadley, 207
Stull, McGrew, Salyers, & Ashburn-Nardo, 242
subjective experience, 38, 145
submission or domination, 34
suboptimal dopaminergic receptors, 74
substance abuse, 12, 33, 164, 168, 172, 203, 242
substance abuse/dependence, 164, 242
substance use, 81, 90, 111, 112, 122, 123, 179, 201, 203, 246, 264
substance use disorder, 81, 90, 111, 112, 123, 203, 264
substance/alcohol use disorders, 117
suicidal, 11, 12, 29, 33, 35, 44, 52, 70, 74, 89, 102, 103, 106, 109, 111, 112, 120, 122, 125, 128, 164, 169, 184, 186, 187, 188, 191, 192, 193, 196, 199, 200, 201, 202, 203, 224, 242, 250, 251, 254, 255, 257, 259, 261, 273
suicidal behavior, 12, 35, 44, 52, 70, 74, 89, 103, 109, 112, 120, 188, 202, 224, 257, 259, 261, 273
suicidal behavior, gestures, or threats, or self-mutilating behavior, 12, 35
suicidal ideation, 29, 106, 111, 169, 186, 188, 196, 255
suicidal ideation, intent and plan, 29
suicidal or homicidal behaviors, 109
suicidal thoughts and behavior, 109
suicidal threats, 188, 193
suicidal urges, 192, 193, 250
suicidality, 26, 35, 58, 66, 114, 115, 119, 120, 168, 188, 221, 259
suicide attempt, 49, 50, 90, 113, 170, 184, 185, 186
suicide attempters, 69, 90
suicide attempts, 49, 113, 170, 186
suicide rate, 109
suicide risk assessment and management, 170
suicide risk assessments, 196
Sulzer et al., 251
Sulzer, Muenchow, Potvin, Harris, & Gigot, 255
superego, 135, 136, 144, 216
supervision, 165, 206, 237, 252
support groups, 11, 248
suppressing emotions, 181
suspicious and paranoid ideation, 41
Swenson and Choi-Kain, 9
symptom overlap, 258
symptom reduction, 11, 34, 48, 95, 103, 106, 115, 170, 197, 261, 282
symptom remission, 48, 49, 50, 62, 256, 261
symptom specificity, 27
symptomology, 5, 34, 47, 110, 113, 115
symptoms, 1, 2, 3, 4, 5, 6, 7, 8, 9, 11, 12, 13, 15, 20, 21, 22, 23, 24, 25, 26, 27, 29, 33, 34, 40, 42, 43, 44, 45, 46, 47, 48, 49, 50, 55, 60, 61, 62, 69, 74, 77, 79, 81, 98, 99, 101, 102, 103, 104, 105, 107, 108, 109, 110, 111, 112, 113, 115, 116, 117, 118, 120, 121, 168, 169, 185, 192, 193, 200, 204, 212, 213, 215, 216, 223, 226, 242, 243, 244, 245, 249, 253, 258, 259, 260, 261, 264, 267, 269, 272, 273, 274, 279, 281
syndrome, 18, 22, 23, 55, 147, 160, 162, 276, 278

systematic meta-analysis, 243
systems of consciousness, 136
systems training for emotional predictability and problem solving (STEPPS), 98, 123

T

target, 167, 171, 172, 173, 174, 176, 193, 229, 248
target behavior, 167, 173, 174
Taylor et al., 35
Tebbett-Mock, Saito, McGee, Woloszyn, & Venuti, 170, 261
technique bias, 231
technique-centric, 206
techniques, 9, 21, 67, 78, 95, 100, 104, 106, 206, 210, 211, 212, 213, 214, 217, 218, 220, 221, 223, 230, 231, 232, 233, 235, 236, 256, 260
techniques lack inherent power, 206, 213, 231
telephone, 107, 123, 127, 128, 183, 195
telephone skills coaching, 183
television, 190, 247, 250, 262, 268, 274, 278
Temes & Zanarini, 50, 261
testing, 6, 9, 22, 27, 41, 99, 148, 153, 220
theories of psychotherapy, 206
theory of mind, 15, 267
therapeutic change, 156, 160
therapeutic interventions, 75, 79
therapeutic process, 155
therapeutic relationship, 144, 158, 163, 165, 172, 173, 192, 195, 198, 212, 255, 260
therapeutics, 264
therapist, vii, 11, 31, 98, 99, 100, 143, 152, 155, 156, 165, 170, 176, 177, 183, 184, 185, 187, 188, 189, 190, 194, 195, 197, 206, 208, 209, 210, 212, 217, 222, 223, 224, 225, 226, 227, 228, 229, 230, 231, 232, 233, 252, 254, 281
therapy, 6, 18, 61, 82, 89, 95, 96, 97, 98, 99, 100, 102, 103, 104, 105, 106, 107, 108, 110, 112, 116, 121, 123, 125, 126, 127, 129, 131, 132, 154, 159, 162, 168, 169, 171, 172, 177, 183, 185, 187, 191, 194, 200, 201, 204, 206, 209, 210, 211, 214, 216, 224, 225, 227, 228, 229, 230, 231, 232, 237, 238, 239, 243, 282
therapy for the therapist, 185, 194
therapy-interfering behaviors, 172, 185, 194
thoughts, 22, 30, 34, 39, 40, 41, 42, 44, 96, 109, 139, 152, 166, 174, 176, 178, 185, 188
THP2 haplotype, 74
THP2 isoform genotype, 74
threatening behavior, 170, 171, 174, 182
threats, 12, 21, 27, 28, 35, 41, 164, 171, 172, 182, 188, 192, 193, 242
three clusters of impaired thought processes, 40
topographic model, 135, 136
Torgersen, Kringlen, & Cramer, 20
training, 95, 97, 98, 104, 121, 123, 130, 165, 169, 194, 206, 207, 208, 211, 213, 214, 226, 236, 237, 244, 247, 252, 253, 260, 261
training effect, 207, 211, 213
training programs, 207
traits, 9, 15, 27, 28, 47, 72, 73, 81, 164, 264, 267
transference, 99, 100, 126, 145, 148, 161
transference-countertransference relationship, 145
transference-focused psychotherapy (TFP), 99, 101, 218, 221
transgender clients, 107
transient psychotic organization, 150
transient, stress-related paranoid ideation or severe dissociative symptoms, 12, 25, 40
transition, 4, 110, 114
transport genes, 74

trauma, viii, ix, 4, 8, 10, 15, 42, 61, 66, 77, 83, 85, 90, 97, 105, 120, 126, 160, 165, 193, 200, 218, 219, 231, 244, 255, 259, 262, 267, 268, 281
trauma-related disorders, 77
traumatic childhood, 101, 225
traumatic childhood experiences, 101
traumatic events, 76
traumatic events in childhood, 76
traumatic experiences, 42, 257
treating borderline personality disorder, 102, 223
treatment as usual (TAU), 98, 102, 103, 104, 105, 107, 168, 170, 204, 221, 278
treatment compliance, 111, 112
treatment decisions, 117
treatment drop out, 107
treatment effectiveness, 115
treatment methods, xi, 215
treatment options, 164
treatment outcome, 88, 115, 117, 122, 131, 208, 243, 260, 261
treatment protocol, 115, 117
treatment resistant, 21, 48, 115, 251
treatment team, 115
trial, 98, 102, 103, 106, 107, 123, 125, 126, 130, 200, 202, 204, 236, 264
tricyclic antidepressants (TCA), 118
trigger emotions, 39
triggers, 138, 174, 186, 192
Trull, Stepp, & Durrett, 20
tryptophan hydroxylase, 74
tryptophan hydroxylase 2 (TPH2), 74
turbulent relationships, 49
twin studies, 73
two worlds example, 213
two-factor model of BPD symptom clusters, 26
typical antipsychotics, 119

U

unconscious, 3, 4, 14, 15, 135, 136, 137, 139, 144, 145, 149, 152, 155, 157, 159, 242
unconscious drives, 136
unconscious ego defenses, 3
unconscious experience, 135, 136, 145
uncontrollable emotions, 181
uncus, 68, 256
unintegrated, 6, 143, 144
unintegrated ego states, 144
unpredictability, 25
unprotected sexual activity, 119
unreification, 223
unstable interpersonal relationships, 25
unstable patterns, 109
unstable patterns of interpersonal relationships, 109
unstable reality testing, 99
unstable relationships, 26, 30, 32, 44, 258
unstable self-image, 12, 32, 43, 109
unstable self-image or sense of self, 12, 32
unstable sense of self, 8
unstable, intense interpersonal relationships, 8
untreatable client, 164
urethral, 138
urges to harm others, 171

V

Valera, Faraone, Murray, & Seidman, 78
validation strategies, 166
Van Duijvenvoorde, Peters, & Braams, 47
Van Vreeswiik, Spinhoven, Eurelings-Bontekoe, and Broersen, 104
Vega et al., 72
ventral amygdala, 72
ventral cingulate gyrus, 68
victims, 42, 250, 273

violence, 42, 87, 168, 268
vision, 215, 226, 234
vlogs, 255
vocation, 245, 254
vocational barriers, 246
vocational support, 246
volatility component, 25
volumetric and functional differences, 76
volumetric decreases, 74
vulnerability, 9, 30, 31, 33, 39, 174, 176, 180, 194, 266
vulnerability factors, 174, 176
Vythilingam et al., 77

W

Wahlstrom et al., 47
Wahlstrom, Collins, White, & Luciana, 46
Wall & Messier, 70
Wampold & Imel, 207, 219, 220
Wampold and Brown, 209
Watson, Corrigan, Larson, & Sells, 253
weekly log, 172
western culture, 215, 216, 223
whole other/object, 141, 153
Widiger et al., 27
Widiger, Crego, Rojas, & Oltmanns, 27
Williams & Broadbent, 70
Williams, Hartstone, & Denson, 168
Wingenfeld, Spitzer, Rullkotter, & Lowe, 68
Wingenfled et al., 66
Winnicott, 142, 145, 162
Winsper et al., 46
Winter, Bohus, & Lis, 254
withhold the diagnosis, 254
Wolf et al., 71
work environment, 229
working memory, 82, 84
workplace, 20
workplace environment, 20
Wright, Hopwood, & Zanarini, 27, 45

Y

Yalom & Leszcz, 216
Yalom, Irving, 216
Young, Jeffrey, 100

Z

Zanarini et al., 35, 40, 47, 48, 259
Zanarini, Frankenburg, Khera, & Bleichmar, 243, 258
Zanarini, Frankenburg, Reich, & Fitzmaurice, 48, 109, 260
Zanarini, Frankenburg, Wedig, & Fitzmaurice, 40
Zanarini, Temes, Frankenburg, Reich, & Fitzmaurice, 48
Zeki & Romaya, 73
zen meditation techniques, 9
Zeng et al., 35
Zimmerman, Rothschild, & Chelminski, 20, 34
Zittel, Conklin, and Westen, 26
Zutphen et al., 71